全国高等医药院校药学类实验教材

生物化学与分子生物学实验

（第三版）

主　　编　　张　嵘
副 主 编　　刘岩峰
英文主审　　赵雪梅
编　　者　　（以姓氏笔画为序）

王　淼　　王月秋　　刘岩峰

刘晓辉　　杜秉娜　　杨　宇

李　洋　　李相儒　　来琳琳

宋永波　　汪　琳　　张　嵘

林盛国　　金汝天　　赵勇山

赵斯奇　　宾　文　　曾　红

中国健康传媒集团
中国医药科技出版社

内 容 提 要

本书为"全国高等医药院校药学类实验教材"之一。全书分为两大部分，分别为基础生物化学与分子生物学实验和药学生物化学与分子生物学实验。为适应普通高等教育国际化的要求，增加了英文对照内容，以便于学生在阅读英文文献、撰写英文论文时参考。

本书可作为药学、中药学及药学相关各专业本科生或硕士研究生实验技术课程的教材使用，也可供有关科研技术人员参考。

图书在版编目（CIP）数据

生物化学与分子生物学实验/张嵘主编. —3 版. —北京：中国医药科技出版社，2019.3
全国高等医药院校药学类实验教材
ISBN 978 – 7 – 5214 – 0838 – 6

Ⅰ.①生… Ⅱ.①张… Ⅲ.①生物化学 – 实验 – 医学院校 – 教材 ②分子生物学 – 实验 – 医学院校 – 教材 Ⅳ.①Q5 – 33 ②Q7 – 33

中国版本图书馆 CIP 数据核字（2019）第 034134 号

美术编辑 陈君杞
版式设计 郭小平

出版 **中国健康传媒集团** | 中国医药科技出版社
地址 北京市海淀区文慧园北路甲 22 号
邮编 100082
电话 发行：010 – 62227427 邮购：010 – 62236938
网址 www.cmstp.com
规格 787 × 1092mm ¹⁄₁₆
印张 13½
字数 265 千字
初版 2006 年 3 月第 1 版
版次 2019 年 3 月第 3 版
印次 2022 年 5 月第 2 次印刷
印刷 北京市密东印刷有限公司
经销 全国各地新华书店
书号 ISBN 978 – 7 – 5214 – 0838 – 6
定价 **38.00 元**
本社图书如存在印装质量问题请与本社联系调换

全国高等医药院校药学类规划教材常务编委会

前　言

　　生物化学与分子生物学是生命科学的重要组成部分，其理论与基本实验技术已广泛渗透并常规应用于生命科学乃至药学的各个领域。尤其是 20 世纪 70 年代以来，分子生物学技术完成了发展、成熟与广泛应用的过程，使生命科学步入迅猛发展、日新月异的崭新阶段，展现了惊人的发展潜力和极其广阔的应用前景。科学与技术从来就是密不可分的，理论的突破促进了技术的发展，实验技术方法和手段的不断更新又为理论研究提供了必需的工具和有力保证。二者彼此促进、相互协作，共同推动了生命科学的蓬勃发展。

　　同样，生物化学与分子生物学实验教学也是高等药学教育基本的教学组成，实验教学体现了学生参与、师生互动、加强实践、思维开拓的教学教育理念，是培养学生科学思维方法、创新意识和科研能力的必备手段。在教学过程中，实验教学既依靠理论教学的支持，又具有相对独立性。因此实验教学是学生理论知识学习的必要补充，也是后续专业技能学习与提高的必要手段。

　　生物化学与分子生物学实验技术具有完整而系统的知识体系，为结合高等药学教育的实际需要，使学生不仅能够系统地学习和掌握生物化学与分子生物学的基本实验技能，而且通过实验教学达到创新性教育的目的，本教材对基本实验内容进行了精心选择和取舍，根据不同的教学目标，本着由浅入深、循序渐进、注重应用、培养创新的原则，将实验内容分为基础生物化学与分子生物学实验和药学生物化学与分子生物学实验两个部分。其中，基础生物化学与分子生物学实验主要包括理论验证实验和基本技术实验，前者着重验证学科理论教学内容，突出实验教学和理论教学的密切关系，加强对理论知识的理解；后者则通过实验操作，使学生掌握基本实验技能。药学生物化学与分子生物学实验的内容结合学科理论、技术及其在药学领域的常见应用，主要包括综合性实验和设计性实验两个部分。其中，综合性实验是指一个实验中包含着几个内容，要运用几种不同的技术才能完成一个完整的实验内容，以此强化训练学生的综合实验技能和综合分析能力。设计性实验则根据教师限定的实验题目，学生自选方案、自查文献、自行设计实验以完成指定实验目标和任务，以此培养创新意识、动手能力和基本科研思维，有利于全面素质的提高。此外，本教材采用中文－英文双语体系编写，有助于提高学生的科技英语水平，沈阳药科大学多年实验双语教学实践表明，学生完全能够接受双语教材的教学。

　　本教材适合于作为药学、中药学及药学相关各专业本科生或硕士研究生实验技术课程的教材使用，也可供有关科研技术人员参考。

　　本教材的编写由长期从事生物化学与分子生物学实验教学的中青年教师执笔，他们有着较为丰富的实验教学经验，能够将教学感受及经验有机地融入教材，帮助学生更好地掌握实验要点，规范实验操作。实验一由赵勇山编写，实验二由王淼编写，实验三由金汝天编写，实验七、十七由杜秉娜编写，实验四、十二由刘岩峰编写，实验五由林盛国编写，实验六、十一由杨宇编写，实验八、九、二十五由张嵘编写，实验十由赵斯奇编写，实验十三由刘晓辉编写，实验十四由李相儒编写，实验十五、二十一由王月秋编写，实验十六、十八、十九由宋永波编写，实验二十由汪琳编写，实验二十二由宾文编写，实验二十三由李洋编写，实验二十四由来琳琳编写，附录由曾红编写，全书的英文部分由赵雪梅责任校对。张景海教授在教材编写过程中提出了宝贵的意见和建议，谨表示衷心感谢。

　　本教材中不当或错误之处恳请同行专家和使用者谅解，并衷心希望读者提出宝贵的意见和建议，以便今后不断完善。

编　者
2019 年 2 月

目 录

第一部分 基础生物化学与分子生物学实验

第二部分　药学生物化学与分子生物学实验

第一部分 基础生物化学与分子生物学实验

实验一 氨基酸及蛋白质的性质

【实验目的】

1. 加深对所学相关蛋白质性质理论知识的理解。
2. 掌握氨基酸和蛋白质常用定性、定量分析的方法及其原理。

一、蛋白质呈色反应

蛋白质的呈色反应是指蛋白质所含的某些氨基酸残基及其特殊结构，在一定条件下可与某些试剂生成有色物质的反应。

不同蛋白质分子所含的氨基酸残基不完全相同，因此所发生的呈色反应也不完全一样。另外，呈色反应并不是蛋白质的专一反应，某些非蛋白质类物质（含有—CS—NH、—CH_2—NH_2、—CRH—NH_2、—CHOH—CH_2NH_2 等基团的物质）也能发生类似的颜色反应。因此，不能仅仅根据呈色反应的结果判断被测物质一定是蛋白质。

（一）双缩脲反应

【实验原理】

尿素加热至 180℃左右时，2 分子尿素脱去 1 分子氨，缩合成 1 分子双缩脲。在碱性条件下，双缩脲与铜离子结合生成紫红色络合物，此反应称为双缩脲反应。其反应过程如下。

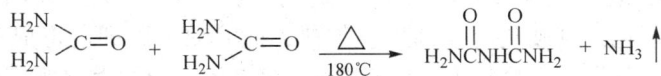

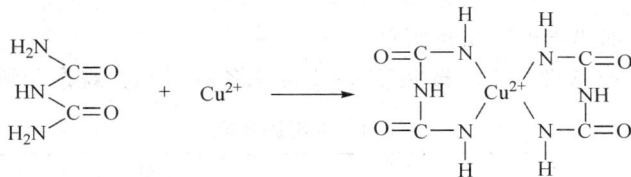

多肽及蛋白质分子结构中均含有许多肽键，其结构与双缩脲分子中的亚酰胺键相同。因此，在碱性条件下与铜离子也能呈现出类似于双缩脲的呈色反应，其反应过程如下。

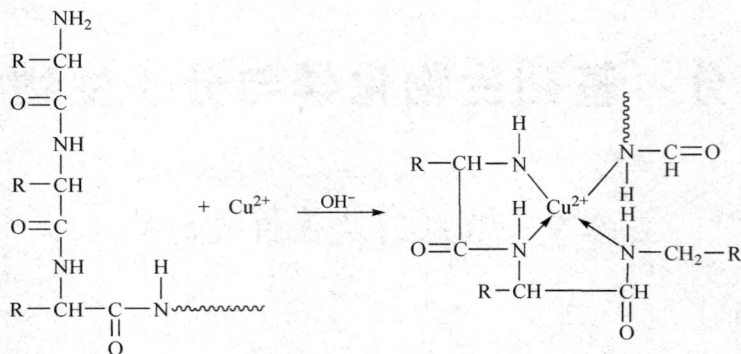

【实验材料】

1. **实验器材**　试管、试管架、移液管、烧杯、煤气灯、胶头滴管。

2. **实验试剂**

（1）蛋白质溶液　鸡蛋清用蒸馏水稀释10倍，通过2~3层纱布滤去不溶物。

（2）0.1%甘氨酸溶液　少量蒸馏水溶解1g甘氨酸后，转移至1000ml容量瓶中，蒸馏水定容至1000ml。

（3）0.01%精氨酸溶液　少量蒸馏水溶解0.1g精氨酸后，转移至1000ml容量瓶中，蒸馏水定容至1000ml。

（4）10%NaOH溶液　少量蒸馏水溶解10g氢氧化钠后，转移至100ml容量瓶中，蒸馏水定容至100ml。

（5）1%CuSO₄溶液　少量蒸馏水溶解1g硫酸铜后，转移至100ml容量瓶中，蒸馏水定容至100ml。

（6）尿素结晶。

【实验步骤】

1. **双缩脲的制备**　取少许尿素结晶（约火柴头大小）放入干燥的试管中，微火加热至尿素熔解至硬化，刚硬化时立即停止加热，此时双缩脲即已形成。冷却后加10%氢氧化钠溶液1ml并振荡，再加入1%硫酸铜溶液2滴，再振荡，观察颜色的变化。

注意：（1）在操作过程中试管不能面向自己或他人，防止烫伤。

（2）控制试管加热程度，防止碳化。

2. **观察现象**　取试管4支，按照表1-1加入各种试剂，观察并解释现象。

表1-1　双缩脲反应

试　剂	管　号			
	1	2	3	4
蛋白质溶液（ml）		1.0		
0.01%精氨酸（ml）			1.0	
0.1%甘氨酸（ml）				1.0
10%NaOH（ml）	2.0	2.0	2.0	2.0
蒸馏水（ml）	1.0			
1%CuSO₄（滴）	2.0	2.0	2.0	2.0
现象				

（二）茚三酮反应

【实验原理】

在弱酸条件下（pH 5～7），蛋白质或氨基酸与茚三酮共热生成蓝紫色缩合物。此反应为一切蛋白质和 α - 氨基酸所共有（亚氨基酸，如脯氨酸和羟脯氨酸产生黄色化合物）。含有氨基的其他化合物亦可发生此反应。

第一步：

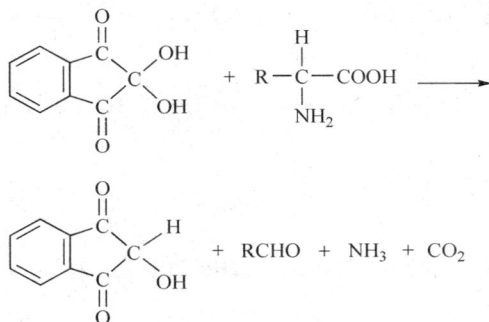

第二步：

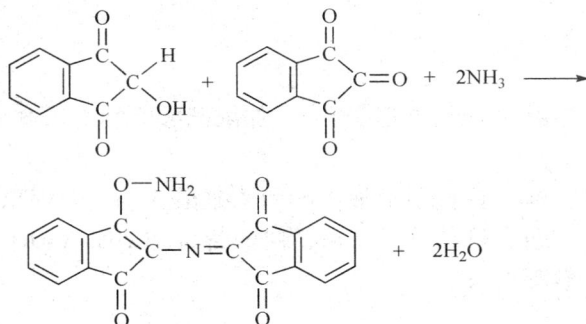

【实验材料】

1. 实验器材 试管、试管架、移液管、烧杯、石棉网、煤气灯。

2. 实验试剂

（1）蛋白质溶液 与双缩脲反应相同。

（2）0.1% 甘氨酸溶液 与双缩脲反应相同。

（3）0.2% 茚三酮乙醇溶液 少量无水乙醇溶解茚三酮 0.2g 后，转移至 100ml 容量瓶中，无水乙醇定容至 100ml。

【实验步骤】

取试管 2 支，分别加入蛋白质溶液及 0.1% 甘氨酸溶液 1ml，然后各加入茚三酮溶液 0.5ml，混匀后置于沸水浴中加热数分钟，观察现象，记录结果并解释原因。

（三）蛋白黄反应

【实验原理】

在蛋白质分子中，具有芳香环的氨基酸（如酪氨酸、色氨酸等）残基上的苯环经硝酸作用可生成黄色的硝基化合物，在碱性条件下硝基化合物可转变为橘黄色的硝醌衍生物，其反应过程如下。

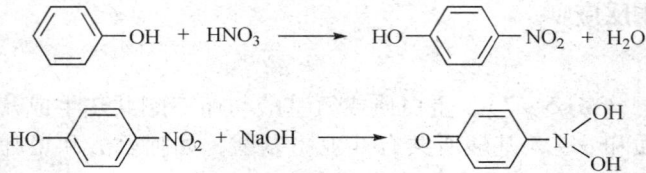

多数蛋白质分子含有带苯环的氨基酸残基，所以都会发生黄色反应。苯丙氨酸不易硝化，需加少量浓硫酸后才能够发生黄色反应。

【实验材料】

1. 实验器材　试管、试管架、移液管、锥形瓶、煤气灯、石棉网、胶头滴管。

2. 实验试剂

（1）蛋白质溶液　与双缩脲反应相同。

（2）浓硝酸。

（3）20% NaOH 溶液　少量蒸馏水溶解 20g 氢氧化钠后，转移至 100ml 容量瓶中，蒸馏水定容至 100ml。

（4）0.1% 苯酚溶液　少量蒸馏水溶解 1g 苯酚后，转移至 1000ml 容量瓶中，蒸馏水定容至 1000ml。

【实验步骤】

（1）取 1% 苯酚溶液约 1ml 放在试管内，加浓硝酸 5 滴，用微火或水浴小心加热，观察结果。

（2）取试管 1 支，加入蛋白质溶液 1ml 和浓硝酸 5 滴，立即出现沉淀，加热，不必至沸腾，沉淀变成黄色，待试管冷却后，向两管各加 20% NaOH 溶液混匀，观察颜色变化，记录结果并解释现象。

（四）坂口反应

【实验原理】

蛋白质在碱性溶液中与次氯酸钠（或次溴酸钠）和 α-萘酚作用生成红色的产物。这是蛋白质分子中精氨酸胍基的特征反应。许多胍的衍生物，如胍乙酸、胍基丁胺等也发生此反应。精氨酸是惟一呈正反应的氨基酸，反应灵敏度达 1:250000。反应式如下。

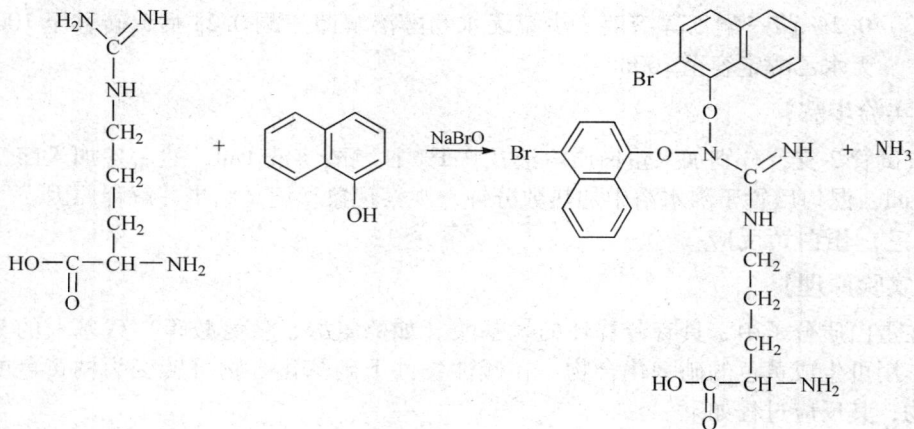

在次溴酸钠缓慢作用下，红色产物继续氧化，引起颜色消失，因此过量的次溴酸钠对反应不利。加入浓尿素，破坏过量的次溴酸钠，能增加颜色的稳定性。此反应可以用来定性鉴定含有精氨酸的蛋白质和定量测定精氨酸的含量。

【实验材料】

1. 实验器材 试管、试管架、移液管、烧杯、胶头滴管。

2. 实验试剂

（1）蛋白质溶液 与双缩脲反应相同。

（2）次溴酸钠溶液 300g NaOH 溶解于 1L 水中，冷却后放在通风橱中，在不断搅拌下，小心地加入纯溴 50g（约 16ml），溶液保存在棕色瓶中。此溶液可保存 2～3 个月。

（3）10% NaOH 溶液 与双缩脲反应相同。

（4）0.2% α-萘酚溶液 0.5g α-萘酚溶于 50ml 乙醇中，使用前以 5 倍水稀释。

（5）0.01% 精氨酸溶液 与双缩脲反应相同。

【实验步骤】

（1）于试管中加入蛋白质溶液 1ml，10% NaOH 溶液 0.5ml，0.2% α-萘酚 2 滴，混合后加入次溴酸钠溶液 2 滴，观察现象。

（2）取 0.01% 精氨酸溶液 1ml，按上述操作，观察现象。

二、蛋白质沉淀反应

蛋白质是亲水胶体，当其稳定因素被破坏或与某些试剂结合成不溶性盐类后，即自溶液中沉淀析出，此现象叫作蛋白质的沉淀反应。

（一）蛋白质的盐析作用

【实验原理】

盐析现象是指向蛋白质溶液中加入大量的中性盐（例如硫酸铵、硫酸钠或氯化钠等），破坏蛋白质的胶体稳定性而聚集沉淀。盐析作用与两种因素有关：①蛋白质分子被浓盐脱水；②分子所带电荷被中和。

蛋白质的盐析作用是可逆过程，用盐析方法沉淀蛋白质时较少引起蛋白质变性，经透析或用水稀释后又可溶解。

盐析不同的蛋白质所需中性盐浓度与蛋白质种类及 pH 有关。分子量大的蛋白质（如球蛋白）比分子量小的（如清蛋白）易于析出。球蛋白在半饱和硫酸铵溶液中即可析出，而清蛋白需在饱和硫酸铵溶液中才能析出。

【实验材料】

1. 实验器材 试管、试管架、移液管、烧杯、漏斗、滤纸。

2. 实验试剂

（1）蛋白质溶液 与双缩脲反应相同。

（2）固体硫酸铵。

（3）10% NaOH 溶液 与双缩脲反应相同。

（4）1% $CuSO_4$ 溶液 与双缩脲反应相同。

【实验步骤】

（1）取蛋白质溶液约 2ml 于试管中，加入硫酸铵粉末，至硫酸铵饱和不再溶解为止，此时溶液颜色为乳白色，用滤纸过滤。

（2）取滤液做双缩脲反应，检查滤液中有无蛋白质存在。

（3）蛋白质沉淀用少量蒸馏水溶解后作双缩脲反应，证明盐析的蛋白质重新溶解于水。

（二）重金属盐类沉淀蛋白质

【实验原理】

当溶液 pH 大于蛋白质等电点时，蛋白质带负电荷，能与带正电荷的重金属（如 Pb^{2+}、Cu^{2+}、Hg^{2+} 及 Ag^+ 等）结合成不溶性盐而沉淀。

重金属盐类沉淀蛋白质通常比较完全，故常用重金属盐除去溶液中的蛋白质。

注意： 在使用某些重金属盐（如硫酸铜或醋酸铅）沉淀蛋白质时，不可过量，否则将引起沉淀再溶解。

【实验材料】

1. **实验器材**　试管、试管架、移液管、烧杯、胶头滴管。

2. **实验试剂**

（1）蛋白质溶液　与双缩脲反应相同。

（2）5% $CuSO_4$ 溶液　少量蒸馏水溶解 5g 硫酸铜后，转移至 100ml 容量瓶中，蒸馏水定容至 100ml。

（3）3% $AgNO_3$ 溶液　少量蒸馏水溶解 3g 硝酸银后，转移至 100ml 容量瓶中，蒸馏水定容至 100ml，转移至棕色瓶中保存。

【实验步骤】

（1）取试管 2 支，各加入蛋白质溶液 1ml。

（2）向两管分别加入 5% $CuSO_4$ 溶液和 3% $AgNO_3$ 溶液 2~3 滴，观察各管所生成的沉淀。

（3）在硫酸铜产生沉淀的试管中，倒掉大部分沉淀，只保留少量沉淀，继续加入 5% $CuSO_4$ 溶液，观察沉淀的溶解。

（三）有机酸沉淀蛋白质

【实验原理】

生物碱是一类含氮的碱性物质。凡能使生物碱沉淀，或能与生物碱发生颜色反应的物质称为生物碱试剂，如三氯醋酸、5-磺基水杨酸、磷钨酸等。当蛋白质溶液 pH 低于其等电点时，蛋白质为阳离子，能与生物碱试剂的阴离子结合，生成不溶性的盐而沉淀。三氯醋酸的作用最为灵敏而且特异，因此广泛应用于沉淀蛋白质。

【实验材料】

1. **实验器材**　试管、试管架、移液管、烧杯、胶头滴管。

2. **实验试剂**

（1）蛋白质溶液　与双缩脲反应相同。

（2）10% 三氯醋酸溶液 少量蒸馏水溶解 10g 三氯醋酸固体，蒸馏水定容至 100ml。

（3）20% 5 - 磺基水杨酸溶液 少量蒸馏水溶解 20g 5 - 磺基水杨酸，蒸馏水定容至 100ml。

【实验步骤】

（1）取蛋白质溶液 1ml 于试管中，加数滴三氯醋酸溶液，观察现象。

（2）取蛋白质溶液 1ml 于试管中，加数滴 5 - 磺基水杨酸溶液，观察现象。

（四）加热沉淀蛋白质

【实验原理】

大多数蛋白质在加热时，由于空间结构被破坏而丧失其稳定性而变性沉淀。蛋白质的热变性作用与加热时间平行，并随温度的升高而加快。短时间加热即可引起沉淀。加热时，盐类的存在及溶液酸碱度对蛋白质的沉淀有很大影响。当蛋白质处于等电点时，加热时沉淀凝固最完全、最迅速。在强酸、强碱溶液中，蛋白质分子由于带有正电荷或负电荷，加热也不沉淀，但溶液中若有中性盐存在，虽在酸性或碱性溶液中，则蛋白质亦可因加热而沉淀。

【实验材料】

1. 实验器材 试管、试管架、移液管、烧杯、石棉网、煤气灯、胶头滴管。

2. 实验试剂

（1）蛋白质溶液 与双缩脲反应相同。

（2）1% 醋酸溶液 量取 1ml 冰醋酸，用蒸馏水定容至 100ml。

（3）10% 醋酸溶液 量取 10ml 冰醋酸，用蒸馏水定容至 100ml。

（4）10% 氢氧化钠溶液 与双缩脲反应相同。

（5）饱和氯化钠溶液 室温下配制过饱和氯化钠溶液，过滤即得饱和氯化钠溶液。

【实验步骤】

取试管 4 支，按表 1 - 2 所示添加试剂。

表 1 - 2 加热沉淀蛋白质反应

试 剂	管 号			
	1	2	3	4
蛋白质溶液（ml）	1.0	1.0	1.0	1.0
1% 醋酸（滴）	1.0			
10% 醋酸（滴）		10.0		
10% NaOH（滴）			10.0	
蒸馏水（滴）	10.0	1.0	1.0	11.0
现象				

加毕混匀，观察各管的情况。放入沸水浴中加热 10 分钟，注意比较各管的沉淀情况。其中 1 号管溶液 pH 接近于蛋白质等电点，在加热之前最先产生沉淀；其次是 4 号管在加热之后产生沉淀；3 号和 2 号管因在较强的酸性或碱性条件下，蛋白质带有大量

的电荷，虽然加热也不沉淀。向 2 号管中加入少许饱和氯化钠溶液，立即出现白色沉淀。

【思考题】

1. 盐析作用的原理是什么？盐析在化学工作中有什么应用？
2. 哪个反应可以用于区别氨基酸与蛋白质？
3. 蛋白质的沉淀试验和颜色反应实验时应注意哪些问题？

Experiment 1　The Properties of Protein and Amino Acid

Purposes

1. To deepen understanding of speculative knowledge about properties of protein which has been learned.

2. To master the methods and principles of quantitative and qualitative experiments of protein and amino acid.

Ⅰ. Color reactions of protein

Color reactions of protein mean that some chemical bonds of protein or chemical groups of amino acid residues can react with specific reagents to form specific colored products under certain condition.

The amino acid residues of different proteins are not quite the same. Therefore, colors of the products are not exactly the same. Color reactions are not the specific reactions of protein. Some non-protein substances (e. g. —CS—NH、—CH$_2$—NH$_2$、—CRH—NH$_2$、—CHOH—CH$_2$NH$_2$) also have similar color reactions. Consequently we cannot judge protein according to the results of the color reactions.

(Ⅰ) Biuret reaction

Principle

Two molecules of carbamide are heated to give a molecule of biuret when the temperature is 180℃ and release a molecule of ammonia. Biuret reacts with an alkaline solution of copper cation can form a purple-colored complex, This reaction is called biuret reaction. The process of biuret reaction is as follows.

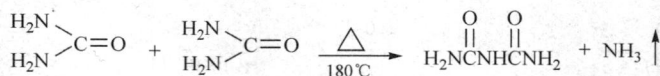

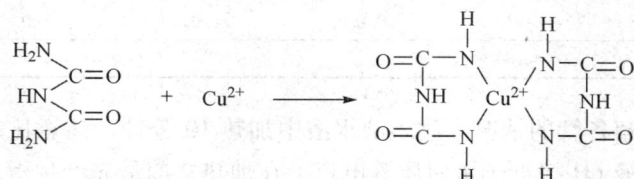

There are many peptide bonds in polypeptides and proteins. The structure of peptide bond is the same as the imido bond of biuret. Therefore protein or polypeptide can react with alkaline solution of copper cation in a similar way to biuret. The process of reaction is as follows.

Materials

1. Apparatus

Test tubes, test tube shelf, pipette, flask, gas lamp, glue head dropper.

2. Reagents

(1) Protein solution　Egg white is diluted with distilled water to ten volumes and filtrated by 2 ~ 3 layers of gauze.

(2) 0.1% Glycine solution　Dissolve 1g glycine into little water, then dilute to 1000ml.

(3) 0.01% Arginine solution　Dissolve 0.1g arginine into little water, then dilute to 1000ml.

(4) 10% NaOH solution　Dissolve 10g NaOH into little water, then dilute to 100ml.

(5) 1% $CuSO_4$ solution　Dissolve 1g $CuSO_4$ into little water, then dilute to 100ml.

(6) Crystal carbamide.

Procedures

1. Preparation of biuret　Add a little crystal carbamide (about the size of a match head) into a dry test tube. Low heat to liquate, stop heating when it begins to vulcanize and biuret can be formed. Cool and add 1ml 10% NaOH solution, mix up, then add 2 drop of 1% $CuSO_4$ solution, mix up again, observe the change of the color.

Cautions: (1) To prevent burns, the tube can not face themselves or others in the process of operation.

(2) To prevent carbonization, the heating degree of the tube should be controlled.

2. Observing the phenomenon　Take four test tubes, in which the reagents as the Table 1-1 are added and mixed, observation and then make an explanation.

Table 1 −1　Biuret reaction

Reagents	Test tube			
	1	2	3	4
Protein solution (ml)		1.0		
0.01% Arginine (ml)			1.0	

(to be continued)

Reagents	Test tube			
	1	2	3	4
0.1% Glycine (ml)				1.0
10 NaOH (ml)	2.0	2.0	2.0	2.0
Distilled H_2O (ml)	1.0			
1% $CuSO_4$ (drop)	2.0	2.0	2.0	2.0
Phenomena				

(Ⅱ) Ninhydrin reaction

Principle

Heating protein or amino acid with ninhydrin in subacid condition (pH 5~7) can get royal purple condensate. This reaction is the mutual property of all proteins and α-amino acids (Amino acids such as proline or hydroxyproline give yellow condensate). Other compounds containing amino groups also have the ninhydrin reaction.

Step1:

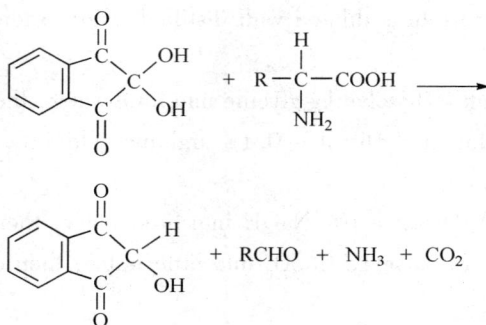

Step2:

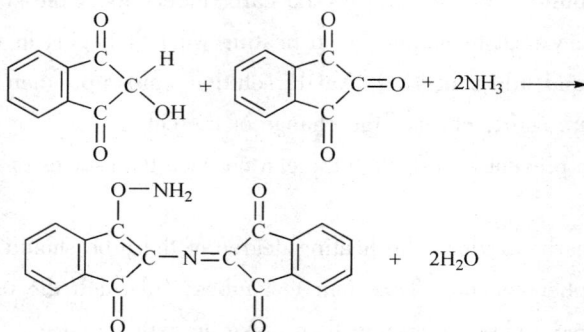

Materials

1. Apparatus

Test tubes, test tube shelf, pipette, flask, asbestos network, gas lamp.

2. Reagents

(1) Protein solution   The same as biuret reaction.

（2）0.1% Glycine solution　The same as biuret reaction.

（3）0.2% Ninhydrin solution　Dissolve 0.2g ninhydrin into absolute ethylalcohol, then dilute to 100ml.

Procedures

Take two test tubes, add 1ml protein solution in one tube and 1ml 0.1% glycine solution in the other, and then add 0.5ml ninhydrin solution in each of the tubes. Mix up and heat them in the boiling water bath for several minutes, observe the phenomena and make an explanation.

(Ⅲ) Yellow reaction

Principle

In protein molecules, the benzene ring of aromatic amino acids (such as tyrosine and tryptophan) can react with nitric acid to produce yellow nitro compound, which can change into saffron nitranilic derivative in basic condition. The reaction is as follows.

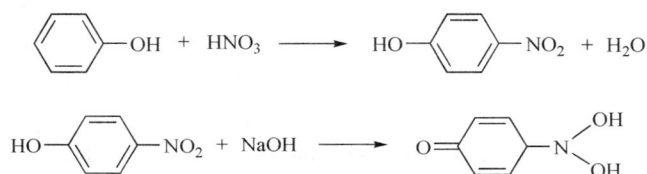

Most proteins have amino acids with aromatic ring, so they have yellow reaction. Phenylalanine is not easy to be nitrified, so, several concentrated sulfuric acid is needed.

Materials

1. Apparatus

Test tubes, test tube shelf, pipette, flask, gas lamp, asbestos network, glue head dropper.

2. Reagents

（1）Protein solution　The same as biuret reaction.

（2）Aquafortis.

（3）20% NaOH solution　Dissolve 20g NaOH into little water, then dilute to 100ml.

（4）0.1% Carbolic acid solution　Dissolve 1g carbolic acid into little water, then dilute to 1000ml.

Procedures

1. Add 1ml 1% carbolic acid solution and 5 drops of aquafortis in the tube, heat carefully with low fire or water bath and observe the result.

2. Take a test tube, add 1ml protein sample solution and 5 drops of aquafortis in it, appear precipitation immediately. Add 20% NaOH solution in each of the tubes, mix up. Observe color varieties, note down the results and explain them.

(Ⅳ) Sakaguohi reaction

Principle

Proteins react with sodium hypochlorite solution (or sodium hypobromite solution) and α-naphthol solution in alkaline condition to produce red component. This is a special reaction of arginine's carbamidine. A lot of guanidine derivatives, such as glucocyamine and agmatine, can also have this reaction. Arginine is the only amino acid which has this reaction and the sensitivity reaches 1 : 250000. The reaction is shown as below.

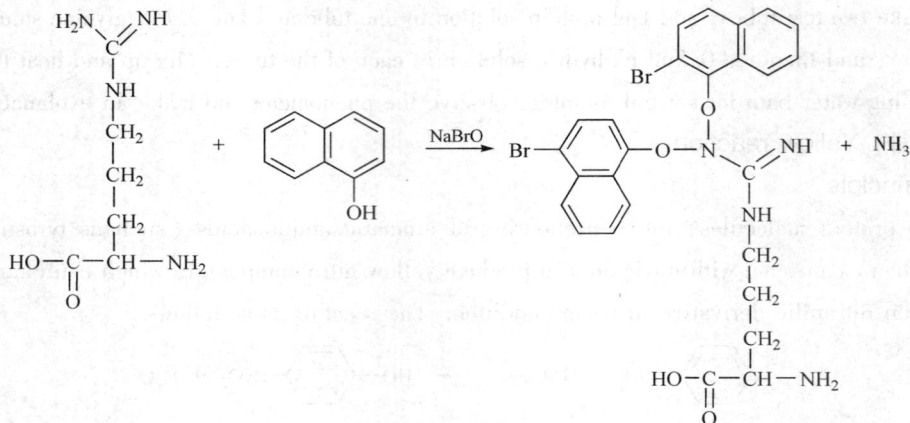

The red products continue to be oxidized under the action of sodium hypobromite, causing the color disappeared. Therefore excess of sodium hypobromite adverse reaction. Adding an excess of concentrated uric acid can destroy the excess of sodium hypobromite and increase the stability of the color. The Sakaguohi reaction is useful in quantitating and determining the natures of protein and the amino acid which contain arginine.

Materials

1. Apparatus

Test tubes, test tube shelf, pipette, flask, glue head dropper.

2. Reagents

(1) Protein solution   The same as biuret reaction.

(2) Sodium bromate solution   Weigh 300g NaOH, dissolve in 1L distilled water, and cool the solution to room temperature in fume hood. Add 50g bromate into the solution while stirred continuously. It can be stored for 2 ~ 3 months in the brown bottle.

(3) 10% NaOH solution   The same as Biuret reaction.

(4) 0.2% α-Naphthol solution   Dissolve 0.5g α-naphthol into 50ml Ethanol. α-naphthol solution was diluted with 5-fold water prior to use.

(5) 0.01% Arginine solution   The same as biuret reaction.

Procedures

1. 1ml of protein solution is added into a test tube, then 0.5ml of 10% NaOH solution and 2 drops of 0.2% α-naphthol are added. After mixing, 2 drops of sodium hypobromite solution are added, and then observe the phenomenon.

2. Add 1ml of 0.01% arginine solution according to the same procedure above, then observe the phenomenon.

Ⅱ. Precipitation reactions of protein

Protein is hydrophilic colloid. Protein can be separated out from solution when the stable factors are damaged or when it combines with some agents to form infusibility salts, which is called precipitation reaction of protein.

(Ⅰ) Salting out of protein

Principle

Salting out refers to the addition of a large number of neutral salt (such as ammonia sulfate, sodium sulfate and sodium chloride) in protein solution, which destroy the colloidal stability of the proteins and result in the precipitation and aggregation.

Two factors relate to salting out: ①Protein molecules are dehydrated by salt. ② The charges of protein molecules are neutralized.

Precipitating protein by salting outdoes not make the denaturation of protein in general. Dialysis or diluted by water can dissolve the precipitation. So salting out is a reversible process.

The neutral salt concentration of precipitating protein by salting out relates to the kind of protein and pH. Large molecule (such as globulin) is easier to be separated out than small molecule (such as albumin). Half saturated ammonium sulfate solution can precipitate out globulin, whereas saturated ammonium sulfate solution is required to precipitate albumin.

Materials

1. Apparatus

Test tubes, test tube shelf, pipette, flask, funnel, filter paper.

2. Reagents

(1) Protein solution   The same as Biuret reaction.

(2) Solid ammonium sulfate.

(3) 10% NaOH solution   The same as Biuret reaction.

(4) 1% $CuSO_4$ solution   The same as Biuret reaction.

Procedures

1. Add 2ml of protein solution in a test tube. Solid ammonium sulfate is added until saturation and the solution is ivory. Leave it stand for several minutes and filtrate by filter paper.

2. Place the filtrate in a test tube for Biuret reaction and check if the protein exists.

3. Dissolve little precipitate in distilled water for biuret reaction, which proves the precipitated protein will be dissolved in water again.

(Ⅱ) Heavy metal salts precipitating protein

Principle

Heavy metal salts (such as Pb^{2+}, Cu^{2+}, Hg^{2+} and Ag^{2+} etc.) are easy to combine with protein to give insoluble salts and precipitate when the pH of solution is above the isoelectric point of the protein.

Heavy metal salts precipitating protein is always complete. So heavy metal salts are often used to remove protein in solution. But we must pay attention not to be excessive while using some heavy metal salts (such as $CuSO_4$ or PbAc) to precipitate protein, or else it will cause the precipitation to dissolve.

Materials

1. Apparatus

Test tubes, test tube shelf, pipette, flask, glue head dropper.

2. Reagents

(1) Protein solution   The same as biuret reaction.

(2) 5% $CuSO_4$ solution   Dissolve 5g $CuSO_4$ into little water, then dilute to 100ml.

(3) 3% $AgNO_3$ solution   Dissolve 3g $AgNO_3$ into little water, then dilute to 100ml and transfer to the brown bottle.

Procedures

1. Take 2 test tubes, add 1ml protein solution.

2. Add 2 ~ 3 drops of 5% $CuSO_4$ and 3% $AgNO_3$ to two test tubes respectively, then observe the phenomenon.

3. Reserve a bit of precipitate which is caused by $CuSO_4$, then add 5% $CuSO_4$ solution to the tube and observe if the precipitation is dissolved, note down the results.

(Ⅲ) Organic acid precipitating protein

Principle

Alkaloid is a kind of nitrogen basic compounds. Substances that can precipitate alkaloid or react with alkaloid to give color products are called alkaloid reagents, such as trichloroacetic acid, 5-sulfosalicylic acid, phosphotungstic acid etc. Alkaloid reagents can combine with cationic proteins to give insoluble salt and precipitate when the pH of solution is under the isoelectric point of the protein. The protein can also be precipitated by organic acid. Trichloroacetic acid is the most sensitive and specific in these acids and is used widely.

Materials

1. Apparatus

Test tubes, test tube shelf, pipette, flask, glue head dropper.

2. Reagents

(1) Protein solution   The same as biuret reaction.

(2) 10% Trichloroacetic acid solution   Dissolve 10g trichloroacetic acid into little water, then dilute to 100ml.

(3) 20% 5-Sulfosalicylic acid   Dissolve 20g 5-sulfosalicylic acid into little water, then dilute to 100ml.

Procedures

1. Add 1ml protein solutions into a test tube, and add several drops of trichloroacetic acid solution. Observe and note down the phenomenon.

2. Add 1ml protein solutions into another test tube, and then add several drops of 5-sulfos-

alicylic acid solution. Observe and note down the phenomenon.

(Ⅳ) Heat precipitating protein

Principle

Most proteins will be denatured while being heated, because the spatial structure of protein is damaged and protein is not stable.

The thermal denaturation of the protein parallels heating time. It increases with the rise of the temperature. Proteins do solidify in short heating time.

Salts and acid-base scale of solution will affect the solidification of protein largely while heating. The solidification of protein is the most complete and quickest at the isoelectric point. Protein does not solidify when being heated if it has positive or negative electric charge in strong acid or strong base solution. But protein can solidify because of being heated while there are neutral salts in solution.

Materials

1. Apparatus

Test tubes, test tube shelf, pipette, flask, gas lamp, asbestos network, glue head dropper.

2. Reagents

(1) Protein solution　The same as biuret reaction.

(2) 1% Acetic acid solution　Dissolve 1ml acetic acid into little water, then dilute to 100ml.

(3) 10% Acetic acid solution　Dissolve 10ml acetic acid into little water, then dilute to 100ml.

(4) 10% NaOH solution　The same as biuret reaction

(5) Saturated NaCl solution　Distribution over saturated sodium chloride solution at room temperature, then filter.

Procedures

Take 4 test tubes, and add reagents according to Table 1 - 2.

Table 1 -2　Heat precipitating protein

Reagents	Test tube			
	1	2	3	4
Protein solution (ml)	1.0	1.0	1.0	1.0
1% Acetic acid solution (drop)	1.0			
10% Acetic acid solution (drop)		10.0		
10% NaOH solution (drop)			10.0	
Distilled H_2O (drop)	10.0	1.0	1.0	11.0
Phenomena				

Mix up, place them in the boiling water bath for 10min, observe and note down the phenomenon and explain them. pH of No. 1 tube close to the isoelectric point and generated precipitation firstly before heating. No. 4 tube generated precipitation after heating. No. 2 and 3 tubes did not generate precipitation after heating, because the proteins have a large number of charges in strong acidic or alkaline condition. Add a little saturated sodium chloride in No. 2 tube, the precipitate appeared immediately.

Questions

1. What is the principle of salting out? In which aspects sdting out be applied in chemical work?

2. What is the difference between amino acids and proteins?

3. What should the students pay attention to when doing precipitation reactions and color reactions of protein?

实验二　蛋白质的定量测定方法

一、Folin – 酚试剂法（Lowry 法）

【实验目的】

1. 学习 Folin – 酚试剂法测定蛋白质含量的原理。

2. 掌握 Folin – 酚试剂法测定蛋白质含量的方法和操作。

【实验原理】

蛋白质中含有酪氨酸和色氨酸残基，能与 Folin – 酚试剂发生氧化还原反应。反应过程分为两步，第一步：在碱性溶液中，蛋白质分子中的肽键与碱性铜试剂中的 Cu^{2+} 作用生成蛋白质 – Cu^{2+} 复合物；第二步：蛋白质 – Cu^{2+} 复合物中所含的酪氨酸或色氨酸残基还原 Folin – 酚试剂中的磷钼酸和磷钨酸，生成蓝色的化合物。呈色反应在 30 分钟内即接近极限，并且在一定浓度范围内，蓝色的深浅度与蛋白质含量呈线性关系，故可用比色的方法确定蛋白质的含量。进行测定时要根据蛋白质含量的不同选用不同的测定波长：若蛋白质含量高时（25 ~ 100μg）在 500nm 波长处进行测定，含量低时（5 ~ 25μg）在 755nm 波长处进行测定。最后根据标准曲线求出未知样品中蛋白质的含量。

Folin – 酚试剂法操作简便，灵敏度高，样品中蛋白质含量高于 5μg 即可，是测定蛋白质含量经常采用的方法之一。

【实验材料】

1. 实验器材　试管、试管架、100ml 容量瓶、移液管、721 型分光光度计。

2. 实验试剂

（1）Folin – 酚试剂甲　将 1g 碳酸钠溶于 50ml 0.1mol/L 氢氧化钠溶液中，再把 0.5g 硫酸铜（$CuSO_4 \cdot 5H_2O$）溶于 100ml 1% 酒石酸钾（或酒石酸钠）溶液，然后将前者 50ml 与后者 1ml 混合。混合后 1 日内使用有效。

（2）Folin – 酚试剂乙　在 1.5L 容积的磨口回流瓶中加入 100g 钨酸钠（$Na_2WO_4 \cdot 2H_2O$）、25g 钼酸钠（$Na_2MoO_4 \cdot 2H_2O$）、700ml 蒸馏水、50ml 85% 磷酸及 100ml 浓盐酸，

充分混匀后回流 10 小时。回流完毕，再加 150g 硫酸锂、50ml 蒸馏水及数滴液体溴，开口继续沸腾 15 分钟，以便驱除过量的溴，冷却后定容到 1000ml。过滤，如果显绿色，可加溴水数滴使其氧化至溶液呈淡黄色。置于棕色瓶中暗处保存。使用前用标准氢氧化钠溶液滴定，酚酞为指示剂，以标定该试剂的酸度，一般为 2mol/L 左右（由于滤液为浅黄色，滴定时滤液需稀释 100 倍，以免影响滴定终点的观察）。使用时适当稀释，使最后浓度为 1mol/L。

（3）标准蛋白质溶液　取牛（或人）血清白蛋白 100mg，精密称定，用少量蒸馏水完全溶解后，转移至 100ml 量瓶中，准确稀释至刻度，使蛋白质浓度为 1mg/ml。

（4）样品溶液　配制约 0.5mg/ml 的酪蛋白溶液作为未知样品溶液。

【实验步骤】

1. 绘制标准曲线　取 7 支试管，按表 2－1 加入试剂，然后混匀。

表 2－1　制作标准曲线

试　剂	管　号						
	0	1	2	3	4	5	6
标准蛋白质溶液（ml）	0.0	0.1	0.2	0.3	0.4	0.5	0.6
蒸馏水（ml）	1.0	0.9	0.8	0.7	0.6	0.5	0.4
Folin－酚试剂甲（ml）	5.0	5.0	5.0	5.0	5.0	5.0	5.0
摇匀，室温下放置 10 分钟							
Folin－酚试剂乙（ml）	1.0	1.0	1.0	1.0	1.0	1.0	1.0

各管加入 Folin－酚试剂乙后，立即摇匀，放置 30 分钟后，在 500nm 处测定各管光密度值，以 0 号管为对照，以光密度值为纵坐标，标准蛋白质含量为横坐标，绘制标准曲线。

2. 测定未知样品　取 2 支试管，分别准确吸取 1ml 样品溶液，各加 5ml Folin－酚试剂甲，摇匀，室温放置 10 分钟，再各加 1ml Folin－酚试剂乙，立即摇匀，放置 30 分钟，在 500nm 处测定光密度值。

【实验结果】

根据未知样品溶液的光密度值，利用标准曲线计算出样品溶液中的蛋白质含量。

二、紫外吸收法

【实验目的】

1. 学习紫外吸收法测定蛋白质含量的原理。
2. 掌握紫外分光光度计的操作方法。

【实验原理】

大多数蛋白质分子结构中含有芳香族氨基酸（酪氨酸和色氨酸）残基，使蛋白质在 280nm 的紫外光区产生最大吸收，并且这一波长范围内的光密度值与蛋白质浓度成正比，利用这一特性可定量测定蛋白质的含量。

紫外吸收法可测定 0.1～0.5mg/ml 的蛋白质溶液，此操作简便，测定迅速，不消耗样品，低浓度盐类不干扰测定。因此，此法在蛋白质的制备中广泛应用。

【实验材料】

1. **实验器材**　试管、试管架、50ml 容量瓶、移液管、紫外分光光度计。

2. **实验试剂**

（1）标准蛋白质溶液　精确配制 2mg/ml 的酪蛋白溶液。

（2）样品溶液　配制约 0.5mg/ml 的酪蛋白溶液作为未知样品溶液。

【实验步骤】

1. **绘制标准曲线**　取 7 支试管，按照表 2－2 加入试剂并得到不同浓度的标准蛋白质溶液。

表 2－2　配制不同浓度的标准蛋白质溶液

试　剂	管　号						
	0	1	2	3	4	5	6
标准蛋白质溶液（ml）	0.0	0.5	1.0	1.5	2.0	2.5	3.0
蒸馏水（ml）	8.0	7.5	7.0	6.5	6.0	5.5	5.0
蛋白质浓度（mg/ml）	0.000	0.125	0.250	0.375	0.500	0.625	0.750

摇匀，在紫外分光光度计上，于 280nm 处以 0 号管为对照，分别测定各管溶液的光密度值。以光密度值为纵坐标，标准蛋白质溶液浓度为横坐标，绘制出标准曲线。

2. **样品测定**　取样品溶液 4ml，加蒸馏水 4ml 混匀，在 280nm 下测定其光密度值。

【实验结果】

根据样品溶液的光密度值和标准曲线，计算出样品溶液的蛋白质含量。

三、微量凯氏定氮法

【实验目的】

学习凯氏定氮法的原理和操作技术。

【实验原理】

凯氏定氮法用于测定样品的含氮量，根据含氮量就可以确定样品中蛋白质的含量。

当蛋白质与浓硫酸共热时，其中的碳、氢元素被氧化成二氧化碳和水，而氮则转变成氨，并进一步与硫酸作用生成硫酸铵。此过程通常称为"消化"。但是，这个反应进行得比较缓慢，通常需要加入硫酸钾或硫酸钠，以提高反应液的沸点，并加入硫酸铜作为催化剂，以促进反应的进行。

消化完成后，在凯氏定氮仪中加入浓碱，可使消化液中的硫酸铵分解，游离出氨。借助水蒸气蒸馏法，将产生的氨蒸馏到一定浓度的硼酸溶液中，氨与溶液中氢离子结合，使溶液中的氢离子浓度降低，指示剂颜色改变，然后用标准盐酸滴定，直至恢复溶液中原来的氢离子浓度为止。根据所用标准盐酸的量可计算出待测物中的总氮量。

蛋白质的含氮量为16%，即1g蛋白质中的氮相当于6.25g蛋白质，用凯氏定氮法测出的含氮量乘以6.25，即得样品中蛋白质的含量。

【实验材料】

1. **实验器材**　微量凯氏定氮仪1套、50ml凯氏烧瓶、移液管、锥形瓶、试管、小玻璃珠。

2. **试验试剂**

（1）浓硫酸、30%氢氧化钠溶液、2%硼酸溶液、标准盐酸溶液（0.01mol/L）。

（2）粉末硫酸钾 - 硫酸铜混合物　K_2SO_4 与 $CuSO_4 \cdot 5H_2O$ 以3:1配比研磨混合。

（3）混合指示剂　由50ml 0.1%甲烯蓝乙醇溶液与200ml 0.1%甲基红乙醇溶液混合配成，贮于棕色瓶中备用。

（4）样品溶液　3mg/ml牛血清白蛋白溶液。

【实验步骤】

1. **安装凯氏定氮仪**　正确安装凯氏定氮仪。

2. **消化**　取4个50ml凯氏烧瓶并标号，各加1颗玻璃珠，在1号及2号瓶中各加样品1ml，催化剂（$K_2SO_4 - CuSO_4 \cdot 5H_2O$）200mg，浓硫酸5ml。注意加样品时应直接送入瓶底，而不要沾在瓶口和瓶颈上。在3号及4号瓶中各加1ml蒸馏水和与1、2号瓶相同量的催化剂和浓硫酸，作为对照。在通风橱内进行消化。

在消化开始时应控制火力，不要使液体冲到瓶颈。待硫酸开始分解并放出SO_2白烟后，适当加强火力，继续消化，直至消化液呈透明淡绿色为止。撤掉火力，冷却至室温。

3. **蒸馏**

（1）**蒸馏器的洗涤**　用水洗涤干净微量凯氏定氮仪，在蒸气发生器中加入用几滴硫酸酸化的蒸馏水和几滴甲基红指示剂，用这样的水蒸气洗涤凯氏定氮仪。约15mg/ml后，在冷凝器下端倾斜放好装有硼酸 - 指示剂的锥形瓶，继续蒸汽洗涤2分钟，观察锥形瓶内的溶液是否变色，如不变色则证明蒸馏装置内部已洗涤干净。移走锥形瓶，停止加热，打开夹子。

（2）**蒸馏**　取下棒状玻璃塞，用吸管吸取消化液，插到反应室小玻璃杯的下方，塞紧棒状玻璃塞。将一个含有硼酸和指示剂的锥形瓶放在冷凝器下方，使冷凝器下端浸没在液体内。取30%的氢氧化钠溶液10ml放入小玻璃杯中，轻提棒状玻璃塞使之流入反应室（为了防止冷凝管倒吸，液体流入反应室必须缓慢）。尚未完全流入时，将玻璃塞盖紧，向玻璃杯中加入蒸馏水约5ml。再轻提玻璃塞，使一半蒸馏水慢慢流入反应室，一半留在玻璃杯中作水封。加热水蒸气发生器，沸腾后夹紧夹子，开始蒸馏。氨气进入锥形瓶，瓶中的酸溶液由紫色变成绿色。变色时开始计时，再蒸馏5分钟。移动锥形瓶，使硼酸液面距离冷凝管约1cm，并用少量蒸馏水洗涤冷凝管口外面，继续蒸馏1分钟，移开锥形瓶，用表面皿覆盖锥形瓶。蒸馏完毕后，必须将反应室洗涤干净，再继续下一个蒸馏操作。待样品和对照均蒸馏完毕后，同时进行滴定。

4. **滴定** 用 0.01mol/L 的标准盐酸溶液滴定各锥形瓶中收集的氨，硼酸指示剂溶液由绿色变淡紫色为滴定终点。

【实验结果】

$$样品中氮的含量（g\%）=\frac{(A-B)\times0.01\times14}{C\times1000}\times100\%$$

$$样品中蛋白质的含量（g\%）=\frac{(A-B)\times0.01\times14\times6.25}{C\times1000}\times100\%$$

式中，A——滴定样品用去的盐酸溶液平均毫升数；

$\qquad$ B——滴定对照液用去的盐酸溶液平均毫升数；

$\qquad$ C——所取样品溶液的毫升数。

四、二喹啉甲酸法（BCA 法）

【实验目的】

掌握用 BCA 方法测定蛋白质含量的原理和操作方法。

【实验原理】

BCA 检测法是 Lowry 测定法的一种改进方法。与 Lowry 方法相比，BCA 法的操作更简单，试剂更加稳定，几乎没有干扰物质的影响，灵敏度更高（微量检测可达到 0.5μg/ml），应用更加灵活。

蛋白质分子中的肽键在碱性条件下能与 Cu^{2+} 生成络合物，同时将 Cu^{2+} 还原成 Cu^+。二喹啉甲酸及其钠盐是溶于水的化合物，在碱性条件下，可以和 Cu^+ 结合，生成深紫色的化合物，这种稳定的化合物在 562nm 处具有强吸收，并且化合物颜色的深浅与蛋白质的浓度成正比，故可用比色的方法确定蛋白质的含量。

【实验材料】

1. **实验器材** 721 分光光度计、恒温水浴槽、移液管、微量进样器、试管和试管架。

2. **实验试剂**

（1）BCA 试剂的配制

① 试剂 A（1L） 分别称取 10g BCA（1%）、20g $Na_2CO_3 \cdot H_2O$（2%）、1.6g $Na_2C_4H_4O_6 \cdot 2H_2O$（0.16%）、4g NaOH（0.4%）、9.5g $NaHCO_3$（0.95%）、加水至 1L，用 NaOH 或固体 $NaHCO_3$ 调节 pH 至 11.25。

② 试剂 B（50ml） 取 2g $CuSO_4 \cdot 5H_2O$（4%），加蒸馏水至 50ml。

③ BCA 试剂 取 50 份试剂 A 与 1 份试剂 B 混合均匀。此试剂可稳定 1 周。

（2）标准蛋白质溶液 取 40mg 牛血清白蛋白，精密称定，溶于蒸馏水中，定容至 100ml，制成 400μg/ml 的溶液。

（3）样品溶液 50μg/ml 的牛血清白蛋白溶液。

【实验步骤】

1. **绘制标准曲线**　取 6 支干燥洁净的大试管，编号，按照表 2 - 3 加入试剂。

表 2 - 3　配制不同蛋白质含量的溶液

试　剂	管　号					
	1	2	3	4	5	6
标准蛋白质溶液（μl）	0	50	100	150	200	250
蒸馏水（μl）	250	200	150	100	50	0
BCA 试剂（ml）	5	5	5	5	5	5
蛋白质含量（μg）	0	20	40	60	80	100

混匀，37℃保温 30 分钟，冷却至室温后，以 1 号管为对照，在 562nm 处测定各管光密度值，以牛血清白蛋白含量为横坐标，以光密度值为纵坐标，绘制标准曲线。

2. **样品测定**　准确吸取 250μl 样品溶液于干燥洁净的试管中，加入 BCA 试剂 5ml，摇匀，于 37℃保温 30 分钟，冷却至室温后，以标准曲线 1 号管为对照测定光密度值。

【实验结果】

根据样品的光密度值和标准曲线，计算出样品的蛋白质含量。

五、考马斯亮蓝染料结合比色法

【实验目的】

掌握用考马斯亮蓝染料结合比色法测定蛋白质含量的原理和操作方法。

【实验原理】

考马斯亮蓝 G - 250 是一种染料，在游离状态下呈红色，最大吸收峰在 465nm。当它与蛋白质结合后变成深蓝色，最大吸收峰变为 595nm。蛋白质含量在 1 ~ 1000μg 范围内，蛋白质 - 染料复合物在 595nm 处的光密度值与蛋白质含量成正比。

蛋白质 - 染料复合物具有很高的光密度值，因此大大提高了蛋白质测定的灵敏度，最低检出量为 1μg 蛋白质。染料与蛋白质结合迅速，大约为 2 分钟，结合物的颜色在 1 小时内稳定。所以本法操作简便，快速，灵敏度高，稳定性好，是一种测定蛋白质含量的常用方法。

【实验材料】

1. **实验器材**　721 型分光光度计、试管、移液管、容量瓶。

2. **实验试剂**

（1）标准蛋白质溶液　取 10mg 牛血清白蛋白，精密称定，溶于蒸馏水中并定容至 100ml，制成 100μg/ml 的溶液。

（2）考马斯亮蓝 G - 250 试剂　称取 100mg 考马斯亮蓝 G - 250，溶于 50ml 95% 乙醇中，加入 85%（M/V）的磷酸 100ml，最后用蒸馏水定容到 1000ml。此溶液可在常温下放置 1 个月。

（3）样品溶液 50μg/ml 牛血清白蛋白溶液。

【实验步骤】

1. 绘制标准曲线 取 6 支干燥洁净的大试管，编号，按表 2-4 加入试剂。

表 2-4 配制不同蛋白质含量的溶液

试 剂	管 号					
	1	2	3	4	5	6
标准蛋白质溶液（ml）	0.0	0.2	0.4	0.6	0.8	1.0
蒸馏水（ml）	1.0	0.8	0.6	0.4	0.2	0.0
考马斯亮蓝 G-250 试剂（ml）	5.0	5.0	5.0	5.0	5.0	5.0
蛋白质含量（μg）	0.0	20.0	40.0	60.0	80.0	100.0

混匀，室温静置 2 分钟，以 1 号管为对照，在 595nm 处测定各管光密度值，以牛血清白蛋白含量为横坐标，以光密度值为纵坐标，绘制标准曲线。

2. 样品测定 准确吸取 1ml 样品溶液于干燥洁净的试管中，加入考马斯亮蓝 G-250 试剂 5ml，摇匀，室温静置 2 分钟。以 1 号管为对照，在 595nm 处测定光密度值。

【实验结果】

根据样品的光密度值和标准曲线计算出样品的蛋白质含量。

【思考题】

1. 试比较 Folin-酚法与考马斯亮蓝染料结合比色法的优缺点。

2. 试比较二喹啉甲酸法与 Folin-酚法的优缺点。

3. 凯氏定氮法在消化样品时，加入浓硫酸、硫酸钾和硫酸铜粉末的目的是什么？

4. 紫外吸收法测定蛋白质含量的原理是什么？

Experiment 2　Protein's Quantification

Ⅰ. Folin-phenol reagent method（Lowry method）

Purpose

1. To learn about the principle of Lowry method to quantitate protein.

2. To master the operational procedures of Lowry method to quantitate protein.

Principle

The principle of Lowry method is that there are tyrosine and tryptophan residues in protein which can perform oxidation-reduction reaction with Folin-phenol reagent. The reaction process can be divided into two steps. The first step is that the peptide bonds of protein can bind with Cu^{2+} to form protein-Cu^{2+} complex in the basic solution. While the second step is that the Tyr or the Trp residue in the protein-Cu^{2+} complex can deoxidize the phosphotungstic acid and phosphomolybdic acid of the alkali phenol reagent, and then form blue products. This reaction approaches limit in 30min. In a definite range, the relationship between absorbance and protein concentration is a straight line. So protein content can be determined by spectroscopic method. When spectroscopic method is used, it is necessary to choose different wavelengths depending on different protein content. If the protein content is high (25 ~ 100μg), the sample is detected at 500nm, but if the protein concentration is low (5 ~ 25μg), the sample is detected at 755nm. Then calculate the protein content of unknown sample from the calibration curve.

Folin-phenol method is easy to perform and has high sensitivity when the protein content in the sample is more than 5μg. It is one of the most widely used methods in quantitation of protein.

Materials

1. Apparatus

Test tubes and test tube shelves, 100ml flasks, pipettes, 721 type spectroscope.

2. Reagents

(1) Folin-phenol reagent A　Dissolve 1g Na_2CO_3 into 50ml of 0.1mol/L NaOH, and then dissolve 0.5g of $CuSO_4 \cdot 5H_2O$ into 100ml of 1% sodium potassium tartrate, mix 50ml of the former and 1ml of the latter. The mixer is useful within one day.

(2) Folin-phenol reagent B　Add 100g of $Na_2WO_4 \cdot 2H_2O$, 25g of $Na_2MoO_4 \cdot 2H_2O$, 700ml of distilled water, 50ml of 85% H_3PO_4 and 100ml of thick HCl into a 1.5L round-bottom stoppered flask, mix well and reflux for 10h. After refluxing, add 150g of Li_2SO_4, 50ml of distilled water, and several drops of liquid Br_2, then boil it for 15min without a cap to get rid of excessive Br_2. After cooling, dilute it to a constant volume of 1000ml with a volumetric flask. Filtrate it, add several drops of bromic water to be oxidized to pale yellow if the filtrate is green. Keep the filtrate in a brown flask in a darkroom. Titrate with calibration NaOH before being used to ascertain the acidity of the reagent with phenolphthalein as the indicator. The acidity of the reagent is about 2mol/L commonly. If the filtrate is pale yellow, dilute 100 times before titrating in order not to affect observing end-point. Dilute properly (about one time) before using to obtain 1mol/L acid.

(3) Standard protein solution　Accurately weigh 100mg of bovine (or human) serum albumin with analytical balance, dissolve it in minimum volume of distilled water, transfer to a 100 ml flask, and accurately dilute to 100ml, which makes the concentration of protein 1mg/ml.

(4) Sample solution　Make 0.5mg/ml casein solution as unknown solution.

Procedures

1. Draw calibration curve

Number 7 test tubes, add reagents as Table 2－1 and mix up.

Table 2 – 1   Draw calibration curve

Reagent	Tube No.						
	0	1	2	3	4	5	6
Standard protein solution（ml）	0.0	0.1	0.2	0.3	0.4	0.5	0.6
Distilled water（ml）	1.0	0.9	0.8	0.7	0.6	0.5	0.4
Folin-phenol reagent A（ml）	5.0	5.0	5.0	5.0	5.0	5.0	5.0
Mix up and keep at room temperature for 10min							
Folin-phonel reagent B（ml）	1.0	1.0	1.0	1.0	1.0	1.0	1.0

Add Folin-phenol reagent B and shake immediately, keep 30min, then determine the optical density at 500nm. The test tube No. 0 is control. Draw the calibration curve while the optical density is y-axis and the standard protein concentration is x-axis.

2. Measure the concentration of sample solution

Take 2 test tubes. Add 1ml of sample solution and Folin-phenol reagent A 5ml in them. Mix up and keep at room temperature for 10min. Add 1ml Folin-phenol reagent B and mix up immediately, keep for 30min, then determine the optical density at 500nm.

Results

Calculate the content of protein of the sample solution according to the optical density of sample solution and the calibration curve.

II. Ultraviolet absorption method

Purpose

1. To learn the principles of ultraviolet absorption method to quantitate protein.

2. To master the operational method of ultraviolet spectrophotometer.

Principle

There are amino acid residues with aromatic ring in protein molecule (such as tyrosine and tryptophan), so there is maximal ultraviolet absorption at 280nm, at which the relationship between optical density and protein concentration is a straight line in a definite range. So protein concentration can be determined by ultraviolet absorption method.

Ultraviolet absorption method can determine the protein concentration ranging from 0.1 to 0.5mg/ml. This method is easy to perform. It determines protein concentration promptly, does not consume samples and cannot be interfered by low salt concentration. So this method is widely used in the preparation of protein.

Materials

1. Apparatus

Test tubes and test tube shelf, 50ml flasks, pipettes, ultraviolet spectrophotometer.

2. Reagents

（1）Standard protein solution   Exactly make 2mg/ml of casein solution.

（2）Sample solution   Make 0.5mg/ml casein solution as unknown sample solution.

Procedures

1. Draw calibration curve

Number 7 test tubes, and add reagents as Table 2 – 2.

Table 2 – 2　Preparing solutions of different protein concentrations

Reagent	Tube No.						
	0	1	2	3	4	5	6
Standard protein solution (ml)	0.0	0.5	1.0	1.5	2.0	2.5	3.0
Distilled water (ml)	8.0	7.5	7.0	6.5	6.0	5.5	5.0
Protein concentration (mg/ml)	0.0	0.125	0.250	0.375	0.500	0.625	0.750

Mix up, measure the optical density at 280nm by ultraviolet spectrophotometer, while the test tube No. 0 is control. Draw optical density-protein concentration curve, while the optical density is y-axis, and the standard protein concentration is x-axis.

2. Sample determination

Take 4ml sample solution, add 4ml distilled water, and measure the optical density at 280nm.

Results

According to the optical density of sample solution and the calibration curve, calculate the protein concentration of the sample solution.

Ⅲ. Kjeldahl method

Purpose

To learn the principles and the operational techniques of Kjeldahl method.

Principle

The Kjeldahl method measures the nitrogen content of a compound and can be used to determine the protein content of a sample provided that the proportion of nitrogen in the protein is known.

When protein is heated with concentrated sulphuric acid, C and H are oxidized to CO_2 and H_2O, while N is oxidized to NH_3, which can change into $(NH_4)_2SO_4$ with sulphuric acid. This process is called digestion. As the digestion stage is slow, potassium or sodium sulphate is usually added to increase the boiling point of the mixture, and $CuSO_4$ is added as catalyst to accelerate the digest reaction.

After digestion, concentrated alkali which is added in Kjelgahl apparatus can decompose $(NH_4)_2SO_4$ in digestive solution to ammonia. Ammonia is distilled by steam distillation and absorbed with boric acid. Ammonia combines with H^+ in boric acid and depresses the concentration of H^+, which causes the color change of indicator. It is titrated with standard hydrochloric acid until it recovers initial concentration of H^+. According to the quantity of standard hydrochloric, the total nitrogen in sample can be determined.

The nitrogen content of protein is usually accepted as 16% of the total weight, namely,

1g nitrogen of protein is equal to 6.25g protein. The quantity of protein in sample is calculated by multiplying 6.25 with the content of nitrogen determined by Kjeldahl method.

Materials

1. Apparatus

A set of Kjeldahl apparatus, 50ml Kjeldahl flasks, pipette, conical flask, test tubes, small beadings.

2. Reagents

(1) Concentrated sulphuric acid, 30% NaOH solution, 2% boric acid, standard hydrochloric acid (0.01mol/L).

(2) K_2SO_4-$CuSO_4$ mixed powder　Mix K_2SO_4 and $CuSO_4 \cdot 5H_2O$ with ratio 3:1 and skive well.

(3) Mixed indicator　Mix 50ml 0.1% alcohol solution of methyl-olefin blueness and 200ml 0.1% methyl red, and then store the mixture in brown flasks.

(4) Sample solution　3mg/ml bovine serum albumin solution.

Procedures

1. Setting up the Kjeldahl apparatus.

2. Digestion

Take four 50ml Kjeldahl flasks and number them, add a beading in each of them. Add 1ml of sample solution and 200mg of catalyst (K_2SO_4-$CuSO_4 \cdot 5H_2O$) and 5ml of concentrated sulphuric acid in No.1 and No.2 Kjeldahl flasks. Be sure to add sample to the bottom of flasks and do not adhere them to flask wall or flask neck. Add 1ml of distilled water to No.3 and No.4 Kjedahl flasks respectively and commensurate catalyst and concentrated sulphuric acid as in No.1 flask, the results of which is control. Digest them in fume hood.

At the beginning of digestion, control the firepower to prevent the digest solution from rushing to the flask neck. After releasing white smoke of SO_2 decomposed by H_2SO_4, enhance the firepower and continue digesting until digestive solution is light green. Put out the fire and place Kjeldahl flasks in fume hood to cool.

3. Distillation

(1) Washing the distillatory　Clean the Kjedahl apparatus with water. Add distilled water which is acidified by several drops of sulphuric acid and methyl red indicator in the steam generator, and then clean the Kjeldahl apparatus with vapor. After about 15min, place a slant conical flask containing boracic acid and indicator under condenser and continue washing with vapor for 2min. Observe the color change of the solution in the conical flask. If the color doesn't change, it proves that the distillatory is clean. Move the conical flask and stop heating, then loosen the clincher.

(2) Distillation　Take off clubbed glass stopple, take digestive solution with pipette and transfer it carefully to the bottom of small glass cup. Stuff up the glass stopple and immerge the bottom of condenser into liquid. Pour 10ml 30% NaOH into a small glass cup, lift up the

clubbed glass stopple so that basic solution will flow slowly into the reaction chamber. (In case that sample will be absorbed conversely, liquid must flow slowly into the reaction chamber.) Stuff up the glass stopple softly before basic solution completes flowing, then add 5ml distilled water into small glass cup. Lift up glass stopple softly to make half of water flow into the reaction chamber, and the other half is still in the small glass cup as waterseal to avoid leakage. Heat the steam generator and clamp the clincher after boiling to begin distillation. Ammonia enters the conical flask, when the acerb solution turns from purple to green, continue distilling for 5min. Move conical flask to keep liquid level of boracic acid about 1cm away from the bottom of condenser, then wash the outside of condenser with water. Continue distilling for one more minute. Move conical flask and cover the conical flask with watch glass. After distilling, clean the reaction chamber. Distill the other samples as the former operation. Titrate after distillation of samples and control is finished.

4. Titration

Titrate the distilled ammonia with 0.01mol/L standard hydrochloric acid solution until the color of boric indicator solution changes from light green to pale purple.

Results

$$\text{Nitrogen content of sample (g\%)} = \frac{(A - B) \times 0.01 \times 14}{C \times 1000} \times 100\%$$

$$\text{Protein content of sample (g\%)} = \frac{(A - B) \times 0.01 \times 14 \times 6.25}{C \times 1000} \times 100\%$$

In this equation:

A—The average volume (ml) of hydrochloric acid which is consumed in titrating samples.

B—The average volume (ml) of hydrochloric acid which is consumed in titrating controls.

C—The volume (ml) of sample.

Ⅳ. Bicinchoninic acid (BCA) method

Purpose

To master the principle and procedures of BCA method to quantitate protein.

Principle

BCA method is a modification of Lowry method. The BCA techniques more simple during manipulation, no effect of interfering substances, greater stability of working reagent, higher sensitivity (the minimum detection can be 0.5μg/ml), and greater flexibility compared to Lowry method.

The peptide bond of amino acids can bind with Cu^{2+} to form a complex in the basic solution and meanwhile Cu^{2+} is deoxidized to Cu^+. Bicinchoninic acid and its sodium salt are water-soluble. In the alkaline environment, it can bind with Cu^{2+} to form a dark purple compound, which has strong absorbance at 562nm. As the depth of color is linear with the content of protein, the matching method can be used to determine protein content.

Materials

1. Apparatus

721 Type spectrophotometer, constant temperature water bath, pipettes, microsyringe, test tubes and test tube shelves.

2. Reagents

（1）BCA reagent

① Reagent A（1L）　Weigh 10g BCA（1%）, 20g $Na_2CO_3 \cdot H_2O$（2%）, 1.6g $Na_2C_4H_4O_6 \cdot 2H_2O$（0.16%）, 4g NaOH（0.4%）, 9.5g $NaHCO_3$（0.95）respectively. Add water to 1L, and then adjust the pH to 11.25 with NaOH or solid $NaHCO_3$.

② Reagent B（50ml）　Take 2g $CuSO_4 \cdot 5H_2O$（4%）, add distilled water to 50ml.

③ BCA Reagent　Take 50 Reagent A and 1 Reagent B, mix up. This reagent can remain stable for a week.

（2）Standard protein solution　Weigh 40mg bovine serum albumin, dissolve in distilled water to 1000ml, so the concentration of standard protein solution is 400μg/ml.

（3）Sample solution　50μg/ml Bovine serum albumin solution.

Procedures

1. Draw calibration curve

Take six dry and clean test tubes, and add reagents as Table 2-3.

Table 2-3　Preparation of different protein concentration solution

Reagents	Tube No.					
	1	2	3	4	5	6
Standard protein solution（μl）	0	50	100	150	200	250
Distilled water（μl）	250	200	150	100	50	0
BCA reagent（ml）	5	5	5	5	5	5
Protein concentration（μg）	0	20	40	60	80	100

Mix up, incubate for 30 min at 37℃, then cool to the room temperature. Determine the optical density at 562nm while tube No.1 is control. Draw optical density-protein concentration calibration curve. The bovine serum albumin concentration is x-axis and the optical density is y-axis.

2. Sample determination

Put 250μl of sample solution in a clean and dry test tube, add 5ml of BCA reagent and shake up, incubate at 37℃ for 30min. Measure the optical density at 562nm while tube No.1 is control.

Results

Calculate the protein concentration of the sample solution according to the optical density of sample solution and the calibration curve.

V. Coomassie brilliant blue dye-binding method

Purpose

To master the principles and method of Coomassie brilliant blue dye-binding method to quantitate protein.

Principle

Coomassie brilliant blue G-250 is a red dye in acidic solution and its absorbance maximun is at 465nm. When combined with protein, it shows a shift in its absorption maximum from 465nm to 595nm. The optical density at 595nm is directly proportional to protein concentration in a definite range of 1 to 1000μg.

As protein-dye has high optical density value, the sensitivity could be improved and the minimum detectable quantity is 1μg. The dye can bind with protein in about 2min, and this complex can be stable within 1h. So this method is easy to perform, quick, highly sensitive and stable. It is a widely used method in protein content determination.

Materials

1. Apparatus

721 Type spectrophotometer, test tubes, pipettes, flasks.

2. Reagents

(1) Standard protein solution　Weigh 10mg bovine serum albumin, dissolve in distilled water, then dilute to 100ml to get the 100μg/ml solution.

(2) Coomassie brilliant blue G-250 solution　Weigh 100mg Coomassie brilliant blue G-250, dissolve in 50ml 95% ethanol, then add 85% (*M/V*) phosphate solution 100ml, finally dilute to 1000ml. This solution can be preserved for 1 month at room temperature.

(3) Sample solution　Prepare 50μg/ml bovine serum albumin solution as sample solution.

Procedures

1. Draw calibration curve

Take 6 clean test tubes, and add reagents as Table 2 − 4.

Table 2 − 4　Preparation of different protein content solution

Reagents	Tube No.					
	1	2	3	4	5	6
Standard protein solution (ml)	0.0	0.2	0.4	0.6	0.8	1.0
Distilled water (ml)	1.0	0.8	0.6	0.4	0.2	0.0
Coomassie brilliant blue G-250 solution (ml)	5.0	5.0	5.0	5.0	5.0	5.0
Protein content (μg)	0.0	20.0	40.0	60.0	80.0	100.0

Mix up, and keep it standing for 2min at room temperature. Determine the optical density at 595nm, tube No. 1 is control. Draw optical density-protein content calibration curve, while the bovine serum albumin content is *x*-axis, and the optical density is *y*-axis.

2. Sample determination

Take 1ml of sample solution to a clear and dry test tube, add 5ml of Coomassie brilliant blue G-250 reagent and shake, and keep it standing for 2min at room temperature. Determine the optical density at 595nm while Tube No. 1 is control.

Results

Calculate protein content of sample solution according to the optical density and the calibration curve.

Questions

1. Compare the advantages and disadvantages of Folin-phenol reagent method with Coomassie brilliant blue dye-binding method.

2. Compare the advantages and disadvantages of Bicinchoninic acid method with Folin-phenol reagent method.

3. What is the function of adding thick sulphuric acid and K_2SO_4-$CuSO_4$ mixed powder while digesting sample in the Kjeldahl method?

4. What is the principle of Ultraviolet absorption method?

实验三　葡聚糖凝胶层析

【实验目的】

1. 学习葡聚糖凝胶的特性及凝胶层析的原理。
2. 掌握凝胶层析的基本操作技术。

【实验原理】

凝胶层析又称为分子排阻层析或凝胶过滤，是以被分离物质的分子量差异为基础的一种层析分离技术。层析的固定相载体是凝胶颗粒，目前应用较广的是葡聚糖凝胶（Sephadex）和琼脂糖凝胶（Sepharose）。

葡聚糖凝胶是由直链的葡聚糖单体和交联剂3-氯-1，2-环氧丙烷交联而成的具有多孔网状结构的高分子化合物。凝胶颗粒中网孔的大小可通过调节葡聚糖和交联剂的比例来控制，交联度越大，网孔越小；交联度越小，网孔越大。被分离物质由于分子量不同而具有不同的直径，当它们通过葡聚糖凝胶层析柱时，直径大于凝胶网孔的大分子物质不能进入凝胶颗粒内部，完全被凝胶排阻，只能随着流动相在凝胶颗粒的间隙中流动，因此流程短，阻力小，流速快，而先流出层析柱；直径小于凝胶网孔的小分子物质可完全进入凝胶颗粒内部，流程长，阻力大，流速慢，而最后从层析柱中流出。若被分离物质的分子量介于完全排阻和完全进入网孔的物质的分子量之间，则在两者之间从柱中流出，由此就可以达到分离目的。

葡聚糖凝胶层析为分离蛋白质等生物大分子提供了一种非常温和的方法。葡聚糖凝胶网孔的大小决定了被分离蛋白质的分子量范围，其可从几百到几十万道尔顿，因此被广泛应用。

　　本实验以葡聚糖凝胶 G-25 作为固定相载体分离蓝色葡聚糖-2000 和溴酚蓝。蓝色葡聚糖-2000 分子量接近 2×10^6，而溴酚蓝分子量为 670，二者分子量相差较大，前者完全排阻，而后者则可完全进入凝胶颗粒网孔内，二者因通过层析柱的时间不同而实现分离。

【实验材料】

　　1. 实验器材　层析柱（1cm×20cm，附有一小段乳胶管及螺旋夹）、洗脱液瓶、试管及试管架、量筒、721 型分光光度计。

　　2. 实验试剂

　　（1）Tris-醋酸缓冲液（pH 7.0）　取 0.01mol/L Tris 溶液（含 0.1mol/L KCl）900ml，用浓醋酸调 pH 至 7.0，加蒸馏水至 1000ml。

　　（2）溴酚蓝溶液　称取溴酚蓝 10mg，溶于 5ml 无水乙醇中，充分搅拌使其溶解，然后逐滴加入 Tris-醋酸缓冲液（pH 7.0）至溶液呈深蓝色。

　　（3）蓝色葡聚糖-2000 溶液　称取蓝色葡聚糖-2000 10mg，溶于 2ml Tris-醋酸缓冲液（pH 7.0）中即成。

　　（4）样品溶液　取溴酚蓝溶液 0.1ml，蓝色葡聚糖-2000 溶液 0.5ml 混匀后为样品溶液。

　　（5）葡聚糖凝胶 G-25。

【实验步骤】

　　1. 凝胶的制备　商品凝胶是干燥的颗粒，使用时需经溶胀处理。称取 4g 葡聚糖凝胶 G-25，加 50ml 蒸馏水，搅拌均匀，在室温溶胀 6 小时，或沸水浴溶胀 2 小时，一般采用后一种方法。倾泻法除去凝胶上层水及细小颗粒，用蒸馏水反复洗涤几次，再以缓冲溶液（pH 7.0 Tris-醋酸溶液）洗涤 2~3 次，使 pH 和离子强度达到平衡，最后抽去溶液及凝胶颗粒内部气泡，凝胶可保存在缓冲液内。

　　2. 装柱　将洗净的层析柱，垂直固定在铁架台上，选择有薄膜的一端作为层析柱下口，将下口连接上乳胶管并用螺旋夹夹紧。层析柱中加入洗脱液，打开下口螺旋夹，让溶液流出，最后保留约 2cm 高度的洗脱液，旋紧螺旋夹。将凝胶轻轻搅动均匀，缓缓注入层析柱中，待凝胶沉积到 2cm 时，打开下口螺旋夹，继续装柱，直到凝胶沉积高度达到 10cm 时关闭螺旋夹。装柱过程中严禁产生气泡，尽可能一次装完，避免出现分层。再用洗脱液平衡 1~2 个柱体积，凝胶胶面上始终保持一定量的洗脱液。平衡后，旋紧下端的螺旋夹。

　　3. 加样　打开螺旋夹，使凝胶胶面上的洗脱液流出，直至胶面与液面刚好平齐为止，关闭下端出口。取溴酚蓝及蓝色葡聚糖-2000 样品液 0.3ml，小心地加于凝胶表面上。打开下端螺旋夹，使样品溶液进入凝胶内部，同时开始用试管收集流出液，此为 1 号测定管。当样品溶液恰好流至与凝胶表面平齐时，关闭下端螺旋夹。用少量洗脱液清洗加样区，共清洗 3 次，每次清洗液应完全进入凝胶柱内后再进行下一次清洗，保证清洗过程的流出液收集到 1 号测定管中。清洗结束后在凝胶表面上加入洗脱液，保持高度为 3~4cm。

4. **洗脱与收集**　连接好洗脱液瓶与凝胶层析柱，调节洗脱液流速为 1ml/min，进行洗脱。仔细观察样品在层析柱内的分离现象，收集洗脱液，每管约 3ml 并进行编号，直至样品被完全洗脱下来。用洗脱液作对照，将各收集管中的洗脱液用 721 型分光光度计在波长 540nm 处测定光密度值。

5. **凝胶回收处理方法**　样品完全洗脱后，继续用 3 倍柱体积的洗脱液冲洗凝胶，然后将层析柱下口放在小烧杯中，慢慢打开，再将上口打开，凝胶全部回收，备用。

【实验结果】

以收集管号为横坐标，以光密度值为纵坐标制作洗脱曲线。分析洗脱曲线并讨论实验结果。

【思考题】

1. 葡聚糖凝胶层析为何能分离不同的样品？
2. 葡聚糖凝胶层析操作时应注意哪些问题？

Experiment 3　Sephadex Gel Chromatography

Purpose

1. To learn the specialties of Sephadex gel and principle of gel chromatography.
2. To master the basic operational techniques of gel chromatography.

Principle

Gel chromatography is also called molecular exclusion chromatography or gel filtration. It is a kind of chromatographic separation technique based on the difference of molecular weight of the materials to be isolated. The stationary phase supporter is gel particle. The most widely used gels are dextran gel (Sephadex) and agarose gel (Sepharose) at present.

Sephadex gel is a kind of porous and reticular macromolecular compound. It is cross-linked by glucan as straight chain and 3 – chlorine – 1, 2 – epoxypropane as cross-linking agent. The pore size of gel particles is controlled by the proportion of glucan and cross-linking agent. The greater the degree of cross linking is, the smaller the pore size is. On the contrary, the less the degree of cross linking is, the bigger the pore size is. The substances being isolated have different diameters because of different molecular weights. When the substances flow through the chromatography column, the substances of macromolecules whose diameters are bigger than the pore size of gel can't enter the gel particle. They are excluded completely and only can flow in the interval of gel particles. Consequently, the distance is short, the resistance force is little and the flow rate is rapid. So they flow out of the chromatography column first. However, micromolecules whose diameters are smaller than the pore size of gel can enter the interior of gel particle completely. Consequently, the distance is long, the resistance force is great and the flow is slow. So they flow out of the chromatography column later. If the molecular sizes is between that of completely excluded and that of completely entering, substance flows out of the column between them. So this method can be used to isolated different substances.

Sephadex gel chromatography is a mild method used to isolate protein. Pore size of gel determines the range of molecular weight of isolated proteins which can be from several hundred to several hundred thousand. It is a widely used method in protein purification.

In this experiment, Sephadex G-25 is stationary phase supporter to separate dextran blue-2000 and bromophenol blue. The molecular weight of Dextran blue-2000 is approximately 2×10^6, while the molecular weight of bromophenol blue is about 670. Because of the obvious molecular weight differences, the former can be excluded completely and the latter can enter the gel particle, so they can be separated by different elution time.

Materials

1. Apparatus

Chromatography column (1cm × 20cm, with latex tubing and clips), elution flask, test tubes and test tube shelf, measuring cylinder, 721 type spectrophotometer.

2. Reagents

(1) Tris-acetate buffer (pH 7.0)　Take 0.01mol/L Tris solution (contains 0.1mol/L KCl) 900ml, adjust pH to 7.0 with acetate, then add distilled water to 1000ml.

(2) Bromophenol blue solution　Weigh 10mg bromophenol blue, dissolve them in 5ml ethanol, stir to make it dissolve completely, then add Tris-acetate buffer (pH 7.0) gradually till the solution becomes dark blue.

(3) Dextran blue-2000 solution　Take 10mg of Dextran blue-2000, dissolve them in 2ml Tris-acetate buffer (pH 7.0).

(4) Sample solution　Mix 0.1ml bromophenol blue and 0.5ml Dextran blue-2000.

(5) Sephadex G-25.

Procedures

1. Gel preparation

The commercial gel is dry particle, should be expanded before using. In this experiment, add 4g Sephadex G-25 to 50ml distilled water and stir, expand for 6h at room temperature or 2h in boiling water. The latter method is use in common. Remove the upper water and small particles with decantation method, wash gel with distilled water several times, then wash them with buffer (Tris-acetate buffer, pH 7.0) 2~3 times to balance the pH and ion concentration. Finally remove bubbles in the gel and solution. The gel can be preserved in the buffer.

2. Packing column

Fix a clean chromatography column on the retort stand vertically, choose the end with membrane as the bottom, then connect the latex tube to the bottom and clamp it. Add eluent, open the screw clamp to let the solution flow out so as to remove the bubbles. When the height of eluent is about 2cm, tighten the screw clamp. Stir the gel particles gently, pour into the column, loosen the screw clamp when the height of the gel deposited at the bottom reaches 2cm, and continue packing till the height reaches 10cm, then tighten the screw clamp. It should be ensured that there is no bubbles or layers of the column bed in the process or again. After packing, wash the gel with eluent (about 1 to 2 column volume) and keep some eluent on the surface of gel. After balancing, tighten the screw clamp.

3. Loading sample

Loosen the screw clamp to make the eluent flow out till the gel surface meets the liquid surface, tighten the screw clamp. Add 0. 3ml sample solution, the mixture of bromophenol blue and Dextran blue-2000, carefully on the surface of gel, do not stir the surface. Open the screw clamp to let the sample solution enter into the gel. As soon as open the screw clamp begin to collect the eluent. This is the sample of No. 1. When the sample solution flows to the surface of gel, turn off the screw clamp. Wash the sample region with a small volume of eluent three times and insure the washing eluent flow completely into the gel each time. The washing eluent must be collected into No. 1 tube. Finally add eluent on the gel surface and keep the height of eluent 3 ~ 4cm higher than the gel surface.

4. Elution and collection

Connect the elution flask and chromatography column. Adjust the flow rate of eluent to about 1ml/min. Observe the separation process of the sample in the chromatography column, collect eluent (about 3ml per test tube) and number them till the sample is totally eluted out. Measure the optical density of eluent in each tube with 721 type spectrophotometer at 540nm.

5. Regeneration of gel

After washing out the sample, wash the gel with eluent about 3 times of column volume. Put a glass beaker under the column bottom, open the bottom end and the upper end slowly, then the gel flows into the beaker for reuse.

Results

The number of test tube is x-axis and the optical density is y-axis. Draw the elution curve. Analysis the elution curve and discuss the results.

Questions

1. Why Sephadex gel chromatography can be used to separate different substances?
2. What problem should us note in Sephadex gel chromatography operation?

实验四 疏水作用层析

【实验目的】
了解疏水作用层析的原理与方法。

【实验原理】
疏水作用层析（hydrophobic interaction chromatography，HIC）是根据分子表面疏水性差别来分离蛋白质和多肽等生物大分子的一种较为常用的方法。蛋白质和多肽等生物大分子的表面常常暴露着一些疏水性基团，我们把这些疏水性基团称为疏水补丁，疏水补丁可以与疏水性层析介质发生疏水性相互作用而结合。不同的分子由于疏水性不同，它们与疏水性层析介质之间的疏水性作用力强弱不同，疏水作用层析就是依据这一原理分离纯化蛋白质和多肽等生物大分子的，疏水作用层析的基本原理如图4－1所示。

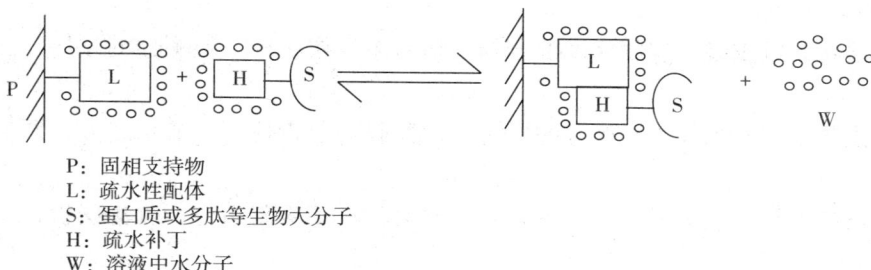

P：固相支持物
L：疏水性配体
S：蛋白质或多肽等生物大分子
H：疏水补丁
W：溶液中水分子

图4－1 疏水作用层析基本原理

溶液中高离子强度可以增强蛋白质和多肽等生物大分子与疏水性层析介质之间的疏水作用，利用这个性质，在高离子强度下将待分离的样品吸附在疏水性层析介质上，然后线性或阶段降低离子强度选择性地将样品解吸。疏水性弱的物质，在较高离子强度的溶液时被洗脱下来，当离子强度降低时，疏水性强的物质才随后被洗脱下来。

Phenyl－Sepharose^{TM} 6 Fast Flow 是疏水性层析介质的一种，这种层析介质是以交联琼脂糖为支持物，交联琼脂糖支持物与苯基共价结合。苯基作为疏水性配体，可以与疏水性物质发生疏水作用，Phenyl－Sepharose^{TM} 6 Fast Flow 结构示意如图4－2。

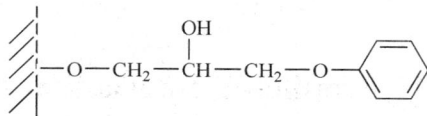

图4－2 Phenyl－Sepharose^{TM} 6 Fast Flow 层析填料结构

【实验材料】

1. 实验器材 层析柱（1.6cm×20cm）、恒流泵、梯度混合器、紫外检测器。

2. 实验试剂

（1）疏水层析介质 Phenyl－Sepharose^{TM} 6 Fast Flow。

（2）溶液A 0.01mol/L pH 7.0 Na_2HPO_4－NaH_2PO_4缓冲溶液，称取4.37g Na_2HPO_4·$12H_2O$ 和1.218g NaH_2PO_4·$2H_2O$，加蒸馏水800ml，溶解后定容至2L。

（3）溶液B 264.28g $(NH_4)_2SO_4$溶于1L溶液A，终浓度2mol/L。

（4）蛋白质样品 溶于溶液B。

【实验步骤】

1. 层析介质准备 Phenyl－Sepharose^{TM} 6 Fast Flow 疏水层析介质保存在20%乙醇中，取出层析介质后，倾出乙醇溶液。加入溶液A，溶液的体积约占总体积的1/4。

2. **装柱** 将层析柱洗净，固定在铁架台上，层析柱下口用螺旋夹夹紧。加入溶液B，打开下口让溶液流出，排出残留气泡，柱中保留高度约2cm的溶液。将准备好的层析介质轻轻搅匀，缓慢加进柱中。层析介质在柱中沉积高度超过1cm时，打开下口。柱床高度达到6~8cm时关闭下口，装柱尽可能一次装完，避免出现界面。

3. **柱平衡** 用溶液B平衡1~2个柱床体积。注意始终保持层析介质处于溶液中，避免干柱。

4. **层析系统安装** 按照梯度混合器、恒流泵、层析柱、检测器的顺序，连接层析系统。

5. **上样** 取样品加入平衡好的层析柱，并收集层析柱下口流出组分，调节流速为1ml/min。

6. **洗涤** 用溶液B洗涤1个床体积，洗去上样不吸附组分，收集层析柱下口流出成分。

7. **洗脱与收集** 按照100%溶液B→100%溶液A（总体积500ml梯度洗脱），收集洗脱液。

8. **层析介质的清洗与保存** 层析介质先用水清洗，然后用0.5mol/L NaOH洗脱，最后用水洗至中性。处理好的层析介质放在20%乙醇中，4℃保存。

【实验结果】

以洗脱时间为横坐标，280nm处紫外吸收值为纵坐标绘图，得到洗脱曲线。分析实验结果，得出实验结论并讨论。

【思考题】

疏水作用层析与反相层析有什么不同？

Experiment 4　Hydrophobic Interaction Chromatography

Purpose

To understand the principle and method of hydrophobic interaction chromatography.

Principle

Hydrophobic interaction chromatography (HIC) is a versatile method for the purification and separation of macromolecules, such as protein and polypeptide, based on differences in their surface hydrophobicity. Many macromolecules have some hydrophobic groups exposed on the surface of it, which is called hydrophobic patch. Hydrophobic patch can bind with resin depend on the interaction with hydrophobic ligand. As is shown in the Fig. 4 – 1, substances are separated on the basis of their varying strength of their hydrophobic interaction with hydrophobic groups attached to the matrix.

Hydrophobic interaction between a macromolecule and the resin is enhanced by high ionic strength buffer. Depend on this property, sample can be adsorb to hydrophobic ligand in the presence of moderately high concentrations of salts. Substance with less hydrophobicity is elu-

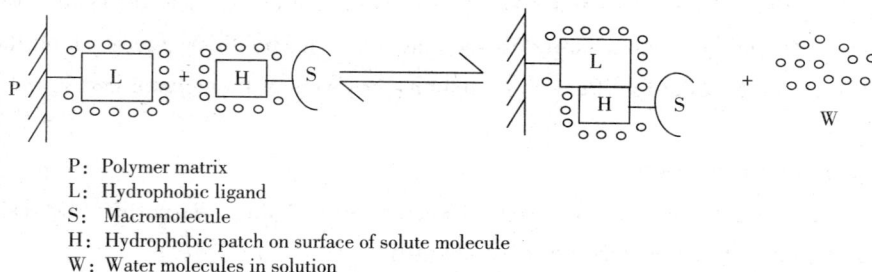

P: Polymer matrix
L: Hydrophobic ligand
S: Macromolecule
H: Hydrophobic patch on surface of solute molecule
W: Water molecules in solution

Fig. 4 – 1　The basic principle of hydrophobic interaction chromatography

ted in higher ionic strength solution, and substance with stronger hydrophobicity is eluted in weaker ionic strength solution.

Phenyl-Sepharose^{TM} 6 Fast Flow is one of the HIC resin. In Phenyl-Sepharose^{TM} 6 Fast Flow, phenyl groups are as HIC ligand which have interaction with hydrophobic biomolecules are coupled to the cross-linked agarose matrices via glycidyl ether bonds (shown in Fig. 4 – 2)。

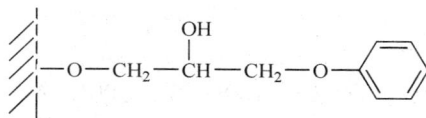

Fig. 4 – 2　The structure of Phenyl-Sepharose^{TM} 6 Fast Flow

Materials

1. Apparatus

Column (1. 6cm × 20cm), pump, gradient mixer, ultraviolet spectrophotometers.

2. Reagents

(1) Hydrophobic chromatography resin　Phenyl-Sepharose^{TM} 6 Fast Flow.

(2) Buffer A　0. 01mol/L pH 7. 0 Na_2HPO_4 and NaH_2PO_4. Weigh 4. 37g $Na_2HPO_4 \cdot 12H_2O$ and 1. 218g $NaH_2PO_4 \cdot 2H_2O$ dissolve in 800ml distilled water, then dilute to 2L with distilled water.

(3) Buffer B　Weigh 264. 28g $(NH_4)_2SO_4$ dissolve in 1L buffer A, the final concentration of $(NH_4)_2SO_4$ is 2. 0mol/L.

(4) Protein sample is dissolved in buffer B.

Procedures

1. Preparing the resin

Phenyl-Sepharose^{TM} 6 Fast Flow resin is preserved in 20% ethanol. Decant the ethanol solution and replace it with buffer A to 1/4 total volume.

2. Packing the column

Fix a clean chromatography column on the retort stand vertically and clamp the bottom. Add buffer B and open the screw clamp to let the solution flow out so as to remove the bubbles. When the height of eluent is about 2cm, tighten the clamp. Stir the resin particles gently, add them into the column, Open the screw clamp when the height of the resin deposited at the bottom reaches 1cm, and continue packing till the height reaches 6~8cm, then turn off the screw clamp. It should be ensured that there is no bubbles or layers of the column bed in the process or again.

3. Equilibration of column
Equilibrate the column with buffer B and keep resin in buffer, do not dry the resin.

4. Assembling the chromatography system
Connect the chromatography system according to the sequence as following, gradient mixer, pump, column and detector.

5. Loading sample
Applied the sample prepared onto the equilibrated column at a flow rate of 1ml/min and collect the solution flowing through.

6. Washing
Wash the column with buffer B to get rid of samples not binding and collect the solutions which have flown out.

7. Elution and collection
Elute the column with a gradient from 100% B to 100% A (total volume is 500ml) and collect the elution.

8. Cleaning and keep of resin
Wash the column with distilled water, 0.5mol/L NaOH, and followed immediately with distilled water to neutrality. Put resin in 20% ethanol and keep at 4℃.

Results
Take the test tube numbered as x axis and the optical density at 280nm as y axis, draw out the elute curve, and analysis the results, give a conclusion and discussion.

Questions
What is the difference between HIC and reverse phase chromatography?

实验五 离子交换层析

【实验目的】
1. 了解离子交换树脂层析的工作原理及操作技术。
2. 学会用离子交换树脂层析法分离混合氨基酸。

【实验原理】
离子交换层析（ion exchange chromatography，IEC），是根据待分离物质电荷的不同来分离不同物质的技术。离子交换层析基质是由带正电荷或负电荷的功能基团与固体支持介质以共价键结合的方式构成的，电荷基团能够分别生成阳离子交换剂和阴离子交换剂。带电荷的物质被带有反相电荷的离子交换剂吸附，而带有中性或相同电荷的物质流过层析柱或被洗脱。带电荷物质的结合是可逆的，当改变盐浓度或 pH 梯度，被吸附的带电物质就能够被洗脱下来。

离子交换层析中，基质是由带电荷的树脂或纤维素组成。通常按所带的基团分为强酸（—SO₃H）、弱酸（—COOH）、强碱［—N(CH₃)₃OH］和弱碱（—NH₂OH）。离子交换树脂是一种合成的高聚物，不溶于水，吸水膨胀。高聚物分子由能电离的极性基团与非极性的树脂组成，极性基团上的离子能与溶液中的离子起交换作用，而非极性的树脂本身物性不变。待分离组分中的离子会与极性基团上的离子发生离子交换，改变盐浓度或 pH，二者的亲和力会发生改变，当洗脱液流过时，样品中的离子按结合力的弱强先后被洗脱，最终实现分离。

本实验用磺酸阳离子交换树脂分离酸性氨基酸（天冬氨酸 pI = 2.97）、中性氨基酸（丙氨酸 pI = 6.0）、碱性氨基酸（赖氨酸 pI = 9.74）的混合液。在低 pH 条件下，天冬氨酸所带电荷少，与树脂结合弱，首先被洗脱下来；pH 4.2 条件下，丙氨酸解离程度小，被洗脱下来；在 pH 12 条件下，因溶液 pH 高于赖氨酸的 pI，赖氨酸解离为阴离子从树脂上被交换下来。通过改变洗脱液的 pH，从而达到 3 种氨基酸被分别洗脱分离。

【实验材料】

1. **实验器材**　层析柱（1.6cm × 25cm）、恒流泵、梯度混合器、试管及试管架、紫外分光光度计、磺酸阳离子交换树脂（Dowex 50）。

2. **实验试剂**

（1）2mol/L HCl、2mol/L NaOH、0.1mol/L HCl、0.1mol/L NaOH。

（2）pH 4.2 枸橼酸缓冲液　0.1mol/L 枸橼酸 54ml 加 0.1mol/L 枸橼酸钠 46ml。

（3）pH 5.0 醋酸缓冲液　0.2mol/L NaAc 70ml 加 0.2mol/L HAc 30ml。

（4）0.2% 中性茚三酮溶液　0.2g 茚三酮加 100ml 丙酮。

（5）氨基酸混合液　丙氨酸、天冬氨酸、赖氨酸各 10ml，分别加入 0.1mol/L HCl 3ml。

【实验步骤】

1. **树脂的处理**　100ml 烧杯中置约 10g 树脂，加 25ml 12mol/L HCl 搅拌 2 小时，倾弃酸液，用蒸馏水充分洗涤树脂至中性。加 25ml 12mol/L NaOH 至上述树脂中搅拌 2 小时，倾弃碱液，用蒸馏水洗涤至中性。将树脂悬浮于 50ml pH 4.2 枸橼酸缓冲液中备用。

2. **装柱**　取直径 0.8 ~ 1.2cm、长度 20 ~ 30cm 的层析柱，底部垫玻璃棉或海绵垫，自顶部注入经处理的上述树脂悬浮液，关闭层析柱出口，待树脂沉降后，放出过量的溶液，再加入一些树脂，至树脂沉积至 8 ~ 10cm 高度即可。于柱子顶部继续加入 pH 4.2 枸橼酸缓冲液洗涤，使流出液 pH 为 4.2 为止，关闭柱子出口，保持液面高出树脂表面 1cm 左右。

3. **加样、洗脱及洗脱液收集**　打开出口使缓冲液流出，待液面几乎与树脂表面齐平时关闭出口，不可使树脂表面干燥。用长滴管将 15 滴氨基酸混合液仔细直接加到树脂顶部，打开出口使其缓慢流入柱内。当液面刚好与树脂表面齐平时，加入 0.1mol/L

HCl 3ml，以 10～12 滴/分的流速洗脱，收集洗脱液，每管 20 滴，逐管收存。当 HCl 液面刚好与树脂表面齐平时，用 1ml pH 4.2 枸橼酸缓冲液冲洗柱壁 1 次，接着用 2ml pH 4.2 枸橼酸缓冲液洗脱，保持流速 10～12 滴/分并注意勿使树脂表面干燥。

在收集洗脱液的过程中，逐管用茚三酮检验氨基酸的洗脱情况，方法是：于各管洗脱液中加 10 滴 pH 5.0 醋酸缓冲液和 10 滴中性茚三酮溶液，沸水浴中煮 10 分钟，如溶液呈紫蓝色，表示已有氨基酸洗脱下来。显色的深度可代表洗脱的氨基酸浓度，可比色测定。

再用 pH 4.2 枸橼酸缓冲液把第二个氨基酸洗脱下来之后，再收集两管茚三酮反应阴性部分，关闭层析柱出口，将树脂顶部剩余的 pH 4.2 枸橼酸缓冲液移去。

于树脂顶部加入 2ml 0.1mol/L NaOH，打开出口使其缓慢流入柱内，继续用 0.1mol/L NaOH 洗脱并逐管收集，注意仍然保持流速 10～12 滴/分，每管 20 滴。做洗脱液中氨基酸检验，在第三个氨基酸用 0.1mol/L NaOH 洗脱下来以后，再继续收集两管茚三酮反应阴性部分。

最后以洗脱液管号为横坐标，洗脱液各管光密度（以水作空白，在 570nm 波长读取光密度）或颜色深浅（以 −，±，+，++……表示）为纵坐标作图，即可画出一条洗脱曲线。

【注意事项】

1. 在装柱时必须防止气泡、分层及柱子液面在树脂表面以下等现象发生。
2. 一直保持流速 10～12 滴/分，并注意勿使树脂表面干燥。

【思考题】

1. 为什么混合氨基酸从磺酸阳离子交换树脂上逐个洗脱下来？
2. 树脂如何保存？

Experiment 5   Ion Exchange Chromatography

Purpose

1. To know the principle and operating techniques of ion exchange chromatography.
2. To learn to use ion exchange chromatography to separate the mixed amino acids.

Principle

Ion exchange chromatography (IEC) is a technique for separating compounds based on their net charge. Ion exchange chromatography medium contains negative or positive charged functional groups covalently bound to a solid support, yielding either a cation or anion exchanger, respectively. Charged compounds are absorbed and retained by an ion exchanger having the opposite charge, whereas compounds that are neutral or have the same charge as the media pass through the volume and are eluted from the column. The binding of the charged compounds with ion exchanger is reversible, and absorbed compounds are commonly eluted with a salt or pH gradient.

In IEC, supporting medium is composed of resin or cellulose with charges. Usually the groups carried by ion-exchange resin can be divided into strong acid ($-SO_3H$), weak acid ($-COOH$), strong base ($-N(CH_3)_3OH$) and weak base ($-NH_2OH$). Ion-exchange resin is a kind of synthetic polymer. It isn't soluble in water, but will dilate when absorbing water. Polymer molecule consists of polar groups that can ionize and nonpolar resin. The ions on the polar groups can exchange with the ion in the solution, but the physical property of the nonpolar resin will not change. When ions of substances exchange with ions of polar groups, different substances can be respectively eluted and separated based on the different intensities of affinity strength, which will change with salt concentration or pH.

This experiment uses sulfonic acid cation-exchange resin to separate the mixture of acidic amino acid (aspartic acid, pI = 2.97), neutral amino acid (alanine, pI = 6.0) and basic amino acid (lysine pI = 9.74). With low pH, aspartic acid with few charges is firstly eluted because it weakly bonds to resin. With pH 4.2, alanine is eluted because of low degree of dissociation. With pH 12, due to higher pH in the mixture than pI of lysine, lysine has negative charges and it is eluted from the resin. Thus, the three kinds of amino acids can be respectively eluted and separated by changing pH.

Materials

1. Apparatus

Column (1.6cm × 25cm), pump, gradient mixer, ultraviolet spectrometer, sulfonic acid cation-exchange-resin (Dowex 50).

2. Reagents

(1) 2mol/L Hydrogen chloride, 2mol/L sodium hydroxide, 0.1mol/L hydrogen chloride, 0.1mol/L sodium hydroxide.

(2) Citric acid buffer pH 4.2　　Mix 54ml 0.1mol/L Citric acid with 46ml 0.1mol/L sodium citrate.

(3) Acetate acid buffer pH 5.0　　Mix 70ml 0.2mol/L sodium acetate with 30ml 0.2mol/L acetate acid.

(4) 0.2% Neutral triketohydrindene hydrate solution　　Dissolve 0.2g triketohydrindene hydrate in 100ml acetone.

(5) Mixture of amino acids　　Add 10ml alanine, aspartic acid, lysine in 3ml of 0.1mol/L hydrogen chloride.

Procedures

1. The disposal of resin

Put about 10g of resin in a 100ml flask, add 25ml of 12mol/L hydrogen chloride, and stir them for 2h. Eliminate the acid liquor, and wash the resin completely with distilled water till it's neutral. Add 25ml of 12mol/L sodium hydroxide to the above resin and stir for 2h. Eliminate the alkaline liquor and wash it with distilled water till it's neutral. Suspend the resin in 50ml, pH 4.2 sodium citric acid buffer, for later use.

2. Packing

Take a chromatography column with the diameter of 0.8 ~ 1.2cm and the length of 20 ~ 30cm, put a piece of glass cotton or sponge circular cushion at the bottom, and pour the above prepared resin from the top. Close the exit of chromatography column. When the resin sediment appears, flow out the excessive solution, add more resin until the height of the resin sediment is about 8 ~ 10cm. Add pH 4.2 citric buffer from the top to wash it until the flowing liquor reaches pH 4.2. Close the exit of the column, and keep the level of the liquor surface about 1cm higher than that of the resin.

3. Loading, elution and collection of eluent

Open the exit to make the buffer flow out. When the level of the liquor is at almost the same height with that of resin, close the exit (don't make the surface of resin dry). Use a long dropper to add 15 drops of amino acids mixture to the top of resin directly and carefully, and open the exit to make it flow into the column slowly. When the level of the liquor is just at the same height as that of resin, add 3ml of 0.1mol/L hydrogen chloride, and elute it at the flowing rate of 10 ~ 12 drops/min. Collect the eluent, 20 drops per tube and collect it one by one. When the level of hydrogen chloride solution is just at the same height as that of resin, use 1ml of pH 4.2 citric acid buffer to wash the column wall once, then elute with 2ml of pH 4.2 citric acid buffer. Keep the flowing rate at 10 ~ 12 drops/min. Pay attention not to make the surface of resin dry.

While collecting the eluent, check the amino acid in the eluent with triketohydrindene hydrate tube by tube. The process is: Add 10 drops of pH 5 acetate acid buffer and 10 drops of neutral triketohydrindene hydrate solution into every tube of eluent. Heating for 10min in the boiling water bath. The solution showing royal blue means some amino acid has been eluted out. The degree of the color can show the concentration of amino acid, and it can be determined by color matching.

After eluting out the second amino acid with pH 4.2 critic acid buffer, collect two tubes of the negative parts of the action of triketohydrindene hydrate. Close the exit of chromatography column, and remove the pH 4.2 critic acid buffer left on the top of the resin.

Add 2ml of 0.1mol/L sodium hydroxide from the top of the resin, open the exit to make it flow into the column slowly. Elute with 0.1mol/L sodium hydroxide according to the above operation, and collect it tube by tube (keep the flowing rate at 10 ~ 12 drops/min) with 20 drops per tube. Check up the amino acid in the eluent. After the third amino acid has been eluted out by 0.1mol/L sodium hydroxide, proceed to collect two tubes of the negative parts of the action of triketohydrindene hydrate.

Finally, take the optical density of every tube of eluent (take water as blank and at the wavelength of 570nm) or the degree of color (expressed with " − , + , + , + + ······") as ordinate, and the tube number of eluent as abscissa, then draw an elution curve.

Cautions

1. Avoid bubbles, laying or the level of the liquor in the column lower than that of the resin when packing.

2. Keep the flowing rate at 10 ~ 12 drops/min, and pay attention not to make the surface of the resin dry.

Questions

1. Why can the mixed amino acids be eluted from the sulfonic acid cation-exchange resin one by one?

2. How to preserve the resin?

实验六　SDS – 聚丙烯酰胺凝胶电泳

【实验目的】

1. 掌握 SDS – 聚丙烯酰胺凝胶电泳的原理。
2. 掌握用此种方法测定蛋白质的分子量。

【实验原理】

SDS 是十二烷基硫酸钠（sodium dodecyl sulfate）的简称，它是一种阴离子表面活性剂，加入到电泳系统中可以打开蛋白质的氢键和疏水键，并结合到蛋白质分子上（在一定条件下，大多数蛋白质与 SDS 的结合比为 1.4g SDS/g 蛋白质），这样可使各种 SDS – 蛋白质复合物都带上相同密度的负电荷，负电荷数量远远超过了蛋白质分子原有的电荷量，从而掩盖了不同种类蛋白质间原有的净电荷差别。

另外，蛋白质与 SDS 形成 SDS – 蛋白质复合物后，会呈现椭圆形或棒状结构，此结构的大小与蛋白质的种类无关，只与蛋白质的分子量成正比，这样可以消除由于天然蛋白质形状的不同而对电泳迁移率的影响。

影响带电粒子电泳的内在因素有三点：①分子所带净电荷的多少；②分子量大小；③分子的形状。当体系中加入 SDS 后，SDS 会与蛋白质结合，消除①、③两个因素，使其电泳迁移率在外界条件固定的情况下，只取决于蛋白质分子量的大小，因而可通过比较已知分子量蛋白质分子的迁移率，求出未知蛋白质的分子量。

【实验材料】

1. **实验器材**　微型凝胶电泳装置、电源（电压 220V，电流 500mA）、Eppendorf 管、微量注射器（50μl 或 100μl）、摇床。

2. **实验试剂**

（1）2mol/L Tris – HCl（pH 8.8）　取 24.2g Tris，溶解于 50ml 蒸馏水，缓慢滴加浓盐酸至 pH 8.8（约加 4ml）；待溶液冷却至室温，pH 会有所升高，转移至 100ml 容量瓶，蒸馏水定容至 100ml。

（2）1mol/L Tris – HCl（pH 6.8）　取 12.1g Tris，加 50ml 蒸馏水，缓慢滴加浓盐酸至 pH 6.8（约加 8ml）；让溶液冷却至室温，pH 会有所升高，转移至 100ml 容量瓶，

蒸馏水定容至 100ml。

（3）10%（W/V）SDS　取 10g SDS，蒸馏水溶解并定容至 100ml，室温保存。

（4）50%（V/V）甘油　取 50ml 100% 甘油，加入 50ml 蒸馏水，混匀。

（5）1%（W/V）溴酚蓝　取 100mg 溴酚蓝，加蒸馏水至 10ml，搅拌，直到完全溶解，过滤除去聚合的染料。

（6）A 液——丙烯酰胺储备液［含 30%（W/V）丙烯酰胺和 0.8%（W/V）甲叉双丙烯酰胺的溶液 100ml］在通风柜中操作，取 29.2g 丙烯酰胺，0.8g 甲叉双丙烯酰胺，加蒸馏水至 100ml，缓慢搅拌直至丙烯酰胺粉末完全溶解，用封口膜封口，可在 4℃ 存放数月。

（7）B 液——4× 分离胶缓冲液　取 75ml 2mol/L Tris – HCl（pH 8.8），加入 4ml 10% SDS，加 21ml 蒸馏水，混匀，可在 4℃ 存放数月。

（8）C 液——4× 浓缩胶缓冲液　取 50ml 1mol/L Tris – HCl（pH 6.8），加入 4ml 10% SDS，加 46ml 蒸馏水，混匀，可在 4℃ 存放数月。

（9）10% 过硫酸铵（APS）　取 0.5g 过硫酸铵，加入 5ml 蒸馏水，可保存在密封的管内，于 4℃ 存放数月。

（10）电泳缓冲液　取 3g Tris，14.4g 甘氨酸，1g SDS，加蒸馏水至 1L，pH 约为 8.3，也可配制成 10 倍的储备液，在室温下长期保存。

（11）5× 样品缓冲液　取 0.6ml 1mol/L Tris – HCl（pH 6.8），加入 2ml 10% SDS，5ml 50% 的甘油，0.5ml 2 – 巯基乙醇，1ml 1% 溴酚蓝，0.9ml 的蒸馏水混匀，可在 4℃ 保存数周，或在 –20℃ 保存数月。

（12）考马斯亮蓝染色液　称取 1.0g 考马斯亮蓝 R – 250，加入 450ml 甲醇，450ml 蒸馏水及 100ml 冰醋酸即成。

（13）考马斯亮蓝脱色液　将 100ml 甲醇、100ml 冰醋酸、800ml 蒸馏水混匀备用。

【实验步骤】

1. 灌制分离胶

（1）组装凝胶模具　可按照使用说明书装配好灌胶用的模具。对于 Bio – Rad 的微型凝胶电泳系统，在上紧螺丝之前，必须确保凝胶玻璃板和隔片的底部与一个平滑的表面紧密接触，有细微的不匹配就会导致凝胶的渗漏。

（2）将 A 液、B 液及蒸馏水在一个小烧瓶或试管中混匀，加入过硫酸铵（APS）和四甲基乙二胺（TEMED）后，轻轻搅拌使其混匀（过量气泡的产生会干扰聚合）。凝胶很快会聚合，操作要迅速。小心将凝胶溶液用吸管沿隔片缓慢加入模具内，这样可以避免在凝胶内产生气泡。注意：丙烯酰胺（A 液中）是神经毒素，操作时必须戴手套。

（3）当加入适量的分离胶溶液时（对于小凝胶，凝胶液加至约距前玻璃板顶端 1.5cm 或距梳子齿约 0.5cm），轻轻在分离胶溶液上覆盖一层约 5mm 的蒸馏水层，这使凝胶表面变得平整。当凝胶聚合后，在分离胶和水层之间将会出现一个清晰的界面。

2. 灌制浓缩胶

（1）除去覆盖在分离胶面上的水层，如果有少量的小液滴残留不会对浓缩胶造成影响，然后将 A 液、C 液和蒸馏水在锥形瓶或小试管中混合。加入 APS 和 TEMED，并轻轻搅拌使其混匀。

（2）将浓缩胶溶液用吸管加至分离胶的上面，直至凝胶溶液到达前玻璃板的顶端。将梳子插入凝胶内，直至梳子齿的底部与前玻璃板的顶端平齐。必须确保梳子齿的末端没有气泡。将梳子稍微倾斜插入可以减少气泡的产生。

（3）凝胶聚合后，小心拔出梳子（防止将加样孔撕裂）。将凝胶放入电泳槽内，如果使用 Bio－Rad 的微型凝胶系统，可预先接好电极。将电泳缓冲液加入内、外电泳槽中，使凝胶的上、下端均能浸泡在缓冲液中。

3. 制备样品和上样

（1）将 20μl 蛋白质样品与 5μl 5×样品缓冲液在一个 EP 管中混合。100℃加热 2～10 分钟，离心 10 秒，如果有大量蛋白质碎片则应延长离心时间。

（2）用微量注射器将样品加入样品孔中。将蛋白质样品加至样品孔的底部，并随着染料水平的升高而升高注射器针头。避免带入气泡，气泡易使样品混入到相邻的加样孔中。

4. 电泳

（1）将电极插头与适当的电极相接。电流流向阳极。将电流调至 11mA/板，保持恒流，待示踪染料由浓缩胶进入分离胶后，将电流调制 20mA/板。

（2）待染料的前沿迁移至凝胶的底部 1cm 处时，关闭电源，从电极上拔掉电极插头，取出凝胶玻璃板，小心移动两玻璃板之间的隔片，将其插入两块玻璃板的一角。轻轻撬开玻璃板，凝胶便会贴在其中的一块板上。

5. 考马斯亮蓝染色

这种染色方法在单条电泳带中蛋白质最小检出量为 50ng 的蛋白质。通常可以根据所需要的敏感度来选择是使用考马斯亮蓝染色或银染色。

（1）戴上手套避免将手指印留在电泳凝胶上，将凝胶移入一个小的盛有 20ml 考马斯亮蓝溶液的容器内（此步操作小心不要将胶撕破）。

（2）对于 0.75mm 的凝胶，可在摇床上缓慢振荡 5～10 分钟，对于 1.5mm 的凝胶，则需 10～20 分钟，在染色和脱色过程中要用盖子或封口膜密闭容器口。弃去染液，将凝胶在水中漂洗数次。戴手套以避免将双手染色。

（3）加入约 50ml 考马斯亮蓝脱色液，清晰的条带很快会显现出来，大部分凝胶脱色需要 1 小时，用过的脱色液则可用水直接冲洗掉。为了脱色完全，需数次更换脱色液并振过夜。

【实验结果】

根据凝胶中标准品与待测样品的相对迁移率判断待测样品的大致分子量。

【思考题】

1. 利用 SDS－PAGE 法测定蛋白质的分子量与利用凝胶层析测定蛋白质的分子量有何不同？

2. SDS 在该电泳方法中的作用是什么？

Experiment 6　SDS-Polyacrylamide Gel Electrophoresis

Purpose

1. To master the principle of SDS-PAGE (sodium dodecyl sulfate polyacrylamide gel electrophoresis).

2. To master this approach to determine the molecular weight of protein.

Principle

SDS is the short term of sodium dodecyl sulfate. It is a kind of anion surface-active agent. It can open the hydrogen bond and hydrophobic bond in the electrophoresis system and combine with the protein molecule (under a certain condition, most of proteins combine with SDS in a ratio of 1.4 gram of SDS per gram protein). As a result, all kinds of SDS-protein complex carry the same negative charge density that is far more than the native net charge of the protein. In this case, the difference of charge between different kinds of proteins will be covered.

Furthermore, SDS-protein complex presents the oval structure, the size of which is proportional to the molecular weight of protein, but not related to the different kinds of protein. This can eliminate impact on the electrophoretic mobility due to the different shapes of natural protein.

There are three internal factors influencing the charged particle electrophoresis: The number of molecular net charge; the molecular weight; and the shape. When SDS is added to this system, SDS can combine with proteins and eliminate the two factors mentioned above, and the electrophoretic mobility only depends on the molecular weight, so we can determine the molecular weight of unknown protein by comparing it with the electrophoretic mobility of known protein.

Materials

1. Apparatus

Mini-Gel apparatus, power supply (capacity 220V, 500mA), Eppendorf tube, hamilton syringes (50 μl or 100 μl), shaker.

2. Reagents

(1) 2mol/L Tris-HCl (pH 8.8)　Weigh 24.2g Tris, dissolve in 50ml distilled water and add concentrated HCl slowly until it reaches pH 8.8 (about 4ml). Cool the solution to room temperature, pH will increase, then transfer it to a 100ml flask, and add distilled water to a total volume of 100ml.

(2) 1mol/L Tris-HCl (pH 6.8)　Weigh 12.1g Tris, dissolve in 50ml distilled water and add concentrated HCl slowly until it reaches pH 6.8 (about 8ml). Cool the solution to room temperature, pH will increase, then transfer it to a 100ml flask, and add distilled water to a total volume of 100ml.

(3) 10% (*W/V*) SDS　Weigh 10g SDS, dissolve in distilled water, add distilled water until the total volume is 100ml, and then store at room temperature.

(4) 50% (*V/V*) Glycerol　Pour 50ml 100% glycerol into 50ml distilled water, and mix completely.

(5) 1% (*W/V*) Bromophenol blue　Weigh 100mg bromophenol blue, add 10ml distilled water and stir until bromophenol blue dissolves completely, and then remove aggregated dye by filtration.

(6) Solution A—Acrylamide stock solution (contain 30% (*W/V*) acrylamide, 0.8% (*W/V*) bis-acrylamide, 100ml)　Weigh 29.2g acrylamide and 0.8g bis-acrylamide, dissolve in distilled water, and dilute with distilled water to 100ml, stir slowly until acrylamide powder dissolves completely, seal with Parafilm and store at 4℃, the solution can be stored for months.

(7) Solution B—4 × Separating gel buffer　Mix 75ml 2mol/L Tris-HCl (pH 8.8), 4ml 10% SDS and 21ml distilled water together, it can be stored for months in the refrigerator.

(8) Solution C—4 × Stacking gel buffer　Mix 50ml 1mol/L Tris-HCl (pH 6.8), 4ml 10% SDS and 46ml distilled water together, it can be stored for months in the refrigerator.

(9) 10% Ammonium persulfate (APS)　Weigh 0.5g ammonium persulfate, dissolve in 5ml distilled water, it can be stored for months in a capped tube at 4℃.

(10) Electrophoresis buffer　Weigh 3g Tris, 14.4g glycine, and 1g SDS, dissolve in distilled water, and dilute with distilled water to 1000ml, pH should be approximately 8.3. It can also be made to 10 × stock solution, and keep at room temperature for a long time.

(11) 5 × Sample buffer　Mix 0.6ml 1mol/L Tris-HCl (pH 6.8), 5ml 50% glycerol, 2ml 10% SDS, 0.5ml 2-mercaptoethanol, 1ml 1% bromophenol blue and 0.9ml distilled water together, it can be stored for weeks in the refrigerator or for months at −20℃.

(12) Commassie brilliant blue staining solution　Weigh 1.0g Coomassie brilliant blue R-250, add 450ml methanol, 450ml distilled water and 100ml glacial acetic acid, mix up sufficiently.

(13) Commassie brilliant blue destaining solution　Mix 100ml methanol, 100ml glacial acidic acid and 800ml distilled water together sufficiently.

Procedures

1. Pouring the separating gel

(1) Assemble gel mould　Assemble gel sandwich according to the manufacturer's instructions. For Bio-Rad Mini-Gel, be sure that the bottom of both gel plates and spacers are perfectly flush against a flat surface before tightening screw. A slight misalignment will result in leak.

(2) Mix up solution A, solution B and distilled water in a small Erlenmeyer flask or a nest tube. Add ammonium persulfate (APS), tetramethylethy lenediamine (TEMED), and stir gently (excessive aeration will interfere with polymerization). Operate rapidly at this moment because polymerization will be finished in a short time. Carefully introduce solution into gel sandwich descending along a spacer by using a pipette. This minimizes the possibility of air

bubbles being trapped within the gel.

Caution: Acrylamide (in Solution A) is a neurotoxin, so plastic gloves should be worn at all times.

(3) When the appropriate amount of separating gel solution has been added (in the case of the Mini-Gel, about 1.5cm from top of front plate or 0.5cm below level where teeth of comb will reach), gently lay about 5mm of distilled water on top of the separating gel. This can make the gel surface flat. When the gel has polymerized, a distinct interface will appear between the separating gel and the water.

2. Pouring the stacking gel

(1) Pour off the water covering the separating gel. The small droplets remaining will not disturb the stacking gel. Mix up solution A, solution C and distilled water in a small Erlenmeyer flask or a test tube, add APS and TEMED, and stir gently to blend it.

(2) Pipet stacking gel solution onto separating gel until solution reaches top of front plate. Carefully insert comb into gel sandwich until bottom of teeth reaches top of front plate. Be sure no bubbles are trapped on end of teeth. Tilting the comb at a slight angle is helpful for insertion without trapping air bubbles.

(3) After stacking gel has polymerized, remove comb carefully (making sure not to tear the well ears). Place gel into electrophoresis chamber. If using Bio-Rad Mini-Gel system, attach both gels to electrode assembly before inserting into electrophoresis tank. Add electrophoresis buffer to inner and outer reservoirs, making sure that both top and bottom of gel are immersed in buffer.

3. Preparing and loading samples

(1) Combine $20\mu l$ protein sample solution with $5\mu l$ $5 \times$ loading buffer in an Eppendorf tube, heat at $100℃$ for $2 \sim 10min$, centrifuge for 10s. If large quantities of debris are present, extend the time of centrifuging.

(2) Loading sample solution into well using a hamilton syringe. Load protein solution on bottom of well and raise syringe tip as dye level rises. Be careful to avoid introducing air bubbles as this may allow some of sample to be carried to adjacent well.

4. Running a gel

(1) Attach electrode plugs to proper electrodes. Current should flow towards the anode. Turn on power supply to 11mA per plate, keep the current constant, increase current to 20mA per plate when the dye migrates from stacking gel into separating gel.

(2) Turn off power supply when the dye front migrates to 1cm from the bottom of the gel, pull up electrode plugs from electrodes, remove gel plates from electrode assembly, carefully move the spacer, and insert the spacer in one corner between the plates, gently pry apart the gel plates. The gel will stick to one of the plates.

5. Staining gel with Coomassie brilliant blue solution

This staining method can detect about 50ng amount of protein in a single band. Generally a choice is made between using Coomassie brilliant blue staining or silver staining, depending on sensitivity desired.

（1）Wearing gloves to avoid transferring fingerprints to the gel, and pick up the gel and transfer it to a small container containing about 20ml Coomassie brilliant blue staining solution. Take care not to tear the gel in this step.

（2）Agitate for 5 ~ 10min for 0.75mm gel, 10 ~ 20min for 1.5mm gel on shaker. Cover container with lid or plastic wrap while staining and destaining. Pour out staining solution and rinse the gel several times in water. Wear gloves to avoid staining hands.

（3）Add about 50ml Coomassie billiant blue destaining solution. Strong bands are visible immediately on a light box, and the gel is largely destained within 1h. The destaining buffer used can be washed down the sink with ample water. To destain completely, change destaining solution several times and agitate overnight.

Results

Identify the approximate molecular weight of unknown protein according to the electrophoretic mobility of the standard protein and the unknown protein.

Questions

1. What is the difference of molecular weight assay between SDS-PAGE and gel chromatography?

2. What is the biological function of SDS in SDS-PAGE?

实验七 聚丙烯酰胺凝胶等电聚焦

【实验目的】

1. 掌握聚丙烯酰胺凝胶等电聚焦的基本原理。

2. 学习用聚丙烯酰胺等电聚焦测定蛋白质等电点的操作和方法。

【实验原理】

聚丙烯酰胺等电聚焦是在形成了 pH 梯度的聚丙烯酰胺凝胶中分离不同等电点的蛋白质并能测定蛋白质等电点的技术。在制备聚丙烯酰胺凝胶的过程中加入两性电解质载体 Ampholine，当向凝胶施加电场时，Ampholine 就会形成连续稳定的 pH 梯度，其顺序是从正极到负极 pH 逐渐增大。

蛋白质是两性电解质分子，它在大于其等电点的 pH 环境中解离成带负电荷的阴离子，向电场的正极泳动；在小于其等电点的 pH 环境中解离成带正电荷的阳离子，向电场的负极泳动。这种泳动只有在等于其等电点的 pH 环境中，即蛋白质所带静电荷为零时才能停止。将具有不同等电点的蛋白质分子加入凝胶中，在电场作用下，不论这些蛋白质分子的原始分布如何，只要带电荷即会产生泳动，泳动的方向和速度取决于它所带电荷的性质和数量，直到泳动到凝胶的 pH 等于该蛋白质等电点的部位，不再移动，聚焦形成蛋白质区带。这样就可以实现分离不同等电点蛋白质的目的。

在蛋白质聚焦的相应位置测定凝胶的 pH，就可得知该蛋白质的等电点。

【实验材料】

1. **实验器材**　小玻璃管（0.5cm × 10cm）2 支、圆盘电泳槽、注射器和长针头、移液管、pH 计。

2. **实验试剂**

（1）两性电解质载体凝胶　丙烯酰胺 3.5g，N – 甲叉双丙烯酰胺 0.1g，pH 3 ~ 10 的 Ampholine 2.5ml，核黄素溶液（4mg/100ml）12.5ml，加水至 50ml。

（2）蛋白质溶液　牛血清白蛋白 7mg 溶于 1ml 蒸馏水。

（3）5% 磷酸溶液　量取 85% 的浓磷酸溶液 5.9ml 至容量瓶中，用蒸馏水定容至 100ml。

（4）2% 氢氧化钠溶液　称取 10g 氢氧化钠，用少量蒸馏水溶解，用蒸馏水定容至 500ml。

（5）考马斯亮蓝 R – 250 染色液　称取考马斯亮蓝 R – 250 0.25g，加入 50% 甲醇 91ml 和冰醋酸 9ml。

（6）40% 蔗糖溶液　称取 4g 蔗糖溶解于 10ml 蒸馏水中。

（7）12% 三氯醋酸溶液　称取 12g 三氯醋酸固体溶解于 100ml 蒸馏水中。

（8）脱色液　乙醇:冰醋酸:蒸馏水 = 25:10:65（V/V）。

【实验步骤】

（1）取 4ml 两性电解质载体凝胶，加入 0.7ml 蛋白质溶液，轻轻混匀，抽去气泡。

（2）取干净小玻璃管 2 支，垂直放置，底端塞以橡皮塞或用封口膜封住，加入 40% 蔗糖溶液 3 ~ 4 滴，吸取两性电解质载体 – 蛋白质混合溶液 1.8ml 缓缓放入小玻璃管中，立即用注射器封上一薄层水（3 ~ 5mm 高），使混合溶液表面与空气隔绝。放置 0.5 ~ 1 小时，观察凝胶的凝聚情况。

（3）用滤纸将凝胶顶端的水吸去，小心拔去小玻璃管管底的橡皮塞或除去封口膜，让蔗糖溶液流出，并用少量蒸馏水清洗，然后将小玻璃管垂直放入圆盘电泳槽中。上槽加入 5% 磷酸溶液，连接正极，下槽加入 2% NaOH 溶液，连接负极。于 150V 条件下进行聚焦，电流稳定不变时（2 ~ 3 小时，基本为零），聚焦完毕。

（4）取出小玻璃管，迅速用蒸馏水将两端洗净。将注射器装满蒸馏水，针头紧贴玻璃管内壁插至凝胶和管壁之间，转动玻璃管，同时推动注射器，使针头在管壁与凝胶间前进，注入蒸馏水，最终凝胶胶条从玻璃管中脱出。

（5）将其中一根凝胶胶条浸于 12% 三氯醋酸溶液中固定 2h，白色蛋白质区带即出现。再浸于考马斯亮蓝染色液中染色 5 小时。取出后，转移至脱色液中脱去背景颜色。

（6）将另一根凝胶胶条按顺序切成 0.5cm 长的小段，分别浸泡于 1.0ml 蒸馏水中过夜，用 pH 计测定 pH。

【实验结果】

以凝胶胶条长度为横坐标，pH 为纵坐标，作图。量出各蛋白质区带的距离，对照曲线查出其等电点。

【思考题】

1. 聚丙烯酰胺凝胶等电聚焦测定蛋白质等电点的原理是什么？

2. 聚丙烯酰胺凝胶等电聚焦操作时应注意哪些问题？

Experiment 7　Polyacrylamide Gel Isoelectric Focusing

Purpose

1. To master the basic principle of polyacrylamide gel isoelectric focusing.

2. To learn the method and approach to measure the isoelectric point of protein.

Principle

Polyacrylamide gel isoeletric focusing is a kind of technique that can separate proteins with different isoelectric points and determine the isoelectric point of proteins in the polyacrylamide gel with pH gradient. Add ampholyte supporter-ampholine while making the polyacrylamide gel. Ampholine form continuous and stable pH gradient in the gel. The pH gradient gradually increases from the anode to the cathode.

Protein molecules are amphoteric electrolytes. They dissociate to negative ion when the pH of the solution is higher than their pI, and migrate towards the anode. On the contrary, protein molecules dissociate to positive ion when the pH of the solution is lower than their pI, and migrate towards the cathode. The migration ends when the pH of the solution is equal to their pI. At this moment, protein molecules' electrostatic charge is zero. In this experiment, add proteins with different pI into the polyacrylamide gel. Under the effect of electric field, no matter what the original distribution of protein molecules in the gelis, they will migrate because of charges. The direction and migration rate depend on the property and quantity of their charges. When protein molecules migrate to the location where the pH of gel is equal to their pI, they will not move and focus to form protein bands. It can separate proteins with different pI.

The pI of protein can be known by measuring the pH of the region where the protein is focused.

Materials

1. Apparatus

2 glass tubes (0.5cm × 10cm), disc electrophoresis tank, syringe and long needle, pipettes, pH meter.

2. Reagents

(1) Ampholyte supporter gel　Take 3.5g acrylamide, 0.1g *N*-methylene bisacrylamide, 2.5ml Ampholine (pH 3~10), 12.5ml riboflavin solution (4mg/100ml), and add distilled water to 50ml.

(2) Protein solution　Dissolve 7mg bovine serum albumin into 1ml distilled water.

(3) 5% Phosphate solution　Add 85% strong phosphoric acid 5.9ml into a volumetric flask, then dilute with distilled water to 100ml.

（4）2% NaOH solution　Dissolve 10g NaOH into water and dilute to 500ml.

（5）Coomassie brilliant blue R-250 solution　Weigh 0.25g Coomassie brilliant blue, and add 91ml 50% methanol and 9ml glacial acetic acid.

（6）40% Sucrose solution　Weigh 4g sucrose, dissolve in a little water, and then dilute to 10ml.

（7）12% Trichloroacetic acid solution　Weigh 12g trichloroacetic acid and dissolve in 100ml distilled water.

（8）Destainer　Ethanol : acetate : distilled water = 25 : 10 : 65 (*V/V*)

Procedures

1. Take 4.0ml ampholyte supporter gel, add 0.7ml protein solution, mix them up and remove the bubbles.

2. Take 2 clean small glass tubes, place them vertically and plug rubber plugs at the bottoms or seal the bottom with parafilm. Add 3 or 4 drops of 40% sucrose solution, and add 1.8ml ampholyte supporter gel-protein mixture into the glass tubes. Immediately cover the gel with a little distilled water (3 ~ 5mm on the top of gel) to isolate the air from the mixture. Then keep for 0.5 ~ 1h. Observe the polymerization.

3. Absorb the surface water with filtration paper after polymerization. Unplug the rubber plug or parafilm. The sucrose solution flows out. Wash it with a little distilled water. Then insert small glass tubes into the disc electrophoresis tank. Add 5% phosphate buffer to the upper tank and this part is connected to the anode. Add 2% NaOH solution to the bottom tank and this part is connected to the cathode. Regulate the voltage to 150V. After 2 ~ 3h, if the current does not change (almost zero), the focusing is over.

4. Take out the small glass tubes and wash them with distilled water immediately. Fill up the injection syringe with distilled water. Insert the needle between the inner wall of glass tube and the outer surface of gel, and then twirl the glass tube while pushing the syringe. Inject distilled water to force the gel out of the small glass tube.

5. Soak one of the gel columns into 12% trichloroacetic acid solution for 2h and white protein bands appear. Then soak this get into Coomassie brilliant blue for 5h. Take the gel out and transfer it into the destainer to get rid of the background color.

6. Cut another gel column into 0.5cm segment and soak it into 1.0ml distilled water overnight, then measure the pH value with pH meter.

Results

The gel column length is *x*-axis, and the pH value is *y*-axis. Draw the curve. Measure the distance of each protein band and check out the pI from the curve.

Questions

1. What is the principle of polyacrylamide gel isoelectric focusing to determine the pI of protein?

2. What are the attentions of polyacrylamide gel isoelectric focusing?

3. What should be paid attention to for polyacrylamide gel isoelectric focusing?

实验八 聚丙烯酰胺凝胶圆盘电泳

【实验目的】

1. 掌握聚丙烯酰胺凝胶电泳的基本原理。

2. 学习利用盘状聚丙烯酰胺凝胶电泳的操作技术分离与鉴定蛋白质。

【实验原理】

聚丙烯酰胺凝胶电泳是以聚丙烯酰胺作为支持物的一种电泳形式。如图 8 – 1 所示，单体丙烯酰胺和交联剂甲叉双丙烯酰胺相互作用可形成聚丙烯酰胺，该聚合反应以四甲基乙二胺（TEMED）作为催化剂，以过硫酸铵（APS）作为引发剂。丙烯酰胺和甲叉双丙烯酰胺的比例可决定凝胶网孔的大小，交联剂所占比重越大，凝胶的网孔就越小。

利用聚丙烯酰胺凝胶电泳分离蛋白质主要依据以下两个因素：首先，蛋白质所带净电荷。在不同的 pH 条件下，蛋白质所带电荷不同。在一定的电场条件下蛋白质将向与其所带电荷相反的电极方向移动，移动速率取决于蛋白质表面电荷的数量，电压越强或电荷越多则蛋白质移动得越快。其次，蛋白质的形状和大小。蛋白质在电泳中所受的阻力主要取决于样品的大小与凝胶网孔大小之间的关系。蛋白质分子越小或凝胶网孔越大，分离样品所受阻力愈小，在电场中的迁移率就越大。在非变性电泳中，天然蛋白质的分离就是蛋白质所带电荷、分子大小及分子形状等因素共同影响、作用的结果。

$$迁移率 = \frac{电压 \times 样品静电荷}{摩擦力}$$

聚丙烯酰胺凝胶电泳中的浓缩效应可显著提高分离过程的分辨率，该效应可通过引入浓缩胶和不连续缓冲溶液系统而获得。浓缩胶处于分离胶的顶部，由较低浓度的丙烯酰胺构成，当样品经过浓缩胶时由于胶内网孔较分离胶网孔大，样品的移动速度较快，最终使样品"堆积"在浓缩胶和分离胶之间。

另外，浓缩胶还具有比分离胶更低的 pH。浓缩胶内的缓冲溶液是 Tris – HCl（pH 6.7），该 pH 远低于 Tris 的 pK 值（8.1）。分离胶内的缓冲溶液是 pH 8.9 的 Tris – HCl，而电泳正负两极的缓冲溶液均为 pH 8.3 的 Tris – 甘氨酸缓冲溶液。在浓缩胶中，小分子并带有大量负电荷的 Cl^- 在凝胶中的移动速率较快，而电荷较少且分子量较大的甘氨酸的移动速率较慢。由于二者在同一电场中，具有相同的电流，由此形成的电压梯度导致甘氨酸离子始终跟随在 Cl^- 的后面，带有负电荷的蛋白质样品则浓缩在甘氨酸离子和 Cl^- 之间向正极移动。当样品进入 pH 8.9 的分离胶时，甘氨酸的解离度增加，在电场中的迁移率高于样品，蛋白质不再夹于两种离子之间向正极移动，这时的蛋白质依靠分子筛效应和电荷效应进行分离（图 8 – 2）。

【实验材料】

1. **实验器材** 电泳仪、电源（电压 200V，电流 500mA）、100℃ 沸水浴、Eppendorf 管、微量注射器（50μl 或 100μl）、带盖的玻璃或塑料小容器、摇床。

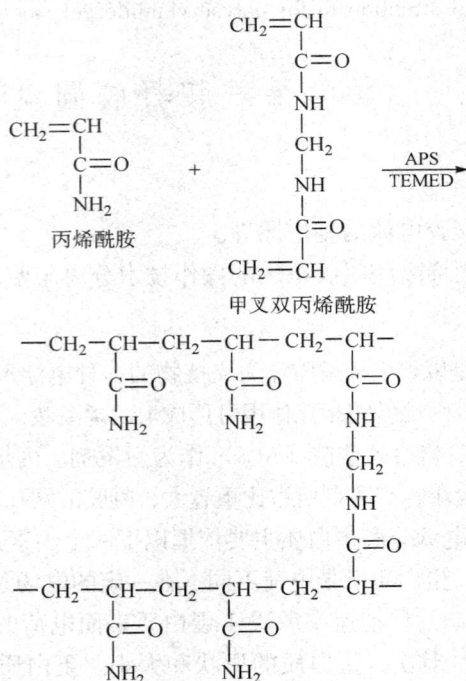

图 8-1　聚丙烯酰胺的形成

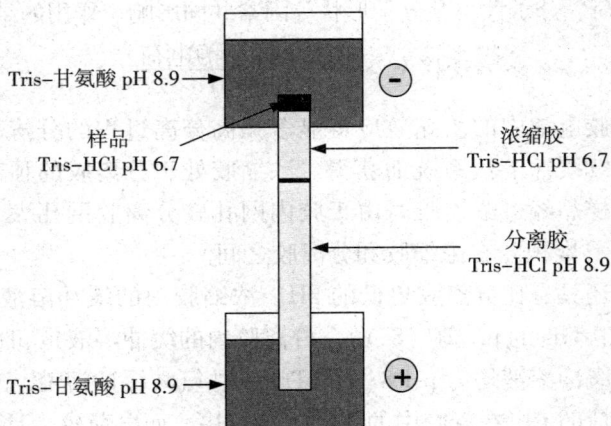

图 8-2　聚丙烯酰胺凝胶电泳缓冲体系示意图

2. **实验试剂**　如表 8-1 和表 8-2 所示。

表 8-1　聚丙烯酰胺凝胶相关试剂及其配方

	试　剂	配　方		pH
1	分离胶缓冲溶液	1mol/L HCl	48.0ml	8.9
		三羟甲基氨基甲烷	36.3g	
		加蒸馏水到 100ml		

续表

	试 剂	配 方		pH
2	单体与交联剂	丙烯酰胺（Acr）	30g	
		甲叉双丙烯酰胺（Bis）	0.8g	
		加蒸馏水到100ml		
3	过硫酸铵	100mg/ml		
4	四甲基乙二胺（TEMED）			
5	浓缩胶缓冲溶液	1mol/L HCl	48ml	
		三羟甲基氨基甲烷（Tris）	5.89g	6.7
		加蒸馏水到100ml		
6	电极缓冲溶液	甘氨酸	28.8g	8.3
		三羟甲基氨基甲烷（Tris）	6.0g	
		加蒸馏水到1000ml，用前稀释10倍		
7	染色液	CBB G - 250 0.1g 溶于95%乙醇		
		加蒸馏水到100ml		
8	示踪染料	溴酚蓝0.05g（溶于100ml 蒸馏水）加蒸馏水到100ml		
9	样品	蛇毒干粉200mg 溶于20ml，pH 6.7 缓冲溶液中		
		再加入25%蔗糖20ml 和溴酚蓝10ml		

表8-2　凝胶配方

试 剂	分离胶（ml）	浓缩胶（ml）
1	1.25	
2	2.5	1
5		1.25
蒸馏水	6.195	7.64
3	0.05	0.1
4	0.005	0.005
总体积	10	10
浓度	7.5	3

【实验步骤】

1. **凝胶柱的制备**　取干净的 10cm×0.6cm 玻璃管，在 7.5cm、8cm 两处画线。底端管口用小块胶布封口，插入橡皮垫中，垂直放置于试管架。用巴斯德滴管吸取分离胶，缓慢贴壁加胶到管内 7.5cm 处，立即加蒸馏水至 8cm 处。待分离胶凝固后，将胶面上的水分甩掉，残留的水分用滤纸条吸干，用滴管快速加浓缩胶到分离胶面上至 8cm 处，再小心地加约 0.5cm 的蒸馏水。

2. **安装电泳槽**　选择无气泡、无裂缝、长度合适的凝胶柱，撕掉胶布，安装到电泳仪上，注意保持垂直并要紧密。向下槽注入电极缓冲液，注意用弯头滴管除去凝胶柱下端的气泡；再向上槽倒入电极缓冲液淹没凝胶柱，同样用滴管除去气泡。

3. **加样**　用微量注射器取样品液 30μl，沿壁缓慢加在浓缩胶面上。

4. **电泳**　连接电极，上槽与负极相连，下槽与正极相连；调节电流至 1mA/管，待示踪染料进入分离胶时调节电流至2mA/管，待示踪染料接近凝胶管底部约0.5cm处，切断电源，电泳时间为2~3小时。

5. **剥胶** 取下凝胶管，用局麻针头注射器吸取一定量的蒸馏水，将针头插入胶柱与管壁之间，边注水边旋转玻管，直至胶柱与管内壁分开，然后用洗耳球轻轻在玻璃管的一端加压，使凝胶柱从玻璃管缓慢滑出，将凝胶置于编号的试管内，用蒸馏水冲洗几次。

6. **染色** 将考马斯亮蓝染色剂倒入放有凝胶条的小试管并没过凝胶条，60℃水浴保温40~50分钟后取出，用水冲洗2~3次。

【实验结果】

观察凝胶条中的蛋白质与考马斯亮蓝染色剂结合后所形成的蓝色复合物，并通过画图记录结果。

【思考题】

1. 聚丙烯酰胺凝胶电泳分离生物大分子的基本原理是什么？
2. 样品液中加入蔗糖和溴酚蓝的目的是什么？

Experiment 8   Polyacrylamide Gel Electrophoresis in Cylindrical Tube

Purpose

1. To master the principle of polyacrylamide gel electrophoresis.

2. To learn the operative technique of cylindrical tube-polyacrylamide gel electrophoresis and its application on protein separation and identification.

Principle

Polyacrylamide gel electrophoresis is a kind of electrophoresis in which the support media is polyacrylamide (PAGE). As is shown in Fig. 8 – 1, the organic monomer, acrylamide can react with cross-linking reagent, methylene bisacrylamide, to form polyacrylamide gel. This polymerizing reaction needs N, N, N', N'-tetramethylethylenediamine (TEMED) as catalyst and ammonium persulfate (APS) as arising agent. The proportions of acrylamide and methylene bisacrylamide determine the size of pores in the gel, and smaller pore sizes are obtained by using a higher concentration of cross-linking reagent to form the gel.

The separation of protein in polyacrylamide gel electrophoresis depends on two aspects: First, net charges on the proteins. Depending on the pH of the buffer, proteins in a sample will carry different charges. When an electric field is applied, proteins will migrate towards their corresponding poles. The rate of migration will depend on the amount of net charges. The higher the voltage or the greater the charge on the protein, the further it will move. Second, shape and size of the proteins: The resistance of a protein is largely determined by the relationship between the effective size of the molecule and the size of the pores in the gel. The smaller the size of the molecule, or the larger the size of the pores in the gel, the lower the resistance and therefore the faster a molecule moves through the gel. In non-denaturing electrophoresis, the native proteins are separated based on a combination of their charge, size and shape.

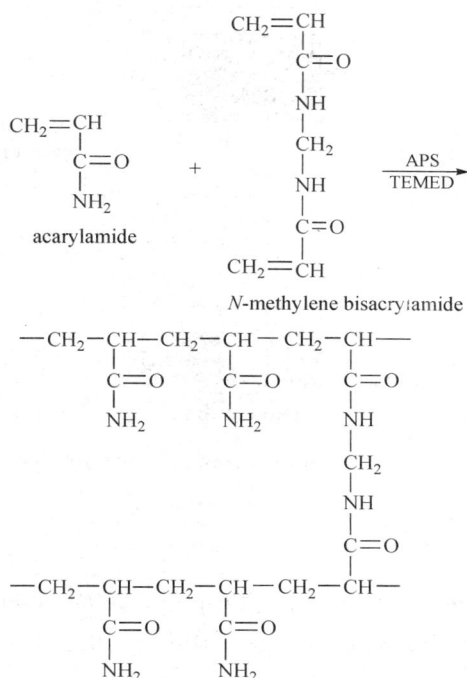

Fig. 8 – 1　The formation of polyacrylamide gel

$$\text{Mobility} = \frac{\text{Applied voltage} \times \text{molecular charge}}{\text{Molecular friction}}$$

The resolution of separation in electrophoresis can be improved by the use of a stacking gel and a discontinuous buffer system, which contributes to the stacking effect. The stacking gel resides on top of the running gel, which is made by using a lower percentage of acrylamide than the running gel, so it has less molecular sieving. After loading samples, the proteins run rapidly through the stacking gel which is highly porous and then "stack" up at the interface between the two gels since the running gel has much smaller pores.

The stacking gel also has a lower pH than the running gel. It is a Tris-HCl buffer at pH 6.7, which is much lower than the pH of Tris (8.1). The running gel is a Tris-HCl buffer at pH 8.9 and the running buffer for the gel is Tris-glycine pH 8.3. In stacking gel, the small and fully-charged chloride will move fast through the porous. The larger and slightly-charged glycine will move slowly. But the current must be the same throughout this electrical circuit, which forms a voltage gradient and allows the glycine to remain just behind the chloride ions. The proteins with negative charges will migrate between the chloride and the glycine in very sharp bands. When the samples enter the running gel with the pH increasing to 8.9, the glycine becomes more significantly deprotonated and it moves ahead of the proteins. The proteins are now not forced to stack between the two ions, and can be separated depending on the molecular sieving and net charges (Fig. 8 – 2).

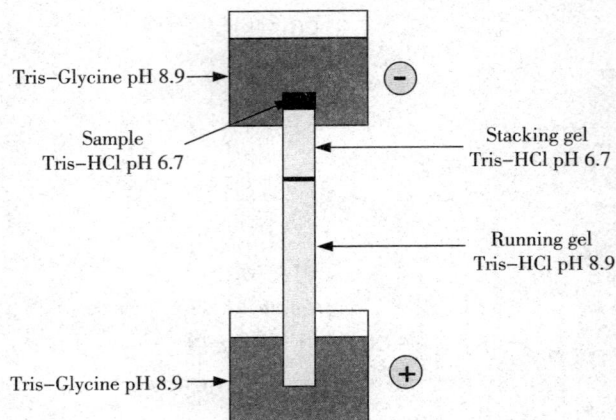

Fig. 8 – 2 The buffer system of polyacrylamide gel electrophoresis

Materials

1. Apparatus

Electrophresis apparatus, power supply (capacity 200V, 500mA), boiling water bath (100℃), Eppendorf tube, Hamilton syringes (50μl or 100μl), small glass or plastic container with lid, shaker.

2. Reagents

As shown in Table 8 – 1 and Table 8 – 2.

Table 8 – 1 The reagent formula of polyacrylamide gel

	Reagent	Formula	pH
1	Separating gel buffer	1mol/L HCl 48.0 ml, Tris 36.3g, add distilled water to 100ml.	8.9
2	Stock acrylamide solution	30g acrylamide, 0.8g bis-acrylamide. Add distilled water to 100ml.	
3	Ammonium persulfate	100mg/ml	
4	N, N, N', N'-tetramethylethyl-enediamine (TEMED)		
5	Stacking gel buffer	48ml 1mol/L HCl, Tris 5.89g. Add distilled water to 100ml.	6.7
6	Electrophoresis buffer	Dissolve 6.0g of Tris base and 28.8g of glycine in water and adjust the volume to 1L. Dilute to 10 times before using.	8.3
7	Gel Staining	Pissolvel 0.1g Coomassie brilliant blue R-250 with 95% ethanol, Add distilled water to 100ml.	
8	Footprint dye	Dissolve bromophenol blue 0.05g in 100ml distilled water.	
9	Sample	Dissolve 200mg snake toxin in 20ml, pH 6.7 stacking gel buffer (5), add 25% sucrose 20ml and bromophenol blue (8) 10ml.	

Table 8 −2 Formula of polyacrylamide gel

Reagent	Separating gel（ml）	Stacking gel（ml）
1	1. 25	
2	2. 5	1
5		1. 25
Distilled water	6. 195	7. 64
3	0. 05	0. 1
4	0. 005	0. 005
Total volume	10	10
Concentration	7. 5	3

Procedures

1. Preparation of the gel

Take a clean glass tube（10cm × 0. 6cm）, make markers at 7. 5cm and 8. 0cm. Cover the bottom with plaster tightly, then put it into cushion, and clamp it in a vertical position. Use a Pasteur（or larger）pipet to transfer separating gel mixture to the tube by running the solution carefully down the edge. Continue to add this solution until it reaches 7. 5cm, and immediately lay distilled water on top of the separating gel gently until it reaches 8. 0cm. When the polymerization has finished in running gel, pour off the overlaying water and then add the stacking gel solution to the tube until the solution reaches 8. 0cm. Gently lay about 0. 5cm of distilled water on top of the stacking gel.

2. Installation of the electrophoresis tank

Select tube with right length but without bubbles or crack. Tear the tape and place the tube into electrophoresis chamber, vertically and airtightly. Fill the inner reservoir with electrophoresis buffer and remove the bubbles with elbow droppers. Add electrophoresis buffer to the outer reservoir, submerge the tube, and get rid of the bubbles.

3. Loading samples

Load 30 μl sample solution with minim syringe, carefully down the edge to the surface of stacking gel.

4. Running a gel

Attach electrode plugs to proper electrodes. Anode should be connected with inner reservoir and current should flow towards the anode. Turn on power supply to 1mA/tube when the dye migrates in stacking gel and change the current to 2mA/tube when the dye migrates to separating gel. When the dye migrates to 0. 5cm from the bottom of the gel, turn off power supply. The time of electrophoresis is 2 ~ 3h.

5. Peeling off the gel

Remove cylindrical tube from electrode assembly firstly and use a syringe with 10cm long pinhead full of water as lube. Put the long pinhead into the spacer between the gel and the inner face of glass, turn while injecting water until the gel is separated from the tube. Blow the tube with rubber pipette bulb gently to make the gel slip out. Put the gel in the numbered tube and clean with distilled water several times.

6. Staining the gel

Fill the tube with Coomassie brilliant blue, and incubate at 60℃ for 40 ~ 50min. Take it out, and wash with water for 2 ~ 3 times.

Results

Observe the blue compound which forms between protein and Coomassie brilliant blue in the gel and draw out the result.

Questions

1. What is the separating principle of polyacrylamide gel electrophoresis?

2. Why are sucrose and bromophenol blue added in the sample solution?

实验九　蛋白质印迹分析

【实验目的】

1. 掌握蛋白质印迹法的基本原理。

2. 了解蛋白质印迹法基本操作和应用。

【实验原理】

蛋白质印迹法又称为免疫印迹法，这是一种可以检测固定在固相载体上蛋白质的免疫化学技术方法。待测蛋白既可以是粗提物也可以经过一定的分离和纯化，该技术需要利用待测蛋白的单克隆或多克隆抗体进行识别。

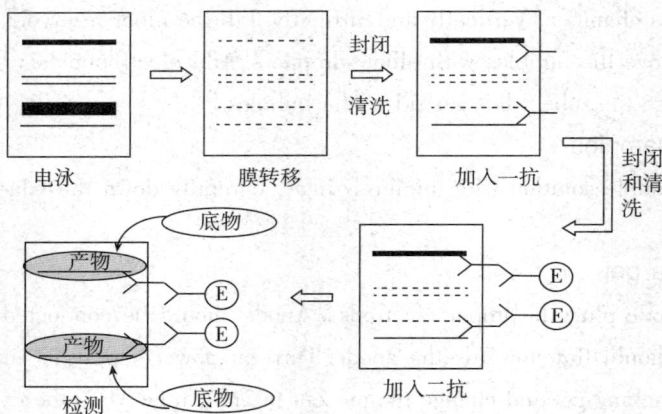

图 9 - 1　蛋白质印迹法基本操作过程

如图 9 - 1 所示，可溶性抗原（待测蛋白）首先要根据其性质，如分子量、分子大小、电荷以及其等电点等采用不同的电泳方法进行分离；通过电流将凝胶中的蛋白质转移到聚偏二氟乙烯膜上；利用抗体（一抗）与抗原发生特异性结合的原理，以抗体作为探针钓取目的蛋白。值得注意的是在加入一抗前应首先加入非特异性蛋白，如牛血清白蛋白对膜进行"封阻"而防止抗体与膜的非特异性结合。

经电泳分离后的蛋白质往往需再利用电泳方法将蛋白质转移到固相载体上，这个过程被称为电泳印迹。常用的两种电转移方法如下。

（1）半干法　凝胶和固相载体被夹在用缓冲溶液浸湿的滤纸之间，通电时间为10~30分钟。

（2）湿法　凝胶和固相载体夹心浸放在转移缓冲溶液中，转移时间可从45分钟延长到过夜进行。

由于湿法的使用弹性更大，并且没有明显浪费更多的时间和原料，因此我们在这里只描述湿法的基本操作过程。

对于目的蛋白的识别需要采用能够识别一抗的第二抗体。该抗体往往是购买的成品，已经被结合或标记了特定的试剂，如辣根过氧化物酶。这种标记是利用辣根过氧化物酶所催化的一个比色反应，该反应的产物有特定的颜色且固定在固相载体上，容易鉴别。因此可通过对二抗的识别而识别一抗，进而判断出目标蛋白所在的位置。

【实验材料】

1. **实验器材**　SDS – PAGE 实验相关材料、电转移装置、供电设备、PVDF 膜、Whatman 3MM 纸、镊子、海绵垫、剪子、手套、小塑料或玻璃容器、浅盘。

2. **实验试剂**

（1）10×转移缓冲溶液　30.3g Tris 碱（0.25mol/L），144g 甘氨酸（1.92mol/L），加蒸馏水至1L，不必调整 pH。

（2）1×转移缓冲溶液　在1.4L 蒸馏水中加入400ml 甲醇及200ml 10×转移缓冲溶液。

（3）TBS 缓冲溶液　将1.22g Tris（10mmol/L）和8.78g NaCl（150mmol/L）加入到1L 蒸馏水中，HCl 调节 pH 至7.5。

（4）TTBS 缓冲液　在1L TBS 缓冲溶液中加入0.5ml Tween 20（0.05%）。

（5）一抗　兔抗待测蛋白抗体。

（6）二抗　辣根过氧化物酶标记羊抗兔抗体。

（7）3%封阻缓冲溶液　牛血清白蛋白15mg 加入 TBS 缓冲溶液并定容至0.5L，过滤，4℃保存，以防止细菌污染。

（8）0.5%封阻缓冲溶液　牛血清白蛋白2.5mg 加入 TTBS 缓冲溶液并定容至0.5L，过滤，4℃保存，以防止细菌污染。

（9）显影试剂　1ml 氯萘溶液（30mg/ml 甲醇配置），加入10ml 甲醇，加入 TBS 缓冲溶液至50ml，加入30μl 30% H_2O_2。

（10）染色液　1g 氨基黑18B（0.1%），250ml 异丙醇（25%）及100ml 醋酸（10%）用蒸馏水定容至1L。

（11）脱色液　将350ml 异丙醇（35%）和20ml 醋酸（2%）用蒸馏水定容至1L。

【实验步骤】

1. **蛋白质的分离**　根据目的蛋白的性质，利用电泳方法将其进行分离。为提高电转移的效率，通常采用 SDS - PAGE 技术（具体实验过程见实验六）。

分离实验结束后，首先将样品墙的上边缘用小刀去除，然后在胶板的右上角切一个小口以便定位，小心放入转移缓冲溶液中待用。

2. 电转移

（1）准备 PVDF 膜　根据胶的大小剪出一片 PVDF 膜，膜的大小应略微小于胶的大小。将膜置于甲醇中浸泡 1 分钟，再移至转移缓冲溶液中待用。

（2）制作胶膜夹心　如图 9 - 2 所示，在一浅盘中打开转移盒，将一个预先用转移缓冲溶液浸泡过的海绵垫放在转移盒的黑色筛孔板上，在海绵垫的上方放置经转移缓冲溶液浸湿的 3MM 纸，小心地将胶板放在 3MM 纸上，并注意排除气泡。将 PVDF 膜放在胶的上方同时注意排除气泡，再在膜的上方放上一张同样用转移缓冲溶液浸湿过的 3MM 纸并赶出气泡，放置另一张浸泡过的海绵垫，关闭转移盒。将转移盒按照正确的方向放入转移槽中，转移盒的黑色筛孔板贴近转移槽的黑色端，转移盒的白色筛孔板贴近转移槽的白色端，填满转移缓冲溶液同时防止出现气泡。

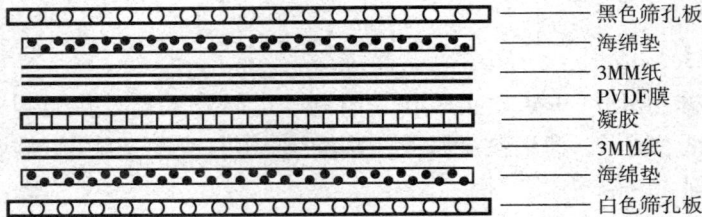

图 9 - 2　夹心放置顺序

（3）电转移　连接电源，在 4℃ 条件下维持恒压 100V 1 小时。

3. 免疫检测

（1）膜染色　断开电源，将转移盒从转移槽中移出，将转移盒的各个部分分开。用镊子将 PVDF 膜小心放入一个干净的容器中，用 10ml TBS 缓冲溶液进行短暂清洗，剪下需要进行染色的膜在染色液中浸泡 1 分钟，然后在脱色液中脱色 30 分钟，确定蛋白质已经转移到 PVDF 膜上。

（2）膜的封闭和清洗　对于没有进行染色的膜，首先倒出 TBS 缓冲溶液，加入 3% 封闭缓冲溶液，轻轻摇动至少 1 小时。倒掉 3% 封闭缓冲溶液，并用 TBS 缓冲溶液清洗 3 次，每次 5 分钟。

（3）加入一抗　倒掉 TBS 缓冲溶液，加入 10ml 0.5% 封闭缓冲溶液及适量的一抗，轻轻摇动 1 小时以上。从容器中倒出一抗及封闭缓冲溶液，用 TTBS 缓冲溶液清洗两次，每次 10 分钟。

（4）加入二抗　倒出 TTBS 缓冲溶液，加入 5ml 0.5% 封闭缓冲溶液及适量的二抗。轻轻摇动 30 分钟，倒出二抗及封闭缓冲溶液，用 TTBS 缓冲溶液清洗两次，每次 10 分钟。

（5）检测　倒掉 TTBS 缓冲溶液并加入显影剂，轻轻摇动 PVDF 膜，观察显影情况，当能够清晰地看到显色带时，用蒸馏水在 30 分钟内分 3 次清洗 PVDF 膜，以终止显色反应的继续进行。

【实验结果】

检查膜上显色结果，蓝紫色带所对应的即是目标蛋白的位置。

【思考题】

1. 蛋白质印迹法的特点是什么？
2. 请解释什么是 BSA，并说明它在本实验中的作用。
3. 请说明二抗在蛋白质印迹法中的生物学功能。
4. 如何保存抗体？

Experiment 9　Western Blot Analysis

Purpose

1. To master the basic principle of western blotting.
2. To understand basic operation and application of western blotting.

Principle

Western blotting is also called immunoblotting. It is a kind of immunochemical techniques which is used to detect a protein immobilized on a matrix. The target protein can be in a crude extract or a more purified preparation and the monoclonal or polyclonal antibody against this protein is necessary to help us to recognize the antigen.

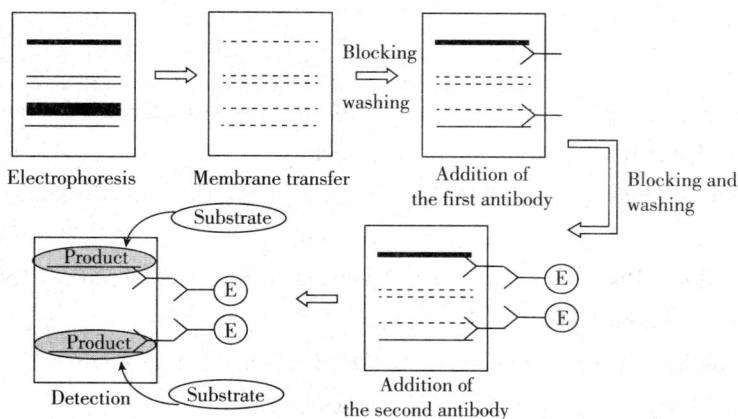

Fig. 9 – 1　The basic procedure of Western blotting

As in Fig. 9 – 1, soluble antigens (the target protein) may be separated by different electrophoresis method based on its molecular weight, size and charge or isoelectric point. After the separation, the proteins are transferred from the gel to a PVDF membrane. Once on the membrane, antibodies (first antibodies) can be used to probe for the presence of particular protein because of the specifically binding of antigen with antibody against it. It should be noted that non-specific binding site can be "blocked" by using other non-specific protein such as bovine

Transferring of protein to a immobilized matrix is most commonly accomplished by electrophoresis. This procedure is called electrotransfer. The two common electrotransfer methods are:

1. Semi-dry method, in which the gel and immobilizing matrix are sandwiched between buffer-wetted filter papers, through which a current is applied for 10 ~ 30min.

2. Wet method, in which the gel-matrix sandwich is submerged in transfer buffer for electrophoresis, which may take as little as 45min or may be allowed to continue overnight.

We only describe the basic procedure of wet method here, since it permits greater flexibility without significant waste in time or materials.

A second antibody is used to detect target protein, which can recognize the first antibody. Typically, the second antibody is purchased product already conjugated to a labeling agent such as horseradish peroxidase. This marker is then visualized by a colorimetric reaction catalyzed by the enzyme which yields a colored product that remains fixed to the membrane. Thus, it is possible to recognize first antibody by recognizing second antibody, and then identify the position of target protein.

Materials

1. Apparatus

Apparatus of SDS-PAGE, electroblotting apparatus, power supply, PVDF membrane, whatman 3MM paper, forceps, sponge pad, scissors, gloves, small plastic or glass container, shallow tray.

2. Reagents

(1) 10 × Transfer buffer　Dissolve 30.3g trizma base (0.25mol/L) and 144g glycine (1.92mol/L) in distilled water without adjusting pH.

(2) 1 × Transfer buffer　Mix 400ml methanol, 200ml 10 × transfer buffer and 1400ml distilled water.

(3) TBS buffer　Dissolve 1.22g Tris (10mmol/L) and 8.78g NaCl (150mmol/L) to 1L distilled water and adjust pH to 7.5 with HCl.

(4) TTBS buffer　Add 0.5ml Tween 20 (0.05%) in 1L TBS buffer.

(5) First antibody　Antibody against the target protein.

(6) Second antibody　Goat anti-rabbit-horseradish peroxidase.

(7) 3% Blocking buffer　Add 15mg bovine serum albumin in TBS buffer to final volume of 0.5L, and keep at 4℃ to prevent bacterial contamination.

(8) 0.5% Blocking buffe　Add 2.5mg bovine serum albumin in TBS buffer to final volume of 0.5L, and keep at 4℃ to prevent bacterial contamination.

(9) Developing reagent　Mix 1ml chloronaphthalene solution (30mg/ml in methanol), 10ml methanol, 39ml TBS buffer and 30μl 30% H_2O_2.

(10) Staining solution　Add 1g amino black 18B (0.1%), 250ml isopropanol (25%)

and 100ml acetic acid（10%）to distilled water with final volume of 1L.

（11）Destaining solution　Add 350ml isopropanol（35%）and 20ml acetic acid（2%）to distilled water with final volume of 1L.

Procedures

1. Separation of protein

The separation of target protein with electrophoresis is decided by its characters, but for normally sufficiently transferring, the most common method is SDS-PAGE.

After separation, remove the upper side of the sample wells with a razor blade. Notch the bottom right-hand corner of the gel for orientation and put the gel in transfer buffer until ready to use.

2. Electrotransfer

（1）Preparation of membrane　Cut a piece of PVDF membrane according to the size of the gel. Incubate in methanol for about 1min on a rocker at room temperature. Remove methanol and equilibrate membrane in 1 × transfer buffer until ready to use.

（2）Arrange gel-membrane sandwich　As in Fig. 9 - 2, in a shallow tray, open the transfer cassette. Put a well-soaked sponge pad on the black piece of the transfer cassette and a wetted 3MM paper on the sponge pad. Place the gel on the paper and arrange well so that all air bubbles are removed. Lay the PVDF membrane on the top of the gel and remove any air bubbles. Place a wetted sheet of 3MM paper over the PVDF membrane and remove the bubbles. Cover it with the second well-soaked pad. Close the sandwich and mount the sandwich in the transfer tank. Put the black sides near the black side of the device. Fill the buffer tank with the transfer buffer.

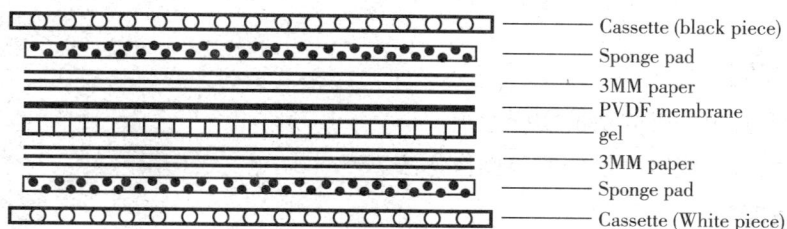

Fig. 9 - 2　The arrangement of sandwich

（3）Electrotransfer　Attach the electrodes. Set the power supply to 100V（constant voltage）for 1h at 4℃.

3. Immunodetection

（1）Membrane staining　Disconnect the transfer apparatus, remove the transfer cassette, and open it. Remove the membrane to a clean container with forcep. Add 10ml TBS buffer and wash for a short time. Cut out the stained stripe and put it in another clean container. Stain this stripe in staining buffer for 1min. Destain for 30min in destaining buffer to check whether protein has been transferred from the gel to the membrane or not.

（2）Membrane blocking and washing　For other part of membrane, pour off TBS buffer. Add 3% blocking buffer, and rock gently for at least 1h. Pour off 3% blocking buffer and rinse briefly with TBS buffer three times, 5min per time.

（3）Adding of first antibody　Pour off TBS buffer. Add first antibody at appropriate dilution in 10ml 0.5% blocking buffer. Rock gently for at least 1h, pour off first antibody solution from membrane and wash twice for 10min with TTBS buffer.

（4）Adding of second antibody　Pour off TTBS buffer. Add second antibody at appropriate dilution in 5ml 0.5% blocking buffer. Rock gently for 30min, pour off second antibody solution from membrane and wash twice for 10min with TTBS buffer.

（5）Detection　Pour off TTBS buffer from membrane and add developing reagent, rock PVDF membrane gently, and monitor the development. When the bands can be seen clearly, stop the development by washing membrane with distilled water for 30min with 3 changes.

Results

Check the bands on membrane, and the band with blue-purple color corresponds to the target protein.

Questions

1. What are the characteristics of western blotting?

2. What is the BSA? And explain its function in this experiment.

3. Please elucidate the function of second antibody during western blotting.

4. How do you reserve antibody?

实验十　酶联免疫吸附法

【实验目的】

1. 学习酶联免疫吸附法的实验原理。

2. 掌握酶联免疫吸附法的实验操作方法。

【实验原理】

酶联免疫吸附法（Enzyme-linked Immunosorbent Assay，ELISA）是在免疫酶技术（immunoenzymatic techniques）的基础上发展起来的一种免疫测定技术。ELISA法综合了抗原、抗体反应的高度特异性与被标记酶的酶促反应的放大作用，使测量的灵敏度可达到纳克（ng）甚至皮克（pg）水平。目前，该技术作为一种诊断方法广泛应用于医疗和病理学领域，同时也在其他各个行业作为一种有效的质量控制方法。

下面将对ELISA原理进行简单的描述。首先将样品抗原固定在一个固相载体表面，然后把一个能与该抗原特异性结合的抗体再覆盖在上面。该抗体已与酶标记连接，最后，将含有酶底物的物质加入系统中，后续发生的酶促反应通常会产生一个有颜色的可检测到的物质，进而达到对样品抗原进行定量测定的目的。三种主要的ELISA方法分别为：直接 ELISA；间接 ELISA；三明治（夹心）ELISA。这三种方法形成了 ELISA 检测的基础，也叫竞争或抑制 ELISA。本实验采用间接 ELISA 法测量某种病毒或蛋白质的效价。

1. **直接 ELISA** 直接 ELISA 被认为是最简单的 ELISA 形式，具体的原理在图 10－1中描述。

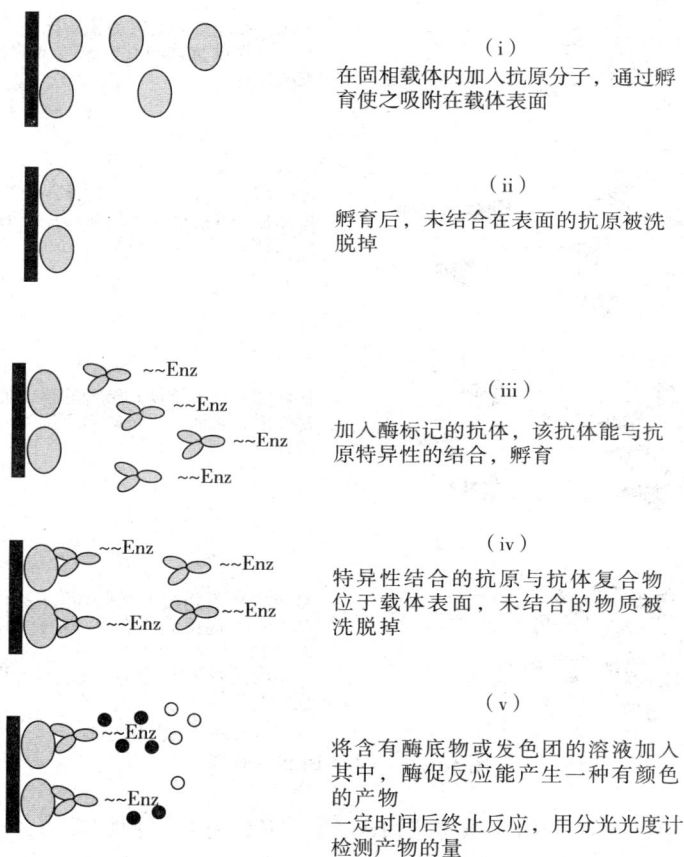

（i）
在固相载体内加入抗原分子，通过孵育使之吸附在载体表面

（ii）
孵育后，未结合在表面的抗原被洗脱掉

（iii）
加入酶标记的抗体，该抗体能与抗原特异性的结合，孵育

（iv）
特异性结合的抗原与抗体复合物位于载体表面，未结合的物质被洗脱掉

（v）
将含有酶底物或发色团的溶液加入其中，酶促反应能产生一种有颜色的产物
一定时间后终止反应，用分光光度计检测产物的量

图 10－1　直接 ELISA 原理

2. **间接 ELISA** 具体原理在图 10－2 中描述。

3. **三明治 ELISA** 三明治 ELISA 被分为直接三明治 ELISA 与间接三明治 ELISA 两个系统，具体原理分别在图 10－3 与图 10－4 中描述。

【实验材料】

1. **实验器材** 聚苯乙烯微量反应板（40 孔或 96 孔）、微量移液器、恒温箱、酶标仪、烧杯、试管、滴管、铝箔纸、滤纸。

2. **实验试剂**

（1）抗原　乙型肝炎病毒、细胞因子等。

（2）待测抗体　免疫后的动物血清。

（3）酶标抗体　根据实验对象选择酶标记抗抗体（二抗）。市售的有辣根过氧化物

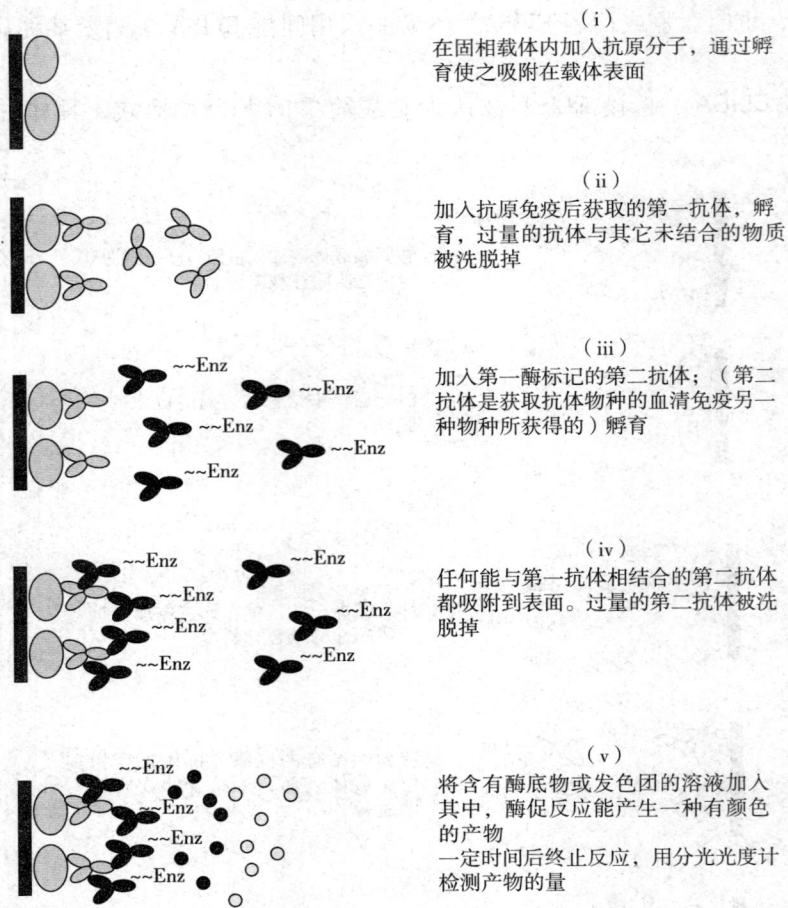

| | （ i ）
在固相载体内加入抗原分子，通过孵育使之吸附在载体表面 |

| | （ ii ）
加入抗原免疫后获取的第一抗体，孵育，过量的抗体与其它未结合的物质被洗脱掉 |

| | （ iii ）
加入第一酶标记的第二抗体；（第二抗体是获取抗体物种的血清免疫另一种物种所获得的）孵育 |

| | （ iv ）
任何能与第一抗体相结合的第二抗体都吸附到表面。过量的第二抗体被洗脱掉 |

| | （ v ）
将含有酶底物或发色团的溶液加入其中，酶促反应能产生一种有颜色的产物
一定时间后终止反应，用分光光度计检测产物的量 |

图 10 - 2　间接 ELISA 原理

酶（HRP）- 羊抗兔 IgG、HRP - 兔抗鼠 IgG 等，按照说明书使用即可。

（4）包被液　0.05mol/L pH 9.6 碳酸盐缓冲液。称取 Na_2CO_3 0.8g，$NaHCO_3$ 1.45g，加少量去离子水溶解后，定容至 500ml。

（5）稀释液　0.01mol/L pH 7.4 磷酸盐 - NaCl 缓冲液（PBS）。称取 NaCl 8.0g，KH_2PO_4 0.2g，$Na_2HPO_4 \cdot 12H_2O$ 2.9g，KCl 0.2g，加去离子水溶解后，定容至 1L。

（6）洗涤液　取 1ml 10% Tween - 20 溶解到 200ml PBS 缓冲液中。

（7）封闭溶液　1% 卵清蛋白（OVA）溶液，取 1g 卵清蛋白溶解于 100ml 稀释液中，此液体最好在临用前根据用量配制。

（8）底物溶液　3，3′，5，5′- 四甲基联苯胺（3，3′，5，5′- tetramethyl benzidine，TMB）作为底物，配制贮备液及应用液。

①底物缓冲液　pH 5.0 ~ 5.4，0.1mol/L 枸橼酸 - 0.2mol/L 磷酸氢二钠。Na_2HPO_4 14.6g，枸橼酸 9.33g，0.75% 过氧化氢 6.4ml，加去离子水溶解后，定容至 1L。

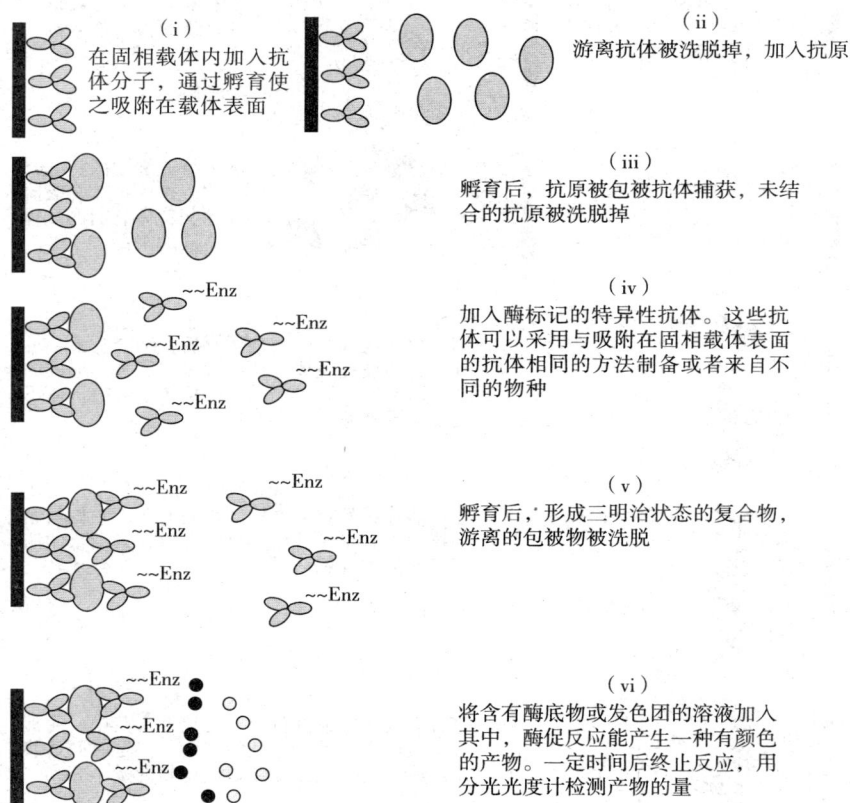

（i）在固相载体内加入抗体分子，通过孵育使之吸附在载体表面

（ii）游离抗体被洗脱掉，加入抗原

（iii）孵育后，抗原被包被抗体捕获，未结合的抗原被洗脱掉

（iv）加入酶标记的特异性抗体。这些抗体可以采用与吸附在固相载体表面的抗体相同的方法制备或者来自不同的物种

（v）孵育后，形成三明治状态的复合物，游离的包被物被洗脱

（vi）将含有酶底物或发色团的溶液加入其中，酶促反应能产生一种有颜色的产物。一定时间后终止反应，用分光光度计检测产物的量

图 10-3　直接三明治 ELISA 原理

②TMB 贮备液　称 TMB 10mg，溶解于 5ml 二甲基亚砜（dimethyl sulfoxide，DMSO），4℃贮存备用。

③底物应用液　临用前，将底物缓冲液与 TMB 贮备液按 1∶1 混合。

（9）终止液　2mol/L H_2SO_4。

【实验步骤】

1. **稀释抗原**　将目的抗原用包被液稀释至 1μg/ml。

2. **包被抗原**　取 96 孔聚苯乙烯检测板，每个孔加 100μl，封盖，4℃过夜，次日倾去孔内液体。

3. **洗涤**　每孔加入 200μl PBS 洗涤液，振荡 3 分钟，倾去液体，重复 3 次，将检测板扣放在洁净的滤纸上，除净液体。

4. **封闭**　每孔中加入 200μl 封闭液，封盖，37℃温箱孵育 1 小时，倾去液体。重复洗涤步骤。

5. **加一抗**　待测血清用稀释液稀释 1000 倍、2000 倍等倍数，阴性血清也稀释成相同的倍数，取不同稀释度的稀释液、阴性血清及待测血清各 100μl 加到对应的孔中，

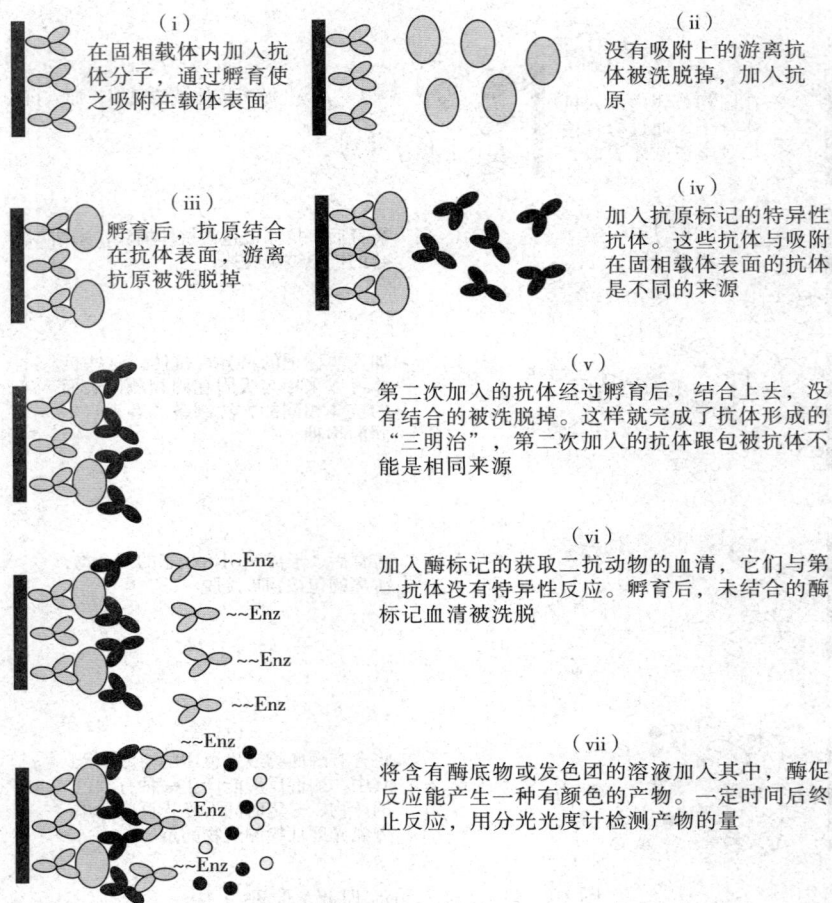

（i）在固相载体内加入抗体分子，通过孵育使之吸附在载体表面

（ii）没有吸附上的游离抗体被洗脱掉，加入抗原

（iii）孵育后，抗原结合在抗体表面，游离抗原被洗脱掉

（iv）加入抗原标记的特异性抗体。这些抗体与吸附在固相载体表面的抗体是不同的来源

（v）第二次加入的抗体经过孵育后，结合上去，没有结合的被洗脱掉。这样就完成了抗体形成的"三明治"，第二次加入的抗体跟包被抗体不能是相同来源

（vi）加入酶标记的获取二抗动物的血清，它们与第一抗体没有特异性反应。孵育后，未结合的酶标记血清被洗脱

（vii）将含有酶底物或发色团的溶液加入其中，酶促反应能产生一种有颜色的产物。一定时间后终止反应，用分光光度计检测产物的量

图 10-4　间接三明治 ELISA 原理

封盖，37℃温箱孵育 1 小时。按照洗涤步骤洗涤，重复 4 次。

6. 加酶标抗体　按照说明书要求用稀释液稀释 HRP - 抗体，每孔加 100μl，封盖，37℃温箱孵育 1 小时，按照洗涤步骤洗涤，重复 5 次。

7. 酶促反应　每孔加入底物 TMB 反应液（现用现配）100μl，37℃避光，反应 15 分钟。每孔加入 50μl 终止液，直到溶液变蓝终止反应。

8. 检测　以稀释液为对照，用酶标仪，测量 450nm 下的各孔光密度，记录结果。

【实验结果】

计算阳性血清与阴性血清吸光度之比（P/N）。当 $P/N \geqslant 2.1$ 时为阳性，$1.5 \leqslant P/N$ 2.1 为可疑，$P/N < 1.5$ 为阴性。

【注意事项】

1. 选择高质量、非特异性吸附小的聚苯乙烯检测板。

2. 向各孔加入的试剂量必须准确，并且加入时不要碰触到检测板。

3. 各个步骤的洗涤一定要充分，尽量除去残留物，减少非特异性吸附。

【思考题】

1. 为什么要用封闭液封闭酶标板?

2. 为何每次都要用洗涤液充分洗涤，若不洗涤或洗涤的不充分会怎样?

3. 酶联免疫吸附法的影响因素有哪些?

Experiment 10　Enzyme-linked Immunosorbent Assay

Purpose

1. To learn about the principle of enzyme-linked immunosorbent assay (ELISA).

2. To master the procedure of ELISA.

Principle

Enzyme-linked immunosorbent assay (ELISA) is one kind of immunoassay techniques based on the immunoenzymatic techniques. The strong specificity of antigen-antibody binding reaction integrates with the amplified effects of marked enzymatic reaction within ELISA, which causes the measurement sensitivity to achieve ng or pg level. The ELISA has been widely used as an diagnostic tool in medicine and plant pathology, as well as an effective quality-control checking method in various industries.

A brief introduction will be made on the principle of ELISA. The sample with an unknown amount of antigen is affixed to a solid surface, and then a specific antibody is applied over the surface so that it can bind to the antigen. This antibody is linked to an enzyme, and, in the final step, a substance containing the enzyme's substrate is added. The subsequent reaction produces a detectable signal, most commonly a color change in the substrate, which indicates the quantity of antigen in the sample. Three main methods form the basis to all ELISAs: Direct ELISA, Indirect ELISA and Sandwich ELISA. All three systems can be used to form the basis of a group of assays called competition or inhibition ELISAs. This experiment uses indirect ELISA to detect the titer of some virus or protein.

1. Direct ELISA　Direct ELISA can be regarded as the simplest form of ELISA, and is illustrated in Fig. 10 – 1.

2. Indirect ELISA　Indirect ELISA is illustrated in Fig. 10 – 2.

3. Sandwich ELISA　Sandwich ELISA can be divided into two systems, which have been named the direct sandwich ELISA and the indirect sandwich ELISA. They are illustrated in Fig. 10 – 3 and Fig. 10 – 4.

The antigen is captured by a solid-phase antibody. Antigen is then detected using antibodies from another species. This in turn is bound by an anti-species conjugate. Thus, the species of serum for the coating and detecting antibodies must be different, and the anti-species conjugate cannot react with the coating antibodies.

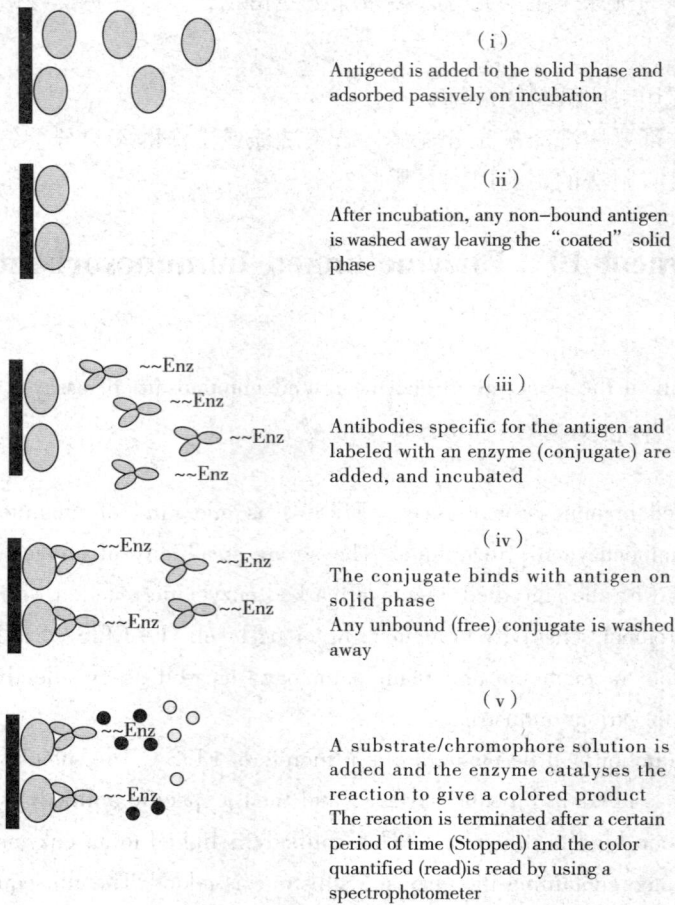

（i）
Antigeed is added to the solid phase and adsorbed passively on incubation

（ii）
After incubation, any non-bound antigen is washed away leaving the "coated" solid phase

（iii）
Antibodies specific for the antigen and labeled with an enzyme (conjugate) are added, and incubated

（iv）
The conjugate binds with antigen on solid phase
Any unbound (free) conjugate is washed away

（v）
A substrate/chromophore solution is added and the enzyme catalyses the reaction to give a colored product
The reaction is terminated after a certain period of time (Stopped) and the color quantified (read)is read by using a spectrophotometer

Fig. 10 – 1   Direct ELISA

Material

1. Apparatus

Polystyrene ELISA plates（40 or 96-well）, micropipette, thermostat box, microplate reader, flask, test tube, burette, aluminum-foil paper, filter paper.

2. Reagents

（1）Antigen   Hepatitis B virus, cytokine and so on.

（2）Antibody   Immuned animal serum.

（3）Enzyme labeled antibody   Select enzyme labeled antibody (secondary antibody) according to the experiment, such as commercial horse radish peroxidase (HRP) marked goat anti-rabbit IgG, HRP marked rabbit anti-mouse IgG and so on, and just follow the instructions.

（4）Coating buffer   0. 05mol/L Carbonic acid buffer （pH 9. 6）   Weigh Na_2CO_3 0. 8g, $NaHCO_3$ 1. 45g. Dissolve in distilled water and dilute to 500ml.

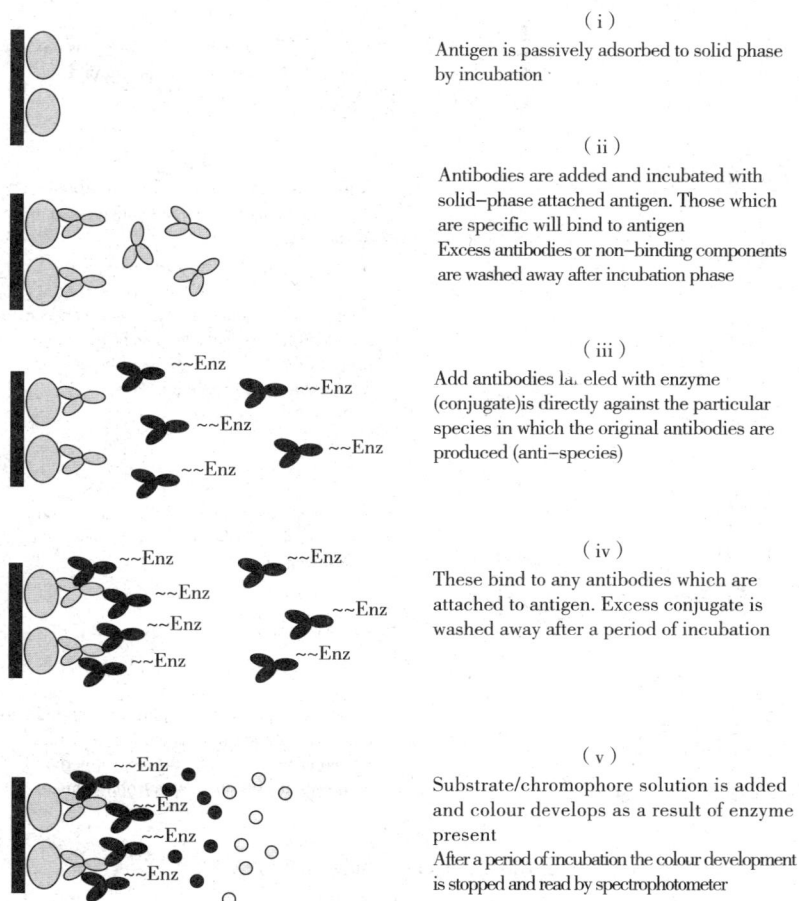

(i)
Antigen is passively adsorbed to solid phase by incubation

(ii)
Antibodies are added and incubated with solid-phase attached antigen. Those which are specific will bind to antigen
Excess antibodies or non-binding components are washed away after incubation phase

(iii)
Add antibodies labeled with enzyme (conjugate)is directly against the particular species in which the original antibodies are produced (anti-species)

(iv)
These bind to any antibodies which are attached to antigen. Excess conjugate is washed away after a period of incubation

(v)
Substrate/chromophore solution is added and colour develops as a result of enzyme present
After a period of incubation the colour development is stopped and read by spectrophotometer

Fig. 10 - 2　Indirect ELISA

(5) Dilution buffer　0.01mol/L Phosphate-NaCl buffer saline (PBS) (pH 7.4)　Weigh NaCl 8.0g, KH_2PO_4 0.2g. $Na_2HPO_4 \cdot 12H_2O$ 2.9g, KCl 0.2g. Dissolve in distilled water and dilute to 1L.

(6) Washing buffer　Dissolve 1ml 10% Tween-20 in 200ml PBS buffer.

(7) Blocking reagent　1% Ovalbumin (OVA) solution. Dissolve 1g ovalbumin in 100ml dilution buffer. It's best to prepare the solution just before using.

(8) Substrate solution　Use 3, 3', 5, 5'-tetramethyl benzidine (TMB) as the substrate, and prepare stock solution and applying solution.

① Substrate buffer　0.1mol/L Citrate - 0.2mol/L Na_2HPO_4 (pH 5.0 ~ 5.4). Dissolve Na_2HPO_4 14.6g, citrate 9.33g, 0.75% hydrogen peroxide adduct 6.4ml in distilled water and dilute to 1L.

② TMB stock solution　Dissolve 200mg 3,3',5,5'-tetramethyl benzidine (TMB) with 5ml dimethyl sulfoxide (DMSO), store at 4℃.

③ Substrate reaction solution　Mix Substrate buffer and TMB stock solution at the propor-

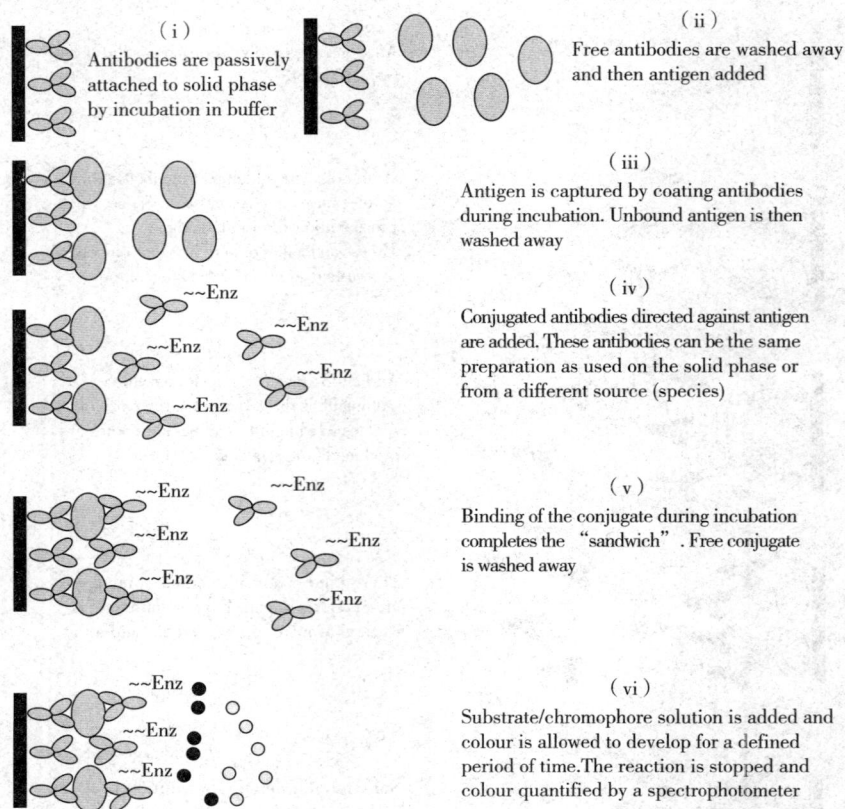

(i) Antibodies are passively attached to solid phase by incubation in buffer

(ii) Free antibodies are washed away and then antigen added

(iii) Antigen is captured by coating antibodies during incubation. Unbound antigen is then washed away

(iv) Conjugated antibodies directed against antigen are added. These antibodies can be the same preparation as used on the solid phase or from a different source (species)

(v) Binding of the conjugate during incubation completes the "sandwich". Free conjugate is washed away

(vi) Substrate/chromophore solution is added and colour is allowed to develop for a defined period of time.The reaction is stopped and colour quantified by a spectrophotometer

Fig. 10 – 3 Direct sandwich ELISA

tion of 1∶1 just before using.

(9) Stop solution   2mol/L H_2SO_4.

Procedures

1. Dilute antigen

Dilute antigen with coating buffer to 1μg/ml.

2. Coating antigen

Add 100μl of antigens per well to 96 well polystyrene ELISA plate. Seal the plate with cover. Incubate it overnight at 4℃. Discard the solution inside well next day.

3. Washing

Add 200μl of PBS wash buffer per well to the plate, oscillate for 3min, discard the liquid and invert the paper onto clean filter paper to remove it thoroughly. Repeat this step two more times.

4. Blocking

Add 200μl of blocking reagent per well to the plate, seal the plate and incubate for 1h at 37℃, discard the solution. Repeat Washing Step 3.

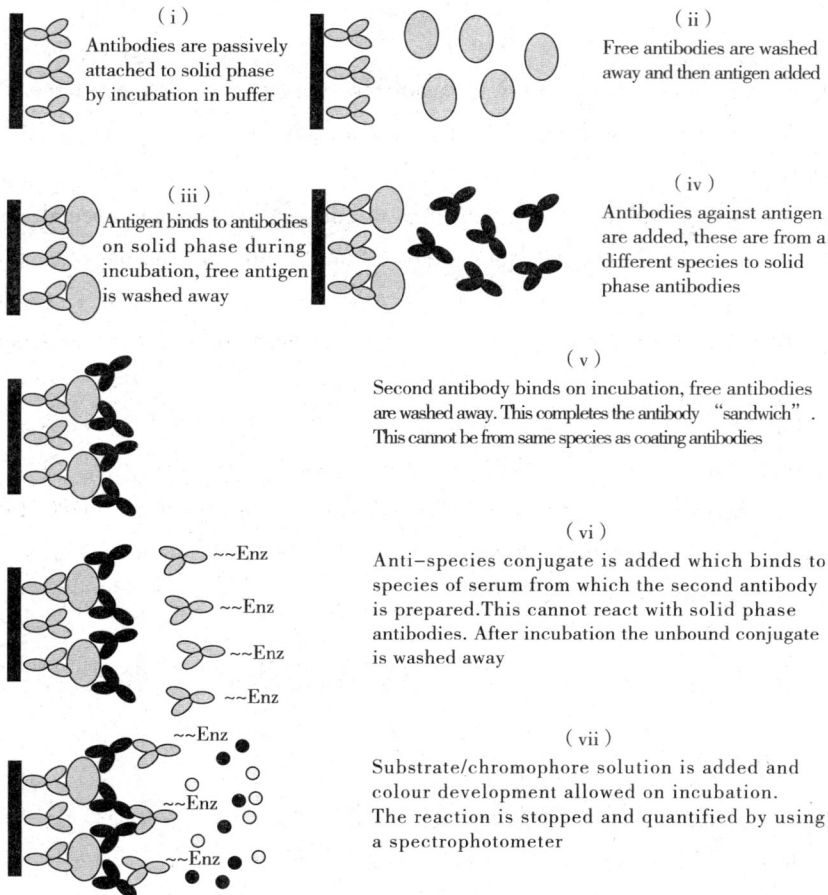

（i）
Antibodies are passively attached to solid phase by incubation in buffer

（ii）
Free antibodies are washed away and then antigen added

（iii）
Antigen binds to antibodies on solid phase during incubation, free antigen is washed away

（iv）
Antibodies against antigen are added, these are from a different species to solid phase antibodies

（v）
Second antibody binds on incubation, free antibodies are washed away. This completes the antibody "sandwich". This cannot be from same species as coating antibodies

（vi）
Anti-species conjugate is added which binds to species of serum from which the second antibody is prepared. This cannot react with solid phase antibodies. After incubation the unbound conjugate is washed away

（vii）
Substrate/chromophore solution is added and colour development allowed on incubation. The reaction is stopped and quantified by using a spectrophotometer

Fig. 10 - 4　Indirect sandwich ELISA

5. Add the first antibody

Detected serum are diluted to 1000 times, 2000 times or any times with dilution buffer such as negative serum. Add 100 μl of dilution buffer, negative serum and detection serum with some diluted times per well to the plate, seal the plate and incubate for 1h at 37℃. Repeat the washing step four times.

6. Add enzyme-labeled antibody

Dilute HRP-antibody according to the instruction. Add 100 μl of diluted HRP-antibody per well, seal the plate and incubate for 1h at 37℃. Repeat the washing step five times.

7. Enzyme reaction

Add 100 μl of TMB reaction solution per well (prepare just before using), seal the plate and incubate it at 37℃. Stop the reaction until the solution becomes blue. Add 50 μl stop solution per well after 15 min.

8. Detection

Read optical density (OD) on microplate reader at 450 nm using dilution buffer as control. Record the results.

Results

Calculate the ratio of positive serum to negative serum (P/N). $P/N \geqslant 2.1$ means positive, $1.5 < P/N < 2.1$ means doubtful. $P/N < 1.5$ means negative.

Cautions

1. Select polystyrene ELISA plates with high quality and weakly non-special absorbance.

2. Add exact quantity of reagents into each well and avoid touching the plate when adding the reagents.

3. Wash the plate thoroughly so as to remove the residues and decrease non-special absorbance.

Questions

1. Why should the plate be blocked with blocking buffer?

2. Why is thoroughly washing with washing solution demanded every time? How would it be with no washing or inadequate washing?

3. What factors will affect ELISA?

实验十一　动物组织中 DNA 的提取与含量测定

【实验目的】

1. 掌握从动物组织中提取 DNA 的原理及操作过程。

2. 熟悉应用二苯胺法测定 DNA 含量的过程。

3. 熟悉微量移液器的使用方法和注意事项。

【实验原理】

1. 从动物肝脏中提取 DNA　细胞中的 DNA 和 RNA，通常会与蛋白质结合，以核蛋白——脱氧核糖核蛋白（DNP）和核糖核蛋白（RNP）的形式存在，且这两种复合物在不同的电解质溶液中的溶解度有较大差异。在低浓度的 NaCl 溶液中，DNP 的溶解度随 NaCl 浓度的增加而逐渐降低，当 NaCl 浓度达到 0.14mol/L 时，DNP 的溶解度约为纯水中溶解度的 1%（几乎不溶）；但当 NaCl 浓度继续升高时，DNP 的溶解度又逐渐增大，当 NaCl 浓度增至 0.5mol/L 时，DNP 的溶解度约等于纯水中的溶解度，当 NaCl 浓度继续增至 1.0mol/L 时，DNP 的溶解度约为纯水中溶解度的 2 倍（溶解度很大）。而 RNP 则不同，它在任意浓度 NaCl 溶液中的溶解度都很大。因此，可以利用不同浓度的 NaCl 溶液将 DNP 和 RNP 进行分离。溶液中游离的 RNA 可以用核糖核酸酶（RNase）除去。在分离过程中，为了防止 DNA 被脱氧核糖核酸酶（DNase）分解，提取时所用溶液中应加入乙二胺四乙酸（EDTA），以螯合 DNase 的辅助因子 Mg^{2+}，抑制其活性。

将提取的 DNP 用十二烷基硫酸钠（SDS）处理，DNA 即与蛋白质分离，变性沉淀的蛋白质可用苯酚 – 三氯甲烷 – 异丙醇混合溶液除去，而 DNA 溶于溶液中，加入适量的乙醇后，DNA 即可从溶液中析出。

2. 二苯胺法测定 DNA 含量　DNA 分子中的 2-脱氧核糖残基，在酸性条件下加热降解，生成 ω-羟基-γ-酮基戊醛，该物质可与二苯胺试剂在加热条件下生成蓝色化合物，此蓝色化合物在 595nm 处有最大吸收，且当 DNA 在 40~400μg 范围内时，吸收值与 DNA 浓度成正比，因此可对 DNA 进行定量。

【实验材料】

1. 实验器材　匀浆机、离心机、离心管、手术剪、吸管、烧杯、量筒、玻璃棒、搪瓷缸、试管、移液管、微量移液器、微量移液器吸头、紫外-可见分光光度计。

2. 实验试剂

（1）新鲜或冷冻动物肝脏。

（2）0.14mol/L NaCl-0.15mol/L EDTA 溶液　称取 4.095g NaCl 及 27.9g EDTANa$_2$·2H$_2$O，用蒸馏水溶解并定容至 500ml。

（3）25% SDS 溶液　称取 25g SDS 溶于 45% 乙醇 100ml 中。

（4）苯酚-三氯甲烷-异丙醇混合液　依次量取 250ml 苯酚、240ml 三氯甲烷及 10ml 异丙醇，于棕色瓶中混匀，冰箱中备用。

（5）5mol/L NaCl 溶液　称取 146.25g NaCl 溶于蒸馏水并定容至 500ml。

（6）二苯胺试剂　称取 1g 二苯胺，溶于 100ml 冰醋酸，再加 1.5ml 浓 H$_2$SO$_4$，于棕色瓶中混匀，冰箱中备用。该溶液使用前新鲜配制。

（7）200μg/ml DNA 标准溶液　称取小牛胸腺 DNA 10mg，以 0.1mol/L NaOH 溶液溶解并定容至 50ml。

（8）50μg/ml 核糖核酸酶（RNase A）　将 10mg/ml RNase A 成品溶液 100μl 用 TE（pH 8.0）溶液定容至 20ml。分装于 Eppendorf 管中，100℃ 加热 15 分钟。室温下缓慢冷却，-20℃ 保存。

（9）95% 乙醇。

【实验步骤】

1. DNA 的提取

（1）称取新鲜或冷冻猪肝 5g，放于离心管中，在冰浴中剪碎，加 10ml 冷的 0.14mol/L NaCl-0.15mol/L EDTA 溶液，利用匀浆机制备匀浆液。

（2）将匀浆液置于离心机中，4000r/min 离心 10 分钟，弃去上清液，收集沉淀（内含 DNP），沉淀中加两倍沉淀体积的冷的 0.14mol/L NaCl-0.15mol/L EDTA 溶液，搅匀，如前所述重复洗涤沉淀 2 次。所得沉淀为 DNP 粗制品。

（3）取 3μl RNase，加入到 DNP 粗制品中，用玻璃棒慢慢搅拌 20 分钟。

（4）向沉淀中加入冷的 0.14mol/L NaCl-0.15mol/L EDTA 溶液，使总体积达到 10ml，在缓慢搅拌的同时滴加 25% 的 SDS 溶液 0.75ml，边加边搅拌，此步骤可使 DNA 与蛋白质分离，注意搅拌要缓慢。

（5）加入 5mol/L NaCl 溶液 2.5ml，使 NaCl 最终浓度约为 1mol/L，缓慢搅拌 10 分

钟，此时溶液略显透明。

（6）加入等体积冷的苯酚－三氯甲烷－异丙醇混合液（约为20ml），于冰浴中搅拌20分钟，3000r/min 离心10分钟。此时离心物分为三层，上层水相含有 DNA，中层为变性的蛋白质沉淀，下层为苯酚－三氯甲烷－异丙醇混合液。

（7）用吸管小心地吸取上层水相，弃去沉淀，再加入等体积的冷的苯酚－三氯甲烷－异丙醇混合液，于冰浴中搅拌10分钟，3000r/min 离心10分钟，取上层水相，根据变性蛋白质层的残留量，选择是否需要在相同条件下重复此步骤。最终将得到的上清液置于干燥小烧杯中。

2. DNA 纯品的制备　取约2倍 DNA 上清液体积的预冷的95% 乙醇，缓慢滴加到含有上清液的烧杯中，边加边用玻璃棒沿一个方向缓慢轻柔地转动，随着乙醇的不断加入可见溶液出现黏稠状物质，并能逐步缠绕于玻璃棒上，直至再无黏稠丝状物出现为止，黏稠丝状物即为制备出的 DNA 纯品。

3. DNA 含量的测定

（1）DNA 标准曲线的制作　取6支洁净干燥试管，编号，按表11－1加入试剂，混合后，于100℃水浴中保温15分钟。冷却至室温后，用紫外－可见分光光度计测定 A_{595}。以 DNA 含量为横坐标，A_{595} 为纵坐标，绘制标准曲线。

表11－1　二苯胺法定量 DNA 标准曲线

	管　号					
	1	2	3	4	5	6
标准 DNA 溶液（200μg/ml）	0.0	0.4	0.8	1.2	1.6	2.0
蒸馏水（ml）	2.0	1.6	1.2	0.8	0.4	
标准 DNA 含量（μg）	0.0	40.0	80.0	120.0	160.0	200.0
二苯胺试剂（ml）	4.0	4.0	4.0	4.0	4.0	4.0
A_{595}						

（2）样品测定　取一干净小试管，加入4ml 0.1mol/L NaOH，将 DNA 样品溶解其中。按照表11－2加入试剂，混合后，于100℃水浴中保温15分钟。冷却至室温后，以1号管为对照测定 A_{595}。根据已得 DNA 标准曲线方程计算 DNA 的量。

表11－2　二苯胺法定量 DNA 样品溶液

	管　号			
	1	2	3	4
DNA 样品溶液（ml）	0.00	0.25	0.50	1.00
蒸馏水（ml）	2.00	1.75	1.50	1.00
二苯胺试剂（ml）	4.00	4.00	4.00	4.00
样品稀释倍数		16.00	8.00	4.00
A_{595}				

4. 结果 选择吸光度在标准曲线范围内的数值，根据标准曲线计算 DNA 含量计算出样品中 DNA 的百分含量。

$$DNA\% = \frac{DNA\ 的量（\mu g）}{猪肝样品的量（\mu g）} \times 100\%$$

【思考题】

在提取核酸过程中，要注意什么问题?

Experiment 11 Extraction and Quantitation of DNA from Animal Tissues

Purpose

1. To master the principle and procedure of extracting DNA from animal tissues.

2. Be familliar with the procedure of diphenylamine method to quantitate DNA.

3. Be familliar with the application method and attentions of micropipette.

Principle

1. Extract DNA from animal livers

A large percentage of DNA and RNA combine with protein to form nucleoprotein, deoxyribonucleoprotein (DNP) and ribonucleoprotein (RNP), in cell. The solubility of DNP and RNP is quite different in various electrolyte solutions. In low concentration of NaCl solution, the solubility of DNP gradually decreases with NaCl concentration increasing. When the concentration arrives at 0. 14mol/L, the solubility of DNP is only 1% of in pure water (nearly insoluble). But when the concentration goes up continually, the solubility of DNP gradually increases. At 0. 5mol/L, it is the same as in pure water. After that, the solubility is twice as much as in pure water when the concentration reaches 1. 0mol/L (high solubility). RNP is different from DNP in that the solubility is large in both high and low concentration of NaCl. So DNP can be separated from RNP according to their different solubility in different concentrations of NaCl. Free RNA can be hydrolyzed by ribonuclease (RNase). During separation, ethylene diamine tetra acetic acid (EDTA) should be added to chelate deoxyribonuclease (DNase)'s cofactor Mg^{2+} in all solution to prevent DNP from being decomposed by enzyme in the procedure of extraction.

DNA will be isolated from DNP after being handled with Sodium dodecyl sulfate (SDS). DNA dissolve in solution and the protein precipitation will be removed by phenol-chloroform-isopropanol mixed solutions. Add some ethanol, DNA will precipitate out from solution.

2. Quantitation of DNA with diphenylamine method

2-Deoxyribose residue in DNA molecule will degrade and then generate ω-hydroxyl-γ-keto amyl aldehyde when being heated in acidic condition. This product can react with diphenylamine to form blue compound under the condition of heating. This blue compound has maximum absorption at 595nm, and the absorbance value is proportional to the concentration of DNA when DNA is within $40 \sim 400 \mu g$. This method can be used to quantitate DNA.

Materials

1. Apparatus

Homogenizer, centrifuge, centrifuge tube, scissors, dropper, glass flask, cylinder, glass rod, enamel, test tube, pipette, micropipette tip, ultraviolet-visible spectrophotometer.

2. Reagents

(1) Fresh or frozen animal liver.

(2) 0.14mol/L NaCl − 0.15mol/L EDTA solution   Weigh 4.095g NaCl and 27.9g ED-TANa$_2$ · 2H$_2$O, dissolve in distilled water, add distilled water to 500ml.

(3) 25% SDS solution   Weigh 25g SDS and, dissolve in 45% ethanol 100ml.

(4) Phenol chloroform-isopropanol mixture   Measure 250ml phenol, 240ml chloroform and 10ml isopropanol successively, mix completely in amber bottle, keep in refrigerator.

(5) 5mol/L NaCl solution   Weigh 146.25g NaCl, dissolve in distilled water and add distilled water to 500ml.

(6) Diphenylamine solution   Dissolve 1g of diphenylamine in 100ml of glacial acetic acid, add 1.5ml concentrated sulfuric acid, mix completely in amber bottle, and keep in refrigerator. The solution must be prepared just before using.

(7) 200μg/ml DNA standard solution   Weigh 10mg calf thymus DNA, dissolve in 0.1mol/L NaOH. Dilute to 50ml with 0.1mol/L NaOH.

(8) 50μg/ml Ribonuclease (RNase)   Dissolve 100μl 10mg/ml RNase A solution in 100μl TE buffer (pH 8.0). After dilute with TE buffer to 20ml, divide in Eppendorf tube and heat in 100℃ for 15min. Cool slowly at room temperature, and keep at −20℃.

(9) 95% ethanol.

Procedures

1. Extraction of DNA

(1) Weigh fresh or frozen pig's liver 5g in the centrifuge tube and cut into small pieces in ice-bath. Add cool 0.14mol/L NaCl − 0.15mol/L EDTA solution 10ml in it. Homogenize the tissue with a homogenizer.

(2) Centrifuge the homogenize at 4000r/min for 10min, discard supernatant and collect precipitate (contain DNP). Add twice volume cool 0.14mol/L NaCl − 0.15mol/L EDTA 10ml in precipitate, stir well, and collect the precipitate by centrifugation as described above and repeat for two times. Gain crude DNP product.

(3) Add 3μl RNase into DNP crude product, and stir slowly for 20min with glass rod.

(4) Add cool 0.14mol/L NaCl − 0.15mol/L EDTA into DNP crude product up to 10ml, drop 0.75ml 25% SDS solution while stirring slowly. This step can separate DNA from protein. Be cautious to stir slowly.

(5) Add 2.5ml 5mol/L NaCl solution, the final concentration of NaCl is 1mol/L, stir

slowly for about 10min, and then the solution is slightly transparent.

(6) Add equal volume cool phenol-chloroform-isopropanol mixture (the volume is about 20ml) and stir for 20min in ice-bath. Then centrifuge at 3000r/min for 10min. There are three layers in the centrifugal tube. DNA sodium salt lies in upper liquid, denatured protein precipitate stays in middle, and chloroform mixture exists in lower layer.

(7) Carefully suck up the upper layer through a pipette, discard precipitate, and add same volume of cool phenol-chloroform-isopropanol stir for 10min in ice-bath, then centrifuge at the same condition mentioned above. Choose whether to repeat this step according to the residual amount of denatured protein precipitate. At last, transfer the supernatant into a clear and dry flask.

2. Preparation of pure DNA product

Drop twice as much cool 95% ethanol as supernatant of DNA into the flask, at the same time, stir slowly with glass rod in the same direction. Ropy material twining round the glass rod is pure DNA.

3. Quantitation of DNA

(1) Draw standard curve of DNA   Take and label six dry test tubes, and add reagents as Table 11 – 1. Mix up, keep at 100℃ water bath for 15min, and cool it to the room temperature. Determine the absorbance at 595nm by UV-VIS spectrophotometer. Draw standard curve of DNA with DNA content as x-axis and A_{595} as y-axis.

Table 11 – 1   DNA standard curve by diphenylamine method

	Test tube					
	1	2	3	4	5	6
Standard DNA solution (200μg /ml)	0.0	0.4	0.8	1.2	1.6	2.0
Distilled water (ml)	2.0	1.6	1.2	0.8	0.4	
Concentration of standard DNA (μg)	0.0	40.0	80.0	120.0	160.0	200.0
Diphenylamine reagent (ml)	4.0	4.0	4.0	4.0	4.0	4.0
A_{595}						

(2) Sample Assay   Take one dry test tube, add 4ml 0.1mol/L NaOH and dissolve the DNA sample completely. Add reagents as the Table 11 – 2. Mix up, keep at 100℃ water bath for 15min, cool it and then determine the absorbance at 595nm with tube No. 1 as control. The content of NDA can be caculated according to the standard curve of DNA.

Table 11-2   Measurement of DNA sample by diphenylamine method

	Test tube			
	1	2	3	4
DNA solution (ml)	0.00	0.25	0.50	1.00
Distilled water (ml)	2.00	1.75	1.50	1.00
Diphenylamine reagent (ml)	4.00	4.00	4.00	4.00
Dilute times of DNA sample		16.00	8.00	4.00
A_{595}				

Results

Choose adaptive absorbance (the value is in the range of DNA standard curve), calculate the content of DNA according to the absorbance and standard curve, and then calculate DNA percentage as formula

$$DNA\% = \frac{DNA\ content\ (\mu g)}{Pig's\ liver\ weight\ (\mu g)} \times 100\%$$

Questions

What should be paid attention to during the extraction of nucleic acid?

实验十二   琼脂糖凝胶电泳

【实验目的】

掌握琼脂糖凝胶电泳鉴定 DNA 的原理与方法。

【实验原理】

琼脂糖是从海藻中提取出来的一种杂聚多糖，是由 D 型和 L 型半乳糖以 α-1,3-糖苷键和 β-1,4-糖苷键相连形成的线状高聚物（图 12-1）。琼脂糖遇冷水膨胀，溶于热水成溶胶，冷却后成为孔径范围从 50nm 到大于 200nm 的凝胶。

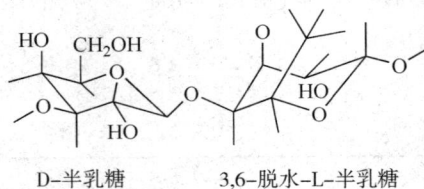

D-半乳糖   3,6-脱水-L-半乳糖

图 12-1   琼脂糖凝胶结构

琼脂糖凝胶电泳是分离、鉴定和纯化 DNA 片段最为常用的方法之一，这种方法简便易行，而且琼脂糖可以灌制成各种形状、大小和孔径，在不同的装置中进行电泳，如果有必要，还能够从凝胶中回收 DNA 谱带。

琼脂糖凝胶的分离范围较广，选择不同凝胶浓度和装置，从 50 个碱基对到几兆不同长度的 DNA 都可以实现分离。使用电场强度和电泳方向恒定的水平板琼脂糖凝胶电泳的方法，可以很好地分离长度在 50~20000bp 的 DNA 片段。

DNA 在琼脂糖凝胶中的迁移率受多种因素影响。例如 DNA 分子的大小，琼脂糖的浓度，所加电压等。DNA 片段越长，泳动速度越慢，而且泳动速度与电场强度成正比。一个给定大小的线性 DNA 片段，在不同浓度的琼脂糖凝胶中迁移率不同，DNA 电泳迁移率的对数与凝胶浓度呈线性关系。

用低浓度的荧光染料如 Golden view™ 或者溴化乙锭染色后，凝胶中的 DNA 可以直接被检测出来，紫外灯下可以直接检测到 20pg 的双链 DNA。

琼脂糖凝胶电泳还可以用于分析 DNA 的纯度，估算 DNA 的含量和对 DNA 进行构象分析。

分子量相同的超螺旋环状（Ⅰ型）、带切口的环状（Ⅱ型）及线状（Ⅲ型）DNA 通过凝胶时的速度不一。这三种 DNA 的相对迁移率主要取决于凝胶的琼脂糖浓度，但也受所使用的电流强度、缓冲液的离子强度及 Ⅰ型 DNA 超螺旋度的影响。在某些条件下，Ⅰ型 DNA 迁移率比Ⅲ型快；在另一些条件下则恰恰相反。

在不断增加溴化乙锭用量的情况下进行电泳，可以确切鉴定不同构象形式的 DNA。随着溴化乙锭浓度的增加，更多的染料结合到 DNA 分子上，Ⅰ型分子的负超螺旋逐渐解开，其分子半径增加，迁移速率减小。达到游离染料的临界浓度时，不再有超螺旋，Ⅰ型 DNA 的迁移速率达最小值。继续增加溴化乙锭，便形成正超螺旋，DNA 分子变得更加致密，迁移速率迅速增加。同时，由于电荷的中和，并且溴化乙锭的嵌入赋予 DNA 较大的刚性，Ⅱ型和Ⅲ型 DNA 的迁移速率会有不同程度的减小，线性 DNA 迁移率可以降低 15%。对于绝大多数 Ⅰ型 DNA，游离溴化乙锭的临界浓度介于 0.1~0.5µg/ml。溴化乙锭是一种强诱变剂，并有中度毒性，取用含有这一染料的溶液时务必戴手套，含有溴化乙锭的凝胶需按照指定方法处理。

【实验材料】

1. **实验器材**　水平电泳装置（包括电泳槽、电泳仪及梳齿）、100℃水浴、沸水浴锥形瓶、微量移液器。

2. **实验试剂**

（1）DNA 样品，DNA 标准分子量标记物，琼脂糖，Golden view™ 染料。

（2）缓冲溶液配制　按照表 12-1 配方。

表 12-1　缓冲液配方

缓冲溶液	工作溶液	储存溶液（每升）
0.5×TBE	0.045mol/L Tris-硼酸	54 g Tris 碱
(Tris 硼酸 EDTA 缓冲溶液)	0.001mol/L EDTA	27.5g 硼酸
		20ml 0.5mol/L EDTA（pH 8.0）
6×样品缓冲液	0.2%溴酚蓝	储存在 4℃
	50%（W/V）蔗糖水溶液	

【实验步骤】

（1）准备好灌胶模具，置于水平面上（实验操作示意图如图 12-2 所示）。

（2）配制 1.5% 琼脂糖凝胶。取 250ml 锥形瓶，加入 50ml 0.5×TBE 缓冲液，称取

0.75g 琼脂糖加入缓冲液中，微波炉加热至完全溶解，然后在 55℃ 水浴中保温。在灌胶模具中插入梳齿，将稍微冷却的凝胶中加入 3μl Golden view™ 混匀，倒入灌胶模具，凝胶厚度 3~5mm，避免气泡产生。

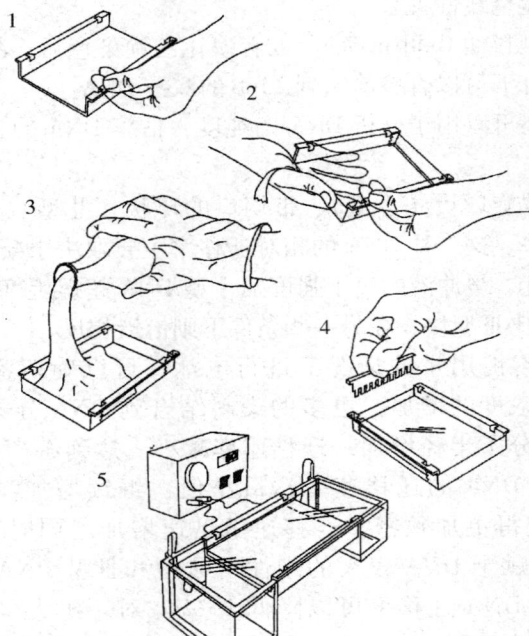

图 12-2　灌胶及电泳操作过程示意

（3）室温放置，待凝胶完全凝固后，按照厂家说明将凝胶放入水平板电泳槽。

（4）在电泳槽中加入足够的 0.5×TBE 电泳缓冲液，电泳缓冲液没过胶面 1mm，拔下梳齿形成样品池。

（5）取样品 20μl 与 4μl 的 6×样品缓冲液混合后，用微量移液器缓慢加入样品池中。

（6）盖上电泳槽并且通电，注意电源正、负极，确保样品向阳极移动。恒压 1~5V/cm（按照两极之间距离计算），至示踪染料溴酚蓝前沿距离凝胶前端 1cm 时，切断电源。

（7）取出凝胶，紫外灯下观察电泳结果并照相，分析实验结果，得出实验结论并进行讨论。

【注意事项】

紫外线对人体，尤其是眼睛有危害性，为减少紫外线照射，必须确保紫外线光源受到遮蔽。

虽然未发现 Golden view™ 有致癌作用，但是各种核酸染料的致癌作用学术界一直存在争议，同时 Golden view™ 对皮肤、眼睛会有一定的刺激。为安全起见，操作时依然应该每次戴手套，不小心接触皮肤后应该立刻清洗，并妥善处理废弃物。

【思考题】

影响琼脂糖凝胶 DNA 迁移率的因素有哪些?

Experiment 12　Agarose Gel Electrophoresis

Purpose

To master the principle and the method of DNA identification with agarose gel electrophoresis.

Principle

Agarose is a linear polymer composed of alternating residues of D-galactose and L-galactose joined by α-$(1 \rightarrow 3)$ and β-$(1 \rightarrow 4)$ glycosidic linkages (as shown in Fig. 12 – 1). Agarose will expand in cold water but become glue in hot water. After cooling, the gel with pores whose diameter is from 50nm to >200nm will be formed.

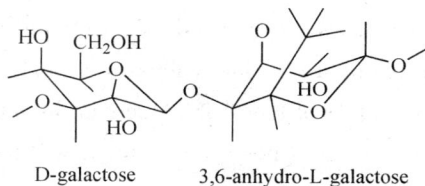

D-galactose　　3,6-anhydro-L-galactose

Fig. 12 – 1　The structure of agarose

Agarose gel electrophoresis is used to separate, identify, and purify DNA fragments. This technique is simple and rapid to perform. Furthermore, agarose gel can be poured in a variety of shapes, sizes, and porosities and can be run in a number of different electrophoresis sapparatus. If necessary, these bands of DNA can be recovered from the gel and used for a variety of purposes.

Agarose gel has a wide range of separation and DNAs from 50bp to several Mb in length can be separated on agarose gels of various concentrations and apparatus. DNA fragments, whose length is from 50bp to 20000bp, are best resolved in agarose gels running in a horizontal electrophoresis sapparatus in an electric field of constant strength and direction.

Several factors determine the rate of migration of DNA through agarose gel, including the molecular size of the DNA, the concentration of agarose, the applied voltage and so on. Larger molecules migrate more slowly, and at low voltages the rate of migration of linear DNA fragments is proportional to the voltage applied. A linear DNA fragment of a given size migrates at different rates through gels containing different concentrations of agarose. There is a linear relationship between the logarithm of the electrophoresis mobility of the DNA and the gel concentration.

The location of DNA within the gel can be determined directly by staining with low concentrations of fluorescent intercalating dyes, such as Golden view™ or ethidium bromide, bands containing as little as 20pg of double-stranded DNA can be detected by direct examination of the gel in UV.

Agarose gel electrophoresis can also be used to analyze the purity of DNA, estimate the content of DNA and conduct DNA conformational analysis.

There are three different kinds of DNA, i. e. supercoiling DNA (type Ⅰ), circular DNA with incision (type Ⅱ), and linear DNA (type Ⅲ). These different types of DNA with the same size will electrophorese at different speeds in an agarose gel. The migration rate of these DNA in an agarose gel are mainly decided by the concentration of the agarose gel, but also affected by the intensity of electric current, ion concentration in the buffer, and the degree of the supercoils in type I DNA. In some circumstances, type I is faster than type Ⅲ. Under other conditions, it is just the opposite.

With the electrophoresis by increasing the ethidium bromide concentration, different conformation of DNA can be detected. With the increase of the ethidium bromide concentration, more dye can bind with DNA, so that the negative supercoils of type I DNA unwind gradually. As the molecular radius increases, the speed of electrophoresis of type I DNA slows down. As the concentration of ethidium bromide reaches a critical concentration, there exist no more supercoils and the migration rate of type I DNA gets to the minimum. If the ethidium bromide concentration continues to increase, positive supercoils will be produced, DNA molecules will get more compact, and the migration rate will increase rapidly. At the same time, due to the charge neutralization and the rigid binding of DNA with ethidium bromide, the migration rate of type Ⅱ and Ⅲ will be reduced to some extent. The migration rate of the linear DNA can be decreased by 15%. As for most type I DNA, the critical concentration of ethidium bromide is between 0. 1 and 0. 5 microgram per milliliter. Ethidium bromide is a powerful mutagen and is toxic. Consult the local institutional safety officer for specific handling and disposal procedures. Wear appropriate gloves when working with solutions that contain this dye.

Materials

1. Apparatus

Horizontal electrophoresis apparatus with chamber, power supply and comb, 100℃ water bath, Erlenmeyer flask, micropipette.

2. Reagents

(1) DNA sample, DNA size standards, agarose, Golden view^{TM}.

(2) Buffer, see Table 12 – 1.

Procedures

1. Seal the edges of the plastic tray supplied with the electrophoresis apparatus with tape to form a mode (as shown in Fig. 12 – 2). Set the mode on a horizontal section of the bench.

2. Prepare 1. 5% (*W/V*) agarose solution in electrophoresis buffer   Add 0. 75g powdered

Table 12 − 1　Buffer formula

Buffer	Working solution	Stock solution/liter
0.5 × TBE	0.045mol/L Tris-boracic acid	54g Tris base
	0.001mol/L EDTA	27.5g Boracic acid
		20ml of 0.5mol/L EDTA (pH 8.0)
6 × Gel buffer	0.2% Bromophenol blue	Storage at 4℃
	50% (W/V) Sucrose in water	

agarose to 50ml 1 × TBE in a 250 ml Erlenmeyer flask. Heat the slurry in a microwave oven until the agarose dissolves. Transfer the flask into a water bath at 55℃. While the agarose solution is cooling, position the comb 0.5 ~ 1.0mm above the plate so that a complete well is formed when agarose is added to the mode. Add 3μl Golden view into the agarose solution, and then pour the warm agarose solution into the mode. The gel should be between 3mm and 5mm thick. Check that no air bubbles are under or between the teeth of the comb.

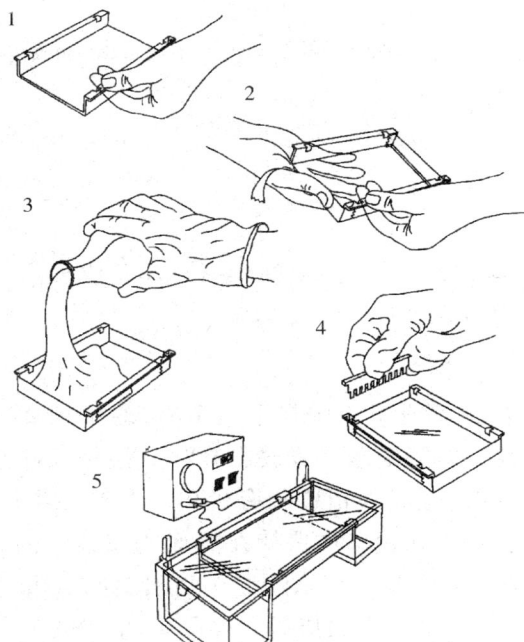

Fig. 12 − 2　Diagram of procedures for gel casting and electrophoresis

3. Allow the gel to set completely and mount the gel in the electrophoresis tank in accordance with the manufacturer's instructions.

4. Add enough 0.5 × TBE electrophoresis buffers to cover the gel to a depth of 1mm. Carefully remove the comb and then form sample cell.

5. Mix 20μl sample with 4μl 6 × gel buffer. Slowly load the sample mixture into the slots of

the submerged gel using micropipette.

6. Close the lid of the gel tank, set up an electric circuit and keep DNA migrating toward the positive anode (red lead). Keep the voltage of $1 \sim 5 V/cm$ (Calculation according to the distance between electrodes). Run the gel until the bromophenol blue have migrated to the position which is about 1cm away from the edge of the gel. Turn off the electric current and remove the leads and lid from the gel tank.

7. Remove the gel, observe under UV light and photographed, analyze the results, and draw conclusions and discussion.

Cautions

Ultraviolet radiation is harmful to human body, especially eyes, so in order to reduce ultraviolet irradiation, make sure that ultraviolet light source are covered.

Even though the Golden view™ were not found to be carcinogenic, but there are controversial of various nucleic acid dyes' carcinogenic effects. And Golden view™ is irritant to the eyes and skin. For security reasons, actions still should wear gloves when accidentally should be cleaned immediately after contact with skin, and properly dispose of waste.

Questions

What determine the rate of migration of DNA through agarose gel?

实验十三　动物组织 RNA 的提取与鉴定

【实验目的】

1. 掌握从动物组织样品中提取、纯化总 RNA 的实验技术。
2. 熟悉微量移液器的使用方法和注意事项。

【实验原理】

TRIzol 试剂是直接从细胞或组织中提取总 RNA 的试剂。它在破碎和溶解细胞时能保持 RNA 的完整性，裂解细胞并释放出 RNA，酸性条件使 RNA 与 DNA 分离，加入三氯甲烷后离心，样品分成水相层和有机层。在酸性条件下，总 RNA 仍然在上层水相，而大多数的 DNA 和蛋白质保持在界面或在较低的有机相。收集上面的水相层后，RNA 可以通过异丙醇沉淀来还原，当抽提的 RNA 用 TE 稀释时其 A_{260}/A_{280} 比值 $\geqslant 2.0$，视为合格。在除水相层后，样品中的 DNA 和蛋白质也能相继以沉淀的方式还原，乙醇沉淀能析出中间层的 DNA，在有机层中加入丙醇能沉淀出蛋白质。

检测 RNA 纯度可通过分光光度计法。RNA 溶液在 260nm、230nm、280nm 下的吸光度分别代表了核酸、杂质浓度和蛋白质等有机物的吸收值，通过 A_{260}/A_{280} 来检测 RNA 纯度，A_{260}/A_{230} 作为参考值。

A_{260}/A_{280} 在 $1.9 \sim 2.1$ 之间，可以认为 RNA 的纯度较好；

A_{260}/A_{280} 小于 1.8，则表明蛋白质杂质较多；

A_{260}/A_{280} 大于 2.2，则表明 RNA 已经降解；

A_{260}/A_{230} 小于 2.0，则表明裂解液中有异硫氰酸胍和巯基乙醇残留。

RNA 样品的浓度（μg/μl）＝ A_{260} × 稀释倍数 × 40/1000

【实验材料】

1. 实验器材　匀浆机、离心机、离心管、手术剪、吸管、烧杯、量筒、玻璃棒、搪瓷缸、试管、移液管、微量移液器、微量移液器吸头、紫外 – 可见分光光度计、组织镊、无菌培养管、90mm 培养皿。

2. 实验试剂　TRIzol 试剂、RNA 酶、75% 乙醇、100% 乙醇、β – 异丙醇、三氯甲烷、RNeasy 试剂盒、TE 缓冲液（pH 8.0）。新鲜动物肝脏。

【实验步骤】

1. RNA 提取

（1）将冷冻保存的小块组织迅速置于装有 1.5ml TRIzol 试剂的无菌培养管中，匀浆。打开匀浆器，加速至全速，分别 1 分钟、30 秒、30 秒，分 3 次匀浆样品，之后放置匀浆液 5 分钟（此间隙润洗匀浆器探头）。

（2）分别取 1ml 匀浆液于 2 个 1.5ml 离心管中，并置于冰上，分别向两个离心管中加入 200μl 三氯甲烷，用力摇动上述装有三氯甲烷和匀浆液的离心管 30s，室温下静置 3 ~ 5 分钟。在 4℃下，以 12000g 转速离心 20 分钟。

（3）倒掉液体部分后，快递合并两个试管中的样品于新的 1.5ml 离心管中，轻微振荡该离心管。将该离心管中的一半样品转移到最初的 1.5ml 离心管中，分别向两个离心管中加入等量的 β – 异丙醇，混匀后室温下静置 15 分钟。

（4）在 4℃下，以 12000g 转速离心 20 分钟。用移液管小心移除上清，用 1ml 75% 乙醇润洗，并轻轻取出沉淀物质。

（5）在 4℃下，以 7500g 转速离心 20 分钟，重新形成沉淀物，用 1ml 乙醇重复上述润洗步骤，然后重复上述离心再沉淀步骤。

（6）移除乙醇，4℃下 7500g 离心 1 分钟，用 100μl 或者 200μl 移液管小心移除残留的乙醇，将沉淀物在室温下风干 5 ~ 10 分钟（留意观察，避免过度干燥，过度干燥会影响再溶解）。将沉淀物再溶解在纯水中，确保总体积 100μl。

2. RNA 检测

（1）取 1μl 纯化的 RNA 于 0.5ml 无 RNA 酶的离心管中，加入 19μl TE 缓冲液（pH 8）按 1∶20 比例稀释。

（2）取 1μl 上述样品分别测定 A_{230}、A_{260} 和 A_{280}，符合下面参数的 RNA 认为其纯度较高。

$$A_{260}/A_{230} > 2.0$$
$$A_{260}/A_{280} > 2.0$$

（3）测 A_{260}，定量 RNA。

RNA 样品的浓度（μg/μl）＝ A_{260} × 稀释倍数 × 40/1000

3. 琼脂糖电泳检测 RNA 质量

（1）吸取含有 1μg RNA 的样品，与 2 ~ 3μl 样品缓冲液混合，上样，电泳。

（2）紫外扫胶后比较电泳条带，通过条带判断 RNA 质量。

【注意事项】

1. 避免 RNA 酶的污染。

2. 实验过程中要自始至终佩戴一次性无菌手套，取用样品和试剂是要保证无菌操作，勤换手套。

3. 使用无菌、一次性塑料器皿和枪头。

4. 开始实验前，擦拭实验台，维持无 RNA 环境。

5. TRIzol 试剂剧毒，使用要小心，在通风橱中使用并佩戴个人防护措施等。

【思考题】

1. 哪些组织中 RNA 含量高？

2. 检测 RNA 纯度时，测 A_{230}、A_{260} 和 A_{280} 的原理是什么？

3. 根据电泳图分析提取的 RNA 质量。

4. 总结防止 RNA 酶污染的实验操作。

Experiment 13　RNA Extraction and Identification from Animal Tissue

Purpose

1. To master the experimental techniques of extraction and purification of total RNA from animal tissue.

2. Be familliar with the application method and attentions of micropipette.

Principle

TRIzol is a reagent for the extraction of total RNA from cells and tissues. It can keep the integrity of the cells while breaking and dissolving cells, lyse cells and release RNA. RNA and DNA can been separated under acidic condition, Addition of chloroform followed by centrifugation, the sample is separated into the aqueous phase and organic phase. Under acidic condition, total RNA remains in the upper aqueous phase, while most of DNA and proteins remain either in the interphones or in the lower organic phase. After collecting the aqueous layer, RNA can be extracted through isopropanol precipitation. RNA is considered pure when the A_{260}/A_{280} of RNA diluted with TE is greater than or equal to 2. 0. DNA and protein in the sample can also be extracted by precipitating. By adding ethanol, DNA in the intermediate layer is precipitated, and the protein in the organic layer is precipitated by adding isopropyl.

RNA purity can be assayed with spectrophotometer. The absorbencies of RNA solution at 260nm, 230nm and 280nm respectively represent the absorption values of nucleic acid, impurity concentration and the protein or other organic matter. A_{260}/A_{280} is detected to represent the purity of RNA, and A_{260}/A_{230} is detected as the reference value.

When A_{260}/A_{280} is between 1.9~2.1, it indicates the RNA is pure.

When A_{260}/A_{280} is less than 1.8, the protein is impure.

When A_{260}/A_{280} is more than 2.2, RNA has degraded.

When A_{260}/A_{230} is less than 2.0, the result indicates there are guanidinium thiocyanate and β-mercaptoethanol remains.

The concentration of RNA samples ($\mu g/\mu l$) = A_{260} × dilution multiple × 40/1000

Materials

1. Apparatus

Homogenizer, centrifuge, centrifuge tube, scissors, dropper, glass flask, measuring cylinder, glass rod, enamel mug, test tube, pipette, micropipette, micropipette tip, ultra-violet-visible spectrophotometer, tissue forceps, culture tube, 90mm petri dish.

2. Reagents

TRIzol reagent, RNAse, 75% ethanol, 100% ethanol, β-isopropanol, chloroform, Qiagen RNeasy mini kit, TE buffer (pH 8.0), Fresh or frozen animal liver.

Procedures

1. RNA extraction

(1) Quickly place the dissected sample into the sterilized culture tube containing 1.5ml TRIzol. Homogenize the tissue. Start the homogenizer and accelerate quickly to full speed. Homogenize the sample three times, for 1min, 30s, and 30s respectively. Allow the homogenized solution to stand for 5min. (Wash the homogenizer probe during this waiting period)

(2) Pipette 1ml TRIzol/Homogenate into two 1.5ml Eppendorf tubes respectively and then put them currently on the ice. Add 200μl chloroform, shake the tubes containing homogenate and chloroform vigorously for 30s and allow standing at room temperature for 3 ~ 5min. Centrifuge at 12000g for 20min at 4℃.

(3) Remove the aqueous phase from each tube and combine them all into a new 1.5ml Eppendorf tube. Mix it briefly. Transfer half of this mixture to the remaining 1.5ml tube. Add an equal volume of isopropanol to each tube and mix thoroughly. Let them stand at room temperature for 15min.

(4) Centrifuge at 12000g for 20min at 4℃. Carefully pipette off the supernatant. Rinse with 1ml 75% ethanol and gently dislodge the precipitate.

(5) Centrifuge at 7500g for 20min at 4℃ to precipitate again. Repeat the rinse with another 1ml 75% ethanol, and then repeat the centrifugation.

(6) Remove the ethanol again. Centrifuge at 7500g for 1min at 4℃ to collect residual ethanol. Carefully remove this ethanol using a 100μl or 200μl micropipette. Allow the precipitate to air dry at room temperature for 5 ~ 10min (Watch the precipitate closely to avoid over drying, which will inhibit redissolving). Redissolve the precipitate in RNAse-free water, RNA resuspend in a total of 100μl.

2. Assaying RNAs

(1) Dilute $1\mu l$ of the purified RNA product in $19\mu l$ of TE buffer pH 8.0. Be sure to use a 0.5ml RNase-free tube for 1:20 dilution.

(2) Use $1\mu l$ of the 1:20 dilution to measure the value of A_{230}, A_{260} and A_{280}, RNA that conforms to the following parameters is considered pure and acceptable.

$$A_{260}/A_{230} > 2.0$$
$$A_{260}/A_{280} > 2.0$$

(3) Measure the value of A_{260} and quantitate RNA.

The concentration of RNA samples $(\mu g/\mu l) = A_{260} \times 40/1000 \times$ dilution multiple

3. Agarose gel electrophoresis for RNA quality assay

(1) Mix $1\mu g$ RNA and $2 \sim 3\mu l$ $6 \times$ loading buffer into gel, and then run agarose gel electrophoresis.

(2) Get the electrophoresis bands under UV and analyze the quality of RNA based on these bands.

Cautions

1. Avoid RNase pollution.

2. Always wear disposable gloves and practice good sterile technique when handling samples and reagents. Change gloves frequently.

3. Always use sterilized, disposable and RNA special-purpose plastic ware and pipettes tips.

4. Before starting, wipe down the work surface to promote an RNAse-free environment.

5. TRIzol reagent is highly toxic and should only be used with caution. Work only in a fume hood with proper personal protective equipment.

Questions

1. Which tissues are rich in RNA?

2. When assaying the purity of extracted RNA, what is the principle of measuring A_{230}, A_{260}, and A_{280}?

3. Talk about the quality of extracted RNA according to your agarose gel.

4. Please summarize the steps of avoiding RNase pollution.

实验十四　PCR 扩增 DNA

【实验目的】

1. 掌握 PCR 扩增 DNA 的原理及技术。

2. 学习 PCR 扩增仪的使用。

【实验原理】

聚合酶链反应（polymerase chain reaction，PCR）是一种体外 DNA 扩增技术，1985

年由 Mullis 等人创立。该技术能在几小时的实验操作中，将 DNA 扩增几百万倍，具有灵敏度高、特异性强、操作简便和应用广泛等优点，目前已成为分子生物学及基因工程中极为有用的研究手段，另外在医学研究和医疗诊断中亦体现出极大的应用价值。

PCR 的工作原理类似于 DNA 的体内复制过程，是将待扩增的 DNA 经变性、退火及延伸三步反应的多次循环，使特定的 DNA 片段在数量上呈指数增加。PCR 扩增首先需要 1 对引物，根据待扩增区域两侧的已知序列合成两个与模板 DNA 互补的寡核苷酸作为引物，引物序列将决定扩增片段的特异性和片段长度。反应体系由模板 DNA、1 对引物、dNTP、耐高温的 DNA 聚合酶、酶反应缓冲体系及必需的离子等所组成。PCR 反应循环的第一步为加热变性，使双链模板 DNA 变性为单链；第二步为复性，每个引物将与互补的 DNA 序列杂交；第三步为延伸，在耐高温的 DNA 聚合酶作用下，以变性的单链 DNA 为模板，从引物 $3'$ 端开始按 $5' \rightarrow 3'$ 方向合成 DNA 链。这样经过一个周期的变性—复性—延伸等三步反应就可以产生倍增的 DNA。假设 PCR 的效率为 100%，反复 n 个循环后，理论上就能扩增 2^n 倍。PCR 反应一般 25～30 次循环，DNA 片段可扩增数百万倍。

常规 PCR 反应用于已知 DNA 序列的扩增，变性温度为 95℃，复性温度为 37℃～55℃，延伸合成温度为 72℃，DNA 聚合酶为 Taq 酶（可耐受 95℃ 左右的高温而不失活），反应循环数为 25～30。

其具体原理如图 14-1。

【实验材料】

1. **实验器材**　PCR 扩增仪、台式高速离心机、移液器、经高压灭菌后的 Eppendorf 管、电泳仪。

2. **实验试剂**

（1）模板 DNA（0.1μg/μl）　含有降钙素基因的重组质粒。

（2）Taq DNA 聚合酶（5U/μl），10×扩增缓冲液，dNTP（2.5mmol/L）：购买。

（3）引物（10μmol/L）　设计并合成与目的 DNA 两侧互补的引物。

引物序列如下：

引物 F　$5'$ - TACCATGGAAGCAGA - $3'$

引物 R　$5'$ - CGAATTCTTAGCCGG - $3'$

【实验步骤】

1. **准备 PCR 反应溶液**

（1）按表 14-1，将下列成分在 0.2ml 灭菌 Eppendorf 管内混合。

表 14-1　PCR 反应体系

组　成	体积（μl）
蒸馏水	14.5
10×Taq PCR 缓冲液	2
dNTP	0.4
引物 F	0.4
引物 R	0.4
模板	2

组 成	体积（μl）
*Taq*DNA 聚合酶	0.3
终体积	20.0

（2）用手指轻弹 Eppendorf 管底部，使溶液混匀。在台式离心机中 10000r/min 离心 2 秒集中溶液于管底。

2. PCR 扩增反应 将加好样品的 Eppendorf 管置于 PCR 扩增仪内，94℃ 5 分钟，使模板 DNA 完全变性，然后按 94℃变性 30 秒，55℃退火 30 秒，72℃延伸 30 秒，重复循环 25 次，循环结束后 72℃延伸 5 分钟。反应完毕，将样品取出置 4℃待用。

3. 琼脂糖凝胶电泳 取出样品，进行琼脂糖凝胶电泳，Godview 染色。具体操作方法见实验十二。

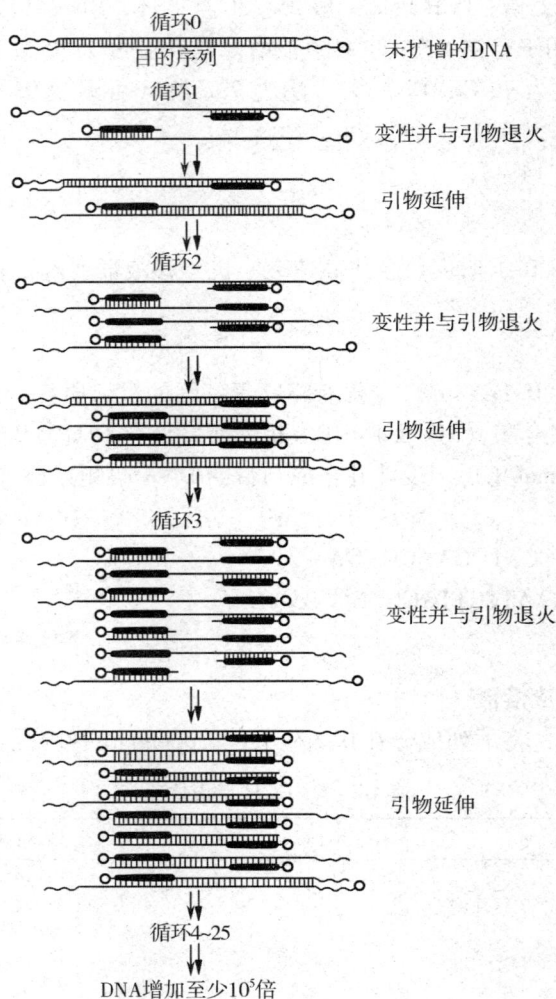

图 14 - 1 PCR 反应过程的原理

【注意事项】

1. PCR 结果若出现非特异性的扩增条带，有必要进一步优化反应条件，包括改变退火温度和时间，调整 Mg^{2+} 浓度等。

2. PCR 反应特异性强，引物浓度、*Taq* DNA 聚合酶和 dNTP 的量不宜过多。

3. 引物设计要合理。一般引物长度为 18 ~ 30 个核苷酸；引物间的 G + C 含量应为 40% ~ 60%，而且避免引物内部产生二级结构；引物 3′ 端不应该互补，避免在 PCR 反应过程中产生引物二聚体；避免引物 3′ 端出现 3 个连续的 G 或 C；理想情况下，成对引物的 G + C 含量应相似，以便以相近的退火温度与互补的模板链相结合，此外，引物 5′ 端序列对于后续操作也是十分有用的，例如对 PCR 产物进行克隆时，可以考虑在引物 5′ 端引入限制性酶切位点。

【思考题】

影响 PCR 的因素有哪些？

Experiment 14　PCR Amplification of DNA

Purpose

1. To master the principle and the techniques of PCR amplification of DNA.

2. To learn how to use the PCR thermal cycler.

Principle

Polymerase chain reaction (PCR) is a technique of amplifying DNA *in vitro*, which was previously established in 1985 by Mullis *et al*. This technique, by which a certain fragment of DNA can be amplified many million-fold in a few of hours under experimental operation, has the advantages of high sensitivity, high specificity, ease of operation, extensive application and so on. Until now PCR has become an essential tool not only in molecular biology but also in genetic engineering. Furthermore, its applications are finding their way into many areas of medical research and medical diagnosis.

The principle of PCR is similar to the natural process of DNA replication *in vivo*. The DNA fragment is amplified with two oligonucleotide primers, each complementary to one end of the DNA target sequence, in a three-step reaction of denaturing, annealing and polymerization. Many cycles can produce the definite DNA fragments increased in quantity by index. A pair of oligonucleotides will serve as PCR primers, which can be designed according to the known sequence information of template DNA. The primers are complementary to one end of the DNA target sequence so that they can decide the length and the location of the amplified DNA fragment. The reaction system comprises template DNA, a pair of primers, dNTPs, thermostable DNA polymerase, reaction buffer, magnesium and optional additives. Each cycle of PCR is as follows: Firstly, denaturation— heat to denature the duplex DNA template at high temperature so that the target DNA is separated into two strands; Secondly, annealing— decrease the temperature of the solution to make the primers and DNA template complement and anneal to partly form double chains; Finally, extension—with thermostable DNA polymerase, the single strand of the DNA template, which is obtained by denaturation, distends to be double strands by addition of nucleotides to primer's 3'end. As a result, by reaction cycle of three steps: denaturation, primer annealing and polymerization, the copy of the definite DNA fragment is doubled over and over again with each cycle. If PCR is 100% efficient, one target mole-cule would become 2^n after n cycles. Usually by 25~30 cycles, DNA fragment is amplified by some million times.

The basic PCR is applied to amplify those DNA fragments whose sequence has been known. The reaction cycle comprises a 95℃ step to denature the duplex DNA, an annealing step of around 37℃~55℃ to allow the primers to bind and a 72℃ polymerization step. *Taq* DNA polymerase is usually used as thermostable DNA polymerase in PCR, which still survives in the denaturation step of 95℃. In addition, 25~30 cycles are used in the basic PCR.

The basic principle of PCR is illustrated in Fig. 14 – 1.

Materials

1. Apparatus

PCR thermal cycler, table high-speed centrifuge, pipette, Eppendorf tubes sterilized by high pressure, electrophoresis apparatus.

2. Reagents

(1) Template DNA (0.1μg/μl) Recombinant plasmid with calcitonin gene.

(2) Purchase *Taq* DNA polymerase (5U/μl), 10 × amplification buffer, dNTPs (2.5 mmol/L).

(3) Primers (10μmol/L) Design and synthesis primers each complementary to one end of the target DNA. The sequence of primers are as follow.

Primer F 5'-TACCATGGAAGCAGA-3'

Primer R 5'-CGAATTCTTAGCCGG-3'

Procedures

1. Preparation of PCR reaction solution

(1) In a sterile 0.2ml Eppendorf tube, add reagents and mix up as Table 14 – 1.

Table 14 – 1 Reaction mixture for PCR

Component	Volume (μl)
Distilled Water	14.5
10 × *Taq* PCR buffer	2.0
dNTP	0.4
Primer F	0.4
Primer R	0.4
Template	2.0
Taq DNA polymerase	0.3
Final volume	20.0

（2）Pellet the bottom of the Eppendorf tube with finger gently in order to mix the solution well. Then the solution is collected by centrifugation, 10000r/min 2s with table high-speed centrifuger.

2. The process of PCR

The Eppendorf tubes containing the reaction mixtures are put into the PCR thermal cycler, the reaction mixtures are kept at 94℃ for 5min to denature DNA fully. Next in turns of denaturing at 94℃ for 30s, annealing at 55℃ for 30s and extending at 72℃ for 30s, repeat for 25 cycles. After these cycles are finished, the reaction mixtures are extended at 72℃ for a further 5min. Finally, take out the sample tubes and store at 4℃.

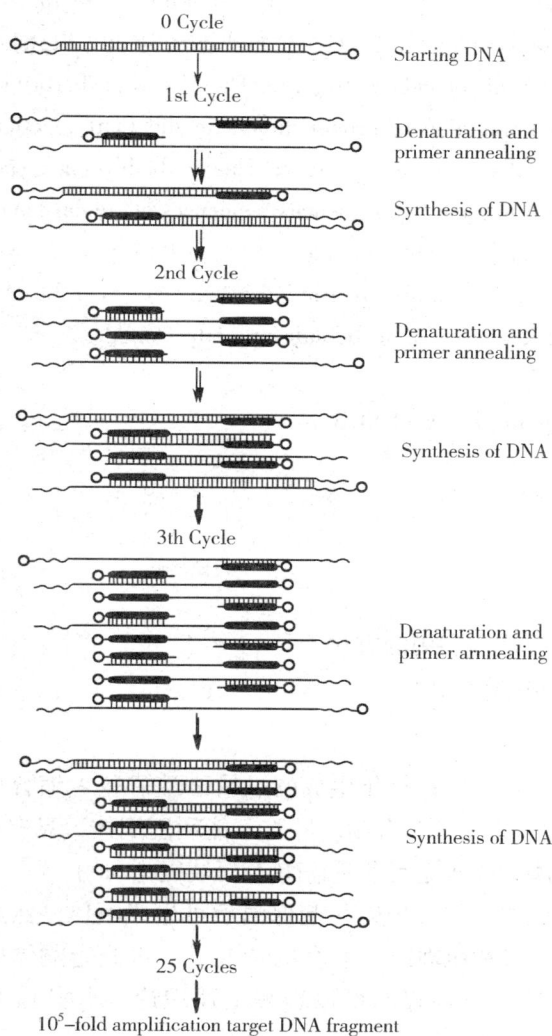

0 Cycle — Starting DNA

1st Cycle — Denaturation and primer annealing / Synthesis of DNA

2nd Cycle — Denaturation and primer annealing / Synthesis of DNA

3th Cycle — Denaturation and primer arnnealing / Synthesis of DNA

25 Cycles

10^5-fold amplification target DNA fragment

Fig. 14 – 1　Principle of the PCR

3. Agarose gel electrophoresis

Withdraw the samples and analyze them by agarose gel electrophoresis. Stain the gel with Godview to visualize the DNA. For the instruction in further details, please see Experiment 12.

Cautions

1. If PCR produces some nonspecific amplification, it may be necessary to optimize the reaction conditions. The parameters to be varied include the annealing temperature, the annealing time and the Mg^{2+} concentration.

2. PCR has high specificity, so the concentration of the primes, *Taq* DNA polymerase and dNTP should not be too high.

3. Design the primes rationally. PCR primers generally range in length from 18 ~ 30 bases. Primers should contain 40% ~ 60% G + C and care should be taken to avoid sequences which would produce internal secondary structure. The 3′ end of the primers should not be complementary to avoid the production of primer-dimers in the PCR reaction. Avoid three G or C nucleotides in a row near the 3′ end of the primer. Ideally, both primers should have similar G + C content so that they anneal to their complementary sequences at similar temperatures. Additionally, the sequence of the primers can also include regions at the 5′ end, which can be useful for downstream applications. For example, restriction enzyme sites can be placed in the primer pair design if the desired PCR product is to be subsequently cloned.

Questions

What is the influencing factor of PCR?

实验十五　酮体的生成和利用

【实验目的】

1. 掌握测定酮体生成与利用的方法。
2. 了解酮体的生成部位。

【实验原理】

在肝脏线粒体中，脂肪酸 β 氧化生成的过量乙酰辅酶 A 缩合成酮体。酮体包括乙酰乙酸、β - 羟丁酸和丙酮三种化合物。肝脏不能利用酮体，只有在肝外组织，尤其是心脏和骨骼肌中，酮体可以转变为乙酰辅酶 A 而被氧化利用。

本实验以丁酸为底物，与肝匀浆一起保温后可生成酮体，然后测定肝匀浆液中酮体的含量。另外，在肝脏和肌肉组织共存的情况下，再测定酮体的含量。在这两种不同条件下，由酮体含量的差别我们可以理解上述理论。本实验主要测定的是丙酮的含量。

酮体测定的原理：在碱性溶液中碘可将丙酮氧化成为三碘甲烷。以硫代硫酸钠滴定剩余的碘，可以计算所消耗的碘，由此也就可以计算出酮体（以丙酮为代表）的含量。反应式如下：

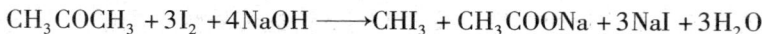

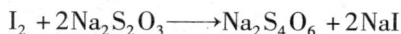

$$CH_3COCH_3 + 3I_2 + 4NaOH \longrightarrow CHI_3 + CH_3COONa + 3NaI + 3H_2O$$
$$I_2 + 2Na_2S_2O_3 \longrightarrow Na_2S_4O_6 + 2NaI$$

【实验材料】

1. 实验器材 试管、移液管、锥形瓶、滴定管及滴定管架。

2. 实验试剂

（1）0.1% 淀粉液 将1g淀粉溶解于蒸馏水中，定容到100ml。

（2）0.9% NaCl 溶液 9g NaCl，加水溶解，定容至1L。

（3）15% 三氯醋酸 15g 三氯醋酸，加水溶解，定容至100ml。

（4）10% NaOH 溶液 10g NaOH，加水溶解，定容至100ml。

（5）10% HCl 溶液 10ml浓盐酸（36.5%）加26.5ml水。

（6）0.5mol/L 丁酸溶液 2gNaOH，加水溶解，定容至100ml，配成0.5mol/L的溶液，取5ml丁酸溶于100ml 0.5mol/L NaOH 中。

（7）0.1mol/L 碘液 I_2 12.5g 和 KI 25g 加水溶解，定容至1L，用0.1mol/L $Na_2S_2O_3$ 标定。

（8）0.02mol/L $Na_2S_2O_3$ 24.82g $Na_2S_2O_3 \cdot 5H_2O$ 和400mg 无水 Na_2CO_3 溶于1L刚煮沸的水中，配成0.1mol/L溶液，用0.1mol/L KIO_3 标定。临用时将标定 $Na_2S_2O_3$ 溶液稀释成0.02mol/L。

【实验步骤】

1. 制备匀浆 将兔处死，取出肝脏，用0.9% NaCl 洗去污血，放滤纸上，吸去表面的水分，称取肝组织5g置研钵中，加少许0.9% NaCl 至总体积为10ml，制成肝组织匀浆。另外再取后腿肌肉5g，按上述方法和比例，制成肌组织匀浆。

2. 酮体的提取 取试管3只，编号，按表15－1操作。

表 15－1 酮体的提取

管号	A	B	C
肝组织匀浆（ml）		2.0	2.0
预先煮沸的肝组织匀浆（ml）	2.0		
pH 7.6 的磷酸盐缓冲液（ml）	4.0	4.0	4.0
丁酸（ml）	2.0	2.0	2.0
43℃水浴保温60分钟			
肌组织匀浆（ml）		4.0	
预先煮沸的肌组织匀浆（ml）	4.0		4.0
43℃水浴保温60分钟			
15% 三氯醋酸（ml）	3.0	3.0	3.0

摇匀后，用滤纸过滤，将滤液分别收集在3支试管中，为无蛋白质滤液。

3. 酮体的测定　取锥形瓶 3 只，按表 15 - 2 所述编号顺序操作。

表 15 - 2　酮体的测定

管　号	1	2	3
无蛋白质滤液（ml）	5.0	5.0	5.0
0.1mol/L I$_2$ - KI（ml）	3.0	3.0	3.0
10% NaOH（ml）	3.0	3.0	3.0

摇匀，静置 10 分钟，向各管中加入 10% HCl 3ml，加 1% 淀粉液 1 滴呈蓝色，分别用 0.02mol/L Na$_2$S$_2$O$_3$ 滴定至溶液呈亮绿色为止。

【实验结果与计算】

肝脏生成的酮体量（mmol/g） = （$C-A$）×Na$_2$S$_2$O$_3$浓度×1/6

肌肉利用的酮体量（mmol/g） = （$C-B$）×Na$_2$S$_2$O$_3$浓度×1/6

式中，A——滴定样品 1 消耗的 Na$_2$S$_2$O$_3$ 体积数；

　　　B——滴定样品 2 消耗的 Na$_2$S$_2$O$_3$ 体积数；

　　　C——滴定样品 3 消耗的 Na$_2$S$_2$O$_3$ 体积数。

【思考题】

为什么只有在肝外组织，酮体才可以被氧化利用？

Experiment 15　Production and Utilization of Ketone Body

Purpose

1. To master the measurement method of production and utilization of ketone body.

2. To understand the production organs of ketone body.

Principle

Within the mitochondria of liver, the excess acetyl CoA produced during fatty acid β-oxidation is converted to acetoacetate, β-hydroxybutyrate, and acetone. This group of molecules is called the ketone body. Liver can not use ketone body as an energy source. Only in extrahepatic tissues, most notably cardiac and skeletal muscle, can ketone body be converted to acetyl CoA, which is then oxidized to generate energy.

Butyric acid is used as initial stuff in this experiment. The butyric acid can be converted to acetyl CoA after heated it with liver homogenate, and then the content of ketone body in liver homogenate is measured. Moreover, the content of ketone body is measured under the condition of coexistence with liver homogenate and skeletal muscle in reaction system. We can comprehend the above theories from the difference of the ketone body content under two different conditions. The content of acetone is measured in this experiment mainly.

The measurement principle of ketone body is shown below: In alkaline solution the iodine can oxidize acetone to iodoform. By titration of the remaining iodine in the reaction system with hyposulphite, the consumption of iodine can be calculated, and then the content of ketone body (with acetone as representative) can be calculated according to the titration results. The equation of reaction is as follows.

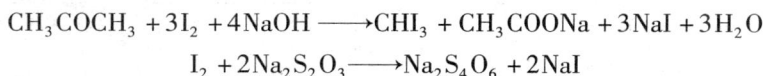

$$CH_3COCH_3 + 3I_2 + 4NaOH \longrightarrow CHI_3 + CH_3COONa + 3NaI + 3H_2O$$

$$I_2 + 2Na_2S_2O_3 \longrightarrow Na_2S_4O_6 + 2NaI$$

Materials

1. Apparatus

Test tubes, pipettes, flasks, Erlenmeyer flask, burettes and burette support.

2. Reagents

(1) 0.1% Starch solution Dissolve 1g starch in distilled water and dilute to 100ml.

(2) 0.9% NaCl solution Dissolve 9g NaCl in distilled water and dilute to 1L.

(3) 15% Trichlorine acetic acid Dissolve 15g trichlorine acetic acid in distilled water and dilute to 100ml.

(4) 10% NaOH solution Dissolve 10g NaOH in distilled water and dilute to 100ml.

(5) 10% HCl solution Add 10ml HCl (36.5%) to 26.5ml distilled water.

(6) 0.5mol/L Butyric acid Dissolve 2g NaOH in 100ml distilled water to get 0.5mol/L NaOH solution. Dissolve 5ml butyric acid in 100ml 0.5mol/L NaOH.

(7) 0.1mol/L Iodine solution Dissolve 12.5g I_2 and 25g KI in distilled water and dilute to 1L, demarcate the solution with 0.1mol/L $Na_2S_2O_3$.

(8) 0.02 mol/L $Na_2S_2O_3$ Dissolve 24.82g $Na_2S_2O_3 \cdot 5H_2O$ and 400mg anhydrous Na_2CO_3 in 1L fresh boiled water to get 0.1mol/L solution, demarcate the solution with 0.1mol/L KIO_3. Dilute the solution to 0.02mol/L just before using.

Procedures

1. Preparation of the specimen

Execute the rabbit, take out the liver and scour off the blood with 0.9% NaCl. Put the liver on filter paper to suck away the surface humidity, weigh 5g of the liver tissue, place it into the mortar, and add a little 0.9% NaCl to a total volume of 10ml. Make liver homogenate. Take 5g muscle of the rear leg, make muscle homogenate according to above-mentioned method and proportion.

2. Extraction of ketone body

Take three tubes, number and operate as the Table 15 – 1.

Table 15 – 1 Extraction of ketone body

Tube No.	A	B	C
The liver homogenate (ml)		2.0	2.0
The pre-boiled liver homogenate (ml)	2.0		
PBS buffer pH 7.6 (ml)	4.0	4.0	4.0

(to be continued)

Tube No.	A	B	C
Butyric acid（ml）	2.0	2.0	2.0
Keep at 43℃ water bath for 60min			
The muscle homogenate（ml）		4.0	
The pre-boiled muscle homogenate（ml）	4.0		4.0
Keep at 43℃ water bath for 60min			
15% Trichlorine acetic acid（ml）	3.0	3.0	3.0

Filter with the filter paper after shaking evenly, collect the filtrate respectively in 3 tubes, and then get the filtrate without protein.

3. Measurement of the ketone body

Take 3 Erlenmeyer flasks, operate as Table 15 – 2 in proper order.

Table 15 – 2　Measurement of the ketone body

Flask No.	1	2	3
Filtrate without protein（ml）	5.0	5.0	5.0
0.1mol/L I_2-KI（ml）	3.0	3.0	3.0
10% NaOH（ml）	3.0	3.0	3.0

Keep statically for 10min after shaking evenly, add 10% HCl 3ml to each tube, and add one drop of 1% starch solution to each tube, then titrate the color of orchid presenting in the solution with 0.02mol/L $Na_2S_2O_3$ until the color of bright green presents in the solution respectively.

Results and calculation

Ketone body produced in liver（mmol/g）＝（$C-A$）× content of $Na_2S_2O_3$ × 1/6

Ketone body consumed in muscle（mmol/g）＝（$C-B$）× content of $Na_2S_2O_3$ × 1/6

In this equation：

A—Volume of the $Na_2S_2O_3$（ml）consumed during titration of sample 1.

B—Volume of the $Na_2S_2O_3$（ml）consumed during titration of sample 2.

C—Volume of the $Na_2S_2O_3$（ml）consumed during titration of sample 3.

Questions

Why is Ketone body oxidized to generate energy only in extrahepatic tissues?

实验十六　转氨作用

【实验目的】

1. 掌握圆盘滤纸层析原理和技术。

2. 了解转氨作用过程。

【实验原理】

转氨基作用是由氨基转移酶（转氨酶）催化的，在这个反应中，α-氨基酸的氨基与 α-酮酸的酮基之间交换，α-氨基酸转变成相应的 α-酮酸，α-酮酸变成一种新的 α-氨基酸。转氨基作用是一种可逆反应，每个转氨基反应均由专一的氨基转移酶所催化，在不同的生物有机体中均有氨基转移酶分布。

本实验将丙氨酸和 α-酮戊二酸与肝匀浆一起水浴反应，肝中的丙氨酸氨基转移酶（ALT，又称谷丙转氨酶 GPT）含量丰富，该酶可将丙氨酸的氨基转移给 α-酮戊二酸，产生丙酮酸和谷氨酸。利用圆盘纸层析可鉴定谷氨酸的存在，并且验证组织中的转氨作用。

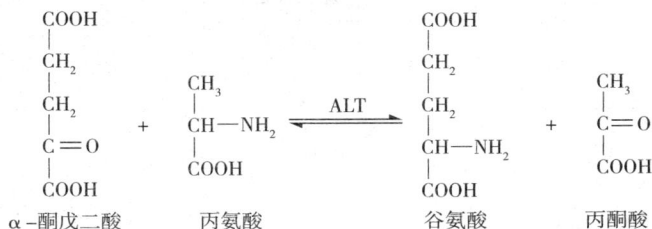

纸层析法（paper chromatography）是生物化学上分离、鉴定氨基酸的常用技术，可用于蛋白质的氨基酸成分的定性鉴定和定量测定。纸层析法是用滤纸作为惰性支持物的分配层析法，纸层析所用展层溶剂大多由有机溶剂和水组成。其中滤纸纤维素上吸附的水是固定相，展层用的有机溶剂是流动相。在层析时，将样品点在距滤纸一端，层析溶剂沿滤纸的一个方向进行展层，这样混合氨基酸在两相中不断分配，由于分配系数（K_d）不同，即不同的氨基酸在相同的溶剂中溶解度不同，氨基酸随流动相移动的速率就不同，结果它们分布在滤纸的不同位置上而形成距点样点距离不等的层析点。物质被分离后在纸层析图谱上的位置可用比移值（rate of flow，R_f）来表示。R_f 是指在纸层析中，从点样点至氨基酸层析点中心的距离与原点至溶剂前沿的距离的比值。R_f 值的大小与物质的结构、性质、溶剂系统、层析滤纸的质量和层析温度等因素有关。在一定条件下，某种物质的 R_f 值是常数。本实验采用纸层析法分离氨基酸。氨基酸是无色的，利用茚三酮反应，可将氨基酸层析点显色作定性、定量用。

【实验材料】

1. 实验器材　培养皿、表面皿、滤纸、匀浆器、试管、试管架、恒温水浴锅、毛细管、移液管、喷雾器、剪刀、铅笔、格尺。

2. 实验试剂

（1）0.01mol/L pH 7.4 磷酸缓冲液　0.2mol/L Na_2HPO_4 溶液 81ml，0.2mol/L NaH_2PO_4 溶液 19ml 混匀，蒸馏水稀释 20 倍。

（2）0.1mol/L 丙氨酸溶液　称取丙氨酸 0.891g 先溶于少量 0.01mol/L pH 7.4 磷酸缓冲液中，1mol/L NaOH 调节至 pH 7.4 后，用磷酸盐缓冲液加至 100ml。

（3）0.01mol/L α-酮戊二酸溶液　称取 α-酮戊二酸 1.461g，溶于少量 0.01mol/L pH 7.4 磷酸缓冲液，1mol/L NaOH 调节至 pH 7.4 后，用磷酸盐缓冲液加至 100ml。

（4）0.1mol/L 谷氨酸溶液　称取谷氨酸 0.735g，溶于少量 0.01mol/L pH 7.4 磷酸缓冲液，1mol/L NaOH 调节至 pH 7.4 后，用磷酸缓冲液加至 100ml。

（5）0.2% 茚三酮溶液　称取茚三酮 0.2g 溶于 100ml 95% 乙醇中。

（6）层析溶剂　水饱和的苯酚。

【实验步骤】

1. 肝匀浆的制备　取新鲜的猪肝 2.5g，加入 8ml 预冷 0.01mol/L pH 7.4 磷酸缓冲液，用捣碎机迅速成匀浆（1 万转大约 30s）。两人一组进行如下的实验。

2. 转氨反应　取大试管 2 支，分别标明测定管与对照管，按表 16-1 进行操作。

表 16-1　转氨反应体系

试　剂（ml）	对照管	测定管
肝匀浆	0.5	0.5
放入沸水中煮 5 分钟，冷却，摇匀		
0.1mol/L 丙氨酸溶液	0.5	0.5
0.01mol/L α－酮戊二酸溶液	0.5	0.5
0.01mol/L pH 7.4 磷酸缓冲液	1.5	1.5
摇匀，37℃水浴保温 50 分钟		
沸水浴 5 分钟，终止反应，取出冷却后摇匀		

取出冷却后，分别用滤纸过滤，滤液分别收集到新的干燥小试管中。

3. 纸层析

（1）取直径 12cm 圆形滤纸 1 张，通过圆心作两条半径 1cm 相互垂直的线，两个线的末端作点样点，分别标定"测定""对照""谷氨酸""丙氨酸"。

（2）取 4 支毛细管，分别吸取测定管溶液、0.1mol/L 谷氨酸溶液、对照管溶液、0.1mol/L 丙氨酸溶液。在点样处点样，注意斑点不可太大，直径要小于 0.3cm，而且每点 1 滴，吹干后方可再点第二滴，每个样品可点 2~3 次。

（3）在滤纸圆心处打一小孔（2~3mm 直径），另取同类滤纸条（1.5cm × 4.0cm），下一半剪成须状，卷成圆筒，如灯芯，从点样相反的一侧插入小孔。

（4）将层析溶剂（水饱和酚溶液）放入直径为 3~5cm 的干燥表面皿正中，表面皿置于直径 10cm 培养皿正中，将滤纸放平在培养皿上，灯芯浸入溶剂中，将另一同样大小培养皿反盖上，溶剂沿灯芯上升到滤纸，再向四周扩展，层析时间 45~60 分钟。溶剂前缘距滤纸边缘约 1cm 时即可取出，用铅笔画出溶剂的边缘，烘箱中干燥。

（5）显色　将滤纸放在培养皿上，喷 0.2% 的茚三酮乙醇溶液，烘箱中干燥，滤纸上会呈现紫色弧状条带。

【实验结果】

用铅笔画出条带的边框，测出表 16-2 中的数值，计算 R_f 值。

表 16 –2 R_f值测定

测定参数	测定样品	谷氨酸	丙氨酸	对照样品
点样点到斑纹中心距离（cm）				
点样点到溶剂前沿距离（cm）				
R_f值				

与已知的标准氨基酸 R_f进行对比，指出条带所对应的氨基酸，并根据结果解释转氨作用。

【注意事项】

1. 层析滤纸不可用手触摸，以免有手印。
2. 在滤纸上画线时只能用铅笔，不可用其他笔。
3. 烘烤时要注意明火。
4. 点样时毛细管不能交叉污染。

【思考题】

1. 如果对照管在沸水浴中煮的时间不够充分，会在层析结果中出现什么现象？
2. 氨基酸滤纸色谱鉴定法操作的关键是什么？

Experiment 16 Transamination

Purpose

1. To master the principles and the basic technological operation of circular paper chromatography.

2. To learn the process of transamination.

Principle

Transamination reactions are catalyzed by aminotransferases (transaminases). In this process the α-amino group is transferred from an α-amino acid to an α-keto acid, and the α-amino acid forms an α-keto acid. In the meantime, the α-keto acid converts to a new amino acid. Transamination reactions are reversible. Every transamination reaction is catalyzed by a specific transaminase. Transaminases are widespread in each organ of an organism.

In this experiment, liver homogenate is under water bath with L-alanine and pyruvate, while alanine aminotransferase (ALT, also called glutamate-pyruvate transaminase, GPT) which is abundant in livers, catalyzes the transfer of the amino group of alanine to α-ketoglutarate, thus yields pyruvate and glutamate. Circular paper chromatography can be used to evaluate the existence of glutamate and prove the transamination reaction in the tissue. The reaction equation is as follows.

$$
\begin{array}{c}
\text{COOH} \\
|\\
\text{CH}_2 \\
|\\
\text{CH}_2 \\
|\\
\text{C}=\text{O} \\
|\\
\text{COOH}
\end{array}
\;+\;
\begin{array}{c}
\text{CH}_3 \\
|\\
\text{CH}-\text{NH}_2 \\
|\\
\text{COOH}
\end{array}
\xrightleftharpoons{\text{ALT}}
\begin{array}{c}
\text{COOH} \\
|\\
\text{CH}_2 \\
|\\
\text{CH}_2 \\
|\\
\text{CH}-\text{NH}_2 \\
|\\
\text{COOH}
\end{array}
\;+\;
\begin{array}{c}
\text{CH}_3 \\
|\\
\text{C}=\text{O} \\
|\\
\text{COOH}
\end{array}
$$

α-ketoglutarate   L-Alanine   L-Glutamate   Pyruvate

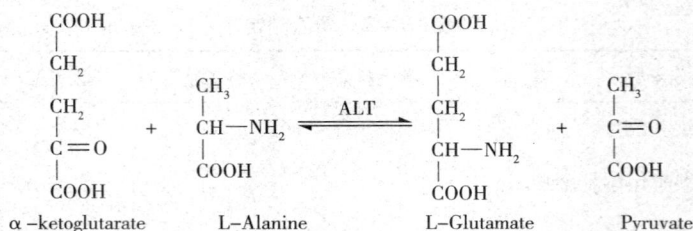

Paper chromatography is an analytical technique for separating and identifying amino acids in biochemistry and can be used to identify and quantify amino acids in protein. In paper chromatography, substances are distributed between a stationary phase and a mobile phase. The stationary phase is usually a piece of high quality filter paper. The mobile phase is a developing solution that travels up the stationary phase, carrying the samples with it. Components of the sample will separate readily according to how strongly they adsorb onto the stationary phase versus how readily they dissolve in the mobile phase. As the solvent slowly travels up the paper, the different components of the mixtures travel at different rates and the mixtures are separated according to the polarities of the molecules and the solvent. The different components of the mixtures can be identified according to the retention factor (R_f). R_f may be defined as the ratio of the distance traveled by the substance to the distance traveled by the solvent. To calculate the R_f value, take the distance traveled by the substance divided by the distance traveled by the solvent. R_f relates to factors such as the structure and property of substance, the solvent system, the temperature and so on. Under certain conditions, R_f value of substance is constant. In this experiment, paper chromatography is used to separate amino acids. Separated amino acids can be colorized and indentified or quantified by ninhydrin ethanol reaction.

Materials

1. Apparatus

Petri dish, watch-glass, a piece of chromatography filter paper, homogenizer, test tubes, test tube shelf, constant temperature water bath, glass capillaries, pipette, sprayer, scissors, pencil, ruler.

2. Reagents

(1) 0.01mol/L pH 7.4 Phosphoric acid buffer   Mix 81ml 0.2mol/l Na_2HPO_4 with 19ml 0.2mol/l NaH_2PO_4, and dilute 20 times with distilled water.

(2) 0.1mol/L Alanine solution   Weigh 0.891g alanine and dissolve it in 0.01mol/L pH 7.4 phosphoric acid buffer. Adjust pH to 7.4 with 1mol/L NaOH and set the volume at 100ml with 0.01mol/L phosphoric acid buffer.

(3) 0.01mol/L α-Ketoglutarate solution   Weigh 1.461g α-ketoglutarate, and dissolve it in 0.01 mol/L pH 7.4 phosphoric acid buffer. Adjust pH to 7.4 with 1mol/L NaOH and set the volume at 100ml with 0.01mol/L phosphoric acid buffer.

(4) 0.1mol/L Glutamate solution   Weigh 0.735g alanine and dissolve it in 0.01mol/L pH 7.4 phosphoric acid buffer. Adjust pH to 7.4 with 1mol/L NaOH and set the volume at

100ml with 0.01mol/L phosphoric acid buffer.

（5）0.2% Ninhydrin ethanol solvent Dissolve 0.2g ninhydrin into 100ml 95% ethanol.

（6）Chromatography solvent Phenol saturated by water.

Procedures

1. The preparation of liver homogenate

Obtain fresh animal liver 2.5g, add 0.01mol/L（pH 7.4）8ml phosphate buffer in icy bath, and then triturate them to be liver homogenate using homogenizer at about 10000r/min for 30s. Working in pairs.

2. Transamination reactions

Take 2 tubes, one is marked as measurement tube, the other is marked as control tube. Perform the experiment according to the Table 16 – 1.

Table 16 – 1 System of transamination reactions

Reagents（ml）	Control tube	Measurement tube
Liver homogenate	0.5	0.5
Bath in boiling water for 5min and cool, mix up		
0.1mol/L Alanine solution	0.5	0.5
0.01mol/L α-Ketoglutarate solution	0.5	0.5
0.01mol/L pH 7.4 Phosphate buffer	1.5	1.5
Mix up and bath at 37℃ for 50min		
Bath in boiling water for 5min and cool, mix up		

After cooling the tubes, filter with filter paper. Transfer filtrate to the new tubes.

3. Paper chromatography

（1）Take a sheet of filter paper 12cm in diameter. Draw two 1cm vertical lines passing its center. Use the terminal points of the two lines as spot application and mark "measurement", "control", "glutamate", "alanine" on the edge of the paper corresponding to each point.

（2）Use 4 capillary tubes, absorb one drop of measurement solution, 0.1mol/L glutamate solution, control solution, and 0.1mol/L alanine solution respectively. Dot the solution at the corresponding points of the lines. Pay attention to the diameter of the spot less than 0.3cm. While the spot is dried, dot the solution again, and each spot may be dotted 2～3 times.

（3）Stab a hole（2～3mm diameter）through the center of the filter paper. Get another filter paper strip（1.5cm×4.0cm）. Roll it into a cylinder, twist it tightly like a lampwick, and insert it into the hole from the reverse side of the dotting spot.

（4）Add chromatography solvent（phenol saturated by water）to a watch-glass 5cm in diameter placed in a Petri dish 10cm in diameter. Put filter paper flatly on the Petri dish in order to soak the lampwick in the chromatography solvent. Cover the Petri dish with another one of the same size. Solvent rises along the lampwick to the filter paper and diffuses in a circle（chromatography time is approximately 45 ~ 60min）. When the solvent diffuses to the position which is about 1cm away from the edge of the filer paper, remove it from the Petri dish. Draw the edge of the solvent with a pencil. Dry it on an electric stove.

（5）Development   Put filter paper flatly on the Petri dish. Spray 0.2% ninhydrin ethanol solvent. Dry it on the electric stove, and purple-arced stripes appear on the filter paper.

Results

Draw the outline of the stripes with a pencil. Record relevant data according to the Table 16 – 2. Calculate the R_f values.

Table 16 – 2   The measurement of R_f values

Parameters	Measurement	Glutamate	Alanine	Control
The distance from the spotting point to the center of the patches（cm）				
The distance from the spotting point to the edge of the solvent（cm）				
R_f				

Contrast the R_f values of the strips of "measurement" and "control" with the R_f values of the known amino acids, and infer what amino acids they are. Explain transamination reactions according to these results.

Cautions

1. Do not touch the chromatography filter paper, or else the fingerprints would be left.

2. Use pencils to draw lines on the filter paper but not other pens.

3. Be cautious of fire when roasting.

4. Prevent cross pollution of capillary tubes when dotting solution.

Questions

1. What is the result if the control tube has not been fully boiled in boiling water?

2. What are the key points of operation of paper chromatography for amino acid identification?

第二部分　药学生物化学与分子生物学实验

实验十七　酶的活力测定和性质研究

【实验目的】

1. 加深对酶的性质的认识。
2. 掌握影响酶活力的各种因素及其作用原理。
3. 掌握测定碱性蛋白酶活力的原理和酶活力的计算方法。
4. 学习测定酶促反应速度的方法和基本操作。

一、碱性蛋白酶活力测定

【实验原理】

酶活力是指酶催化化学反应的能力。酶活力越大，酶促反应速度越快；酶活力越小，酶促反应速度越慢。因此，酶活力的大小可以用在一定条件下它所催化的某一化学反应的速度来表示。测定酶活力实际就是测定酶促反应的速度。

酶促反应的速度可以用单位时间内反应底物的减少量或产物的增加量来表示，为了灵敏起见，通常测定单位时间内产物的生成量。在反应初期，酶促反应速度与酶活力成正比，但随着时间的推移，由于底物浓度降低，产物的增加对酶活力产生抑制等原因，酶促反应速度会逐渐降低。为了正确测定酶活力，就必须测定酶促反应的初速度。

碱性蛋白酶在碱性条件下可以催化酪蛋白水解生成酪氨酸。酪氨酸为含有酚羟基的氨基酸，可与福林试剂发生反应。福林试剂是磷钨酸与磷钼酸的混合物，碱性条件下极其不稳定，容易定量地被酪氨酸还原，生成钨蓝和钼蓝而呈现出不同深浅的蓝色。由于蓝色的深浅与酪氨酸的量成正比，所以可以利用比色法测定出酪氨酸的生成量。碱性蛋白酶的活力就可以用单位时间内酪氨酸的生成量来表示。

【实验材料】

1. **实验器材**　电热恒温水浴槽、分析天平、容量瓶、移液管、漏斗、721 分光光度计。

2. **实验试剂**

（1）福林试剂　在 1L 磨口回流瓶中加入 50g 钨酸钠（$Na_2WO_4 \cdot 2H_2O$）、125g 钼酸钠（$Na_2MoO_4 \cdot 2H_2O$）、350ml 蒸馏水、25ml 85% 磷酸及 50ml 浓盐酸，充分混匀后回流 10 小时。回流完毕，再加 25g 硫酸锂、25ml 蒸馏水及数滴液体溴，开口继续沸腾 15 分钟，以便驱除过量的溴，冷却后定容到 500ml，过滤，置于棕色瓶中暗处保存。使用前加 4 倍蒸馏水稀释。

（2）1% 酪蛋白溶液　称取酪蛋白 1g 于研钵中，先用少量蒸馏水湿润后，慢慢加入 0.2mol/L NaOH 4ml，充分研磨，转移至 100ml 容量瓶中，放入水浴中煮沸 15 分钟，冷却，定容至 100ml，保存于冰箱内。

（3）pH 10 硼砂 - 氢氧化钠缓冲液

甲液（0.05mol/L 硼砂溶液）：取硼砂（$Na_2B_4O_7 \cdot 10H_2O$）19g，用蒸馏水溶解并定容至 1000ml。

乙液：0.2moL/L 氢氧化钠溶液。

pH 10 硼砂 - 氢氧化钠溶液：移取甲液 50ml，加入乙液 21ml，用蒸馏水定容至 200ml。

（4）标准酪氨酸溶液　精确称取酪氨酸 50mg，加入 1ml 1mol/L 盐酸溶解后用蒸馏水定容至 50ml，即得 1mg/ml 酪氨酸标准溶液。

（5）1/2000 碱性蛋白酶溶液　精确称取干酶粉 2g，加入 pH 10 硼砂 - 氢氧化钠缓冲溶液 10ml，溶解，并用玻璃棒搅拌，静置片刻后，将上清液小心倾入容量瓶中，残渣部分再加入少量缓冲溶液，如此反复搅拌溶解 4 次，最后全部移入 200ml 容量瓶中。用缓冲溶液定容至 200ml，充分摇匀，用 2 层纱布或 4 层纱布过滤，吸取滤液 5ml，放入 100ml 容量瓶中，用蒸馏水稀释至 100ml。

（6）0.4mol/L 碳酸钠溶液　称取 42.4g 无水碳酸钠溶解于 1L 蒸馏水中。

（7）0.4mol/L 三氯醋酸溶液　称取 65.4g 三氯醋酸固体溶解于 1L 蒸馏水中。

【实验步骤】

1. 制作酪氨酸标准曲线

（1）取 7 支干燥试管，编号，按表 17 - 1 配制酪氨酸溶液。

表 17 - 1　配制酪氨酸标准溶液

管号	酪氨酸含量（μg）	1mg/ml 酪氨酸标准溶液（ml）	蒸馏水（ml）
0	0	0.0	2.0
1	100	0.1	1.9
2	200	0.2	1.8
3	300	0.3	1.7
4	400	0.4	1.6
5	500	0.5	1.5
6	600	0.6	1.4

（2）在上述试管中，分别加入 1% 酪蛋白溶液 1.0ml，于 40℃ 水浴中保温 15 分钟，取出后，加入 0.4mol/L 三氯醋酸 3.0ml，摇匀，各管分别用滤纸过滤。

（3）分别吸取滤液 1.0ml 放入另 7 支干燥试管中，加入 0.4mol/L 碳酸钠溶液 5.0ml，福林试剂 1.0ml，摇匀，于 40℃ 水浴中保温 15 分钟，然后于每管中各加入 3.0ml 蒸馏水，摇匀。

（4）用 721 型分光光度计，以 0 号管作对照，在 680nm 处测定光密度值。

（5）以酪氨酸含量（微克）为横坐标，光密度值为纵坐标，绘制标准曲线。

2. 样品测定 取 3 支干燥试管，编号，按照表 17 - 2 中顺序加入试剂。

表 17 - 2 样品测定操作及试剂

试 剂	管 号		
	0	1	2
pH 10 硼砂 - 氢氧化钠缓冲液（ml）	1.0	1.0	1.0
1/2000 碱性蛋白酶溶液（ml）	1.0	1.0	1.0
0.4mol/L 三氯醋酸溶液（ml）	3.0	0.0	0.0
1% 酪蛋白溶液（ml）	1.0	1.0	1.0
40℃ 水浴（min）	15.0	15.0	15.0
0.4mol/L 三氯醋酸溶液（ml）	0.0	3.0	3.0

摇匀后，各管分别过滤，各吸取滤液 1.0ml，放入另 3 支干燥试管中，加入 0.4mol/L 碳酸钠溶液 5.0ml，福林试剂 1.0ml，摇匀，于 40℃ 水浴保温 15 分钟，然后于每管中各加入 3.0ml 蒸馏水，摇匀。用 721 型分光光度计在波长 680nm 处，以 0 号管为对照，测定 1、2 号管的光密度值。

【实验结果】

1. 碱性蛋白酶活力单位的定义 碱性蛋白酶在 pH 10、40℃ 的最适条件下水解酪蛋白，每分钟产生 $1\mu g$ 酪氨酸定义为 1 个酶活力单位（U）。

2. 碱性蛋白酶活力计算

$$碱性蛋白酶活力 = (m/t) \times f$$

式中，m——将光密度值代入标准曲线而求得的酪氨酸量（μg）；

t——酶促反应时间（min）；

f——酶的稀释倍数，本实验中 $f = 2000$。

二、酶的特异性

【实验原理】

酶的特异性指的是酶对它所催化的反应以及底物或产物结构有严格的选择性。一种酶只能作用于一种或一类化合物或一定的化学键，促进一定的化学变化，生成一定的产物。

绝大部分酶是蛋白质，结构复杂，在其精细的空间构象中存在一个特殊的活性部位，能专一地与对应的底物结合，从而体现酶的特异性。

本实验以碱性蛋白酶和淀粉酶对相应底物酪蛋白及淀粉的水解作用为例，验证酶的特异性。酪蛋白被酶水解后生成酪氨酸，酪氨酸与福林试剂显现蓝色；若不能被酶水解则无法显现蓝色。淀粉若不能被酶水解则遇碘显现蓝色，若被酶水解则不能显现蓝色。利用颜色反应判断酶是否起到催化作用，以验证酶的特异性。

【实验材料】

1. 实验器材 试管、试管架、移液管、烧杯、恒温水浴锅。

2. 实验试剂

（1）1% 淀粉溶液 将 1g 淀粉溶解于 100ml 蒸馏水中。

（2）1% 酪蛋白溶液 参照"碱性蛋白酶活力测定"。

（3）1/2000 碱性蛋白酶溶液 参照"碱性蛋白酶活力测定"。

（4）pH 10 硼砂 – 氢氧化钠缓冲液 参照"碱性蛋白酶活力测定"。

（5）0.4 mol/L 碳酸钠溶液 参照"碱性蛋白酶活力测定"。

（6）0.4mol/L 三氯醋酸溶液 参照"碱性蛋白酶活力测定"。

（7）福林试剂 参照"碱性蛋白酶活力测定"。

（8）1/2000 淀粉酶溶液 用蒸馏水作稀释溶剂，配制方法同碱性蛋白酶液相同。

（9）碘 – 碘化钾溶液 10g 碘和 20g 碘化钾同时溶解于 100ml 蒸馏水中，贮于棕色瓶内。使用前稀释 10 倍。

【实验步骤】

1. 取 5 支试管，编号，按表 17 – 3 加入试剂。

表 17 – 3 酶的特异性

试 剂	管 号				
	0	1	2	3	4
1% 酪蛋白溶液（ml）	1.0	1.0	1.0		
pH 10 硼砂 – 氢氧化钠缓冲液（ml）		1.0			
蒸馏水（ml）	2.0		1.0	1.0	1.0
1% 淀粉溶液（ml）				1.0	1.0
1/2000 碱性蛋白酶溶液（ml）		1.0			1.0
1/2000 淀粉酶溶液（ml）			1.0	1.0	

2. 摇匀，各管置于 40℃ 水浴中保温 15 分钟。

3. 3、4 号管分别加入碘液 2 滴，观察现象。

4. 向 0、1、2 号管分别加入 3.0ml 0.4mol/L 三氯醋酸溶液，摇匀，过滤，各吸取滤液 1.0ml，加入 0.4mol/L 碳酸钠溶液 5.0ml，福林试剂 1.0ml，摇匀，置于 40℃ 水浴保温 15 分钟。观察现象。

三、激动剂和抑制剂对酶活力的影响

【实验原理】

许多物质对酶活力可以产生影响。能够提高酶活力，加速酶促反应进行的物质称为酶的激动剂。能够抑制酶活力，降低酶促反应速度的物质称为抑制剂。本实验分别考查 $MnCl_2$ 和 $HgCl_2$ 对碱性蛋白酶的激动和抑制作用。

【实验材料】

1. 实验器材 试管、漏斗、恒温水浴锅、温度计、移液管、721 分光光度计。

2．实验试剂

（1）1% 酪蛋白溶液　参照"碱性蛋白酶活力测定"。

（2）1/2000 碱性蛋白酶溶液　参照"碱性蛋白酶活力测定"。

（3）pH 10 硼砂 – 氢氧化钠缓冲液　参照"碱性蛋白酶活力测定"。

（4）8×10^{-3} mol/L $MnCl_2$ 溶液　称取 1g $MnCl_2$ 溶解于 1L 蒸馏水中。

（5）8×10^{-3} mol/L $HgCl_2$ 溶液　称取 2.17g $HgCl_2$ 溶解于 1L 蒸馏水中。

（6）0.4mol/L 碳酸钠溶液　参照"碱性蛋白酶活力测定"。

（7）0.4mol/L 三氯醋酸溶液　参照"碱性蛋白酶活力测定"。

（8）福林试剂　参照"碱性蛋白酶活力测定"。

【实验步骤】

取 3 支试管，按照表 17 – 4 加入试剂。

表 17 – 4　激动剂和抑制剂对酶活力的影响

试　剂	管　号		
	1	2	3
1% 酪蛋白溶液（ml）	1.0	1.0	1.0
pH 10 硼砂 – 氢氧化钠缓冲溶液（ml）	1.0	1.0	1.0
8×10^{-3} mol/L $MnCl_2$ 溶液（ml）			1.0
8×10^{-3} mol/L $HgCl_2$ 溶液（ml）		1.0	
蒸馏水（ml）	1.0		
1/2000 碱性蛋白酶溶液（ml）	1.0	1.0	1.0

混合均匀，于 40℃水浴中保温 15 分钟。各加入 0.4mol/L 三氯醋酸溶液 3.0ml，过滤，各吸取滤液 1.0ml，加入 0.4mol/L 碳酸钠溶液 5.0ml，福林试剂 1.0ml，摇匀，于 40℃水浴保温 15 分钟。显色后，观察实验现象，根据结果判定碱性蛋白酶的激动剂和抑制剂。

四、温度对酶活力的影响

【实验原理】

温度对酶活力有显著影响。一方面，在低温时，提高温度可以增强酶活力，使酶促反应速度加快。通常温度每升高 10℃，反应速度加快 1 倍左右，直至反应速度达到最大值。另一方面，大多数酶是蛋白质，温度过高可引起蛋白质变性，导致酶活力丧失。因此，反应速度达到最大值以后，如果温度继续升高，反应速度反而逐渐下降，以致完全停止反应。因此，酶促反应速度达到最大值时的温度称为酶的最适温度。高于或低于最适温度时，反应速度都降低。

本实验以唾液淀粉酶对淀粉的水解作用为例，观察温度对酶活力的影响。在不同温度下具有不同酶活力的唾液淀粉酶在相同时间内催化淀粉水解生成的产物不同。淀粉初步水解的产物分子量较大，遇碘显现蓝色，称为淀粉糊精；淀粉糊精继续水解得到分子较小的糊精，遇碘显现红色，称为红糊精；红糊精再水解变成分子更小的糊精，遇碘不显色，叫作无色糊精，无色糊精可进一步水解成麦芽糖和葡萄糖，遇碘不显色利用这些颜色反应来判定唾液淀粉酶在不同温度下酶活力的大小。

【实验材料】

1. **实验器材**　参照"酶的特异性"。

2. **实验试剂**

（1）1%淀粉溶液　将1g淀粉溶解于100ml蒸馏水中。

（2）碘-碘化钾溶液　10g碘和20g碘化钾同时溶解于100ml蒸馏水中，贮于棕色瓶内。使用前稀释10倍。

（3）稀释的唾液。

【实验步骤】

1. 收集唾液1ml，用蒸馏水稀释5~10倍（根据个人的酶活性而定），混匀后备用。

2. 取试管2支，各加稀释唾液2.0ml，一支试管直接加热煮沸，另一支试管置于冰浴中预冷5分钟。

3. 另取4支试管，编好序号，按表17-5进行操作。

表 17-5　温度对酶活力的影响

步　骤	管　号			
	1	2	3	4
第一步	加入1%淀粉溶液20滴			
第二步	冰浴5分钟		37℃水浴5分钟	
第三步	加预冷的唾液10滴		加常温唾液10滴	加煮沸唾液10滴
第四步	摇匀，冰浴10分钟	摇匀，冰浴5分钟，移至37℃水浴5分钟	摇匀，37℃水浴10分钟	
第五步	加碘液3滴			

4. 观察各管的实验现象，分析原因。

五、pH对酶活力的影响

【实验原理】

酶活力受环境pH的影响极为显著。通常只在一定pH范围内酶才能表现出活力。当酶活力达到最高时的pH称为该酶的最适pH。高于或低于最适pH时，酶活力都降低。

pH影响酶活力的主要原因有两个方面：首先，pH影响酶活性中心上一些基团的解离情况，也影响底物的解离状态，从而影响酶活性中心与底物的结合或催化作用。其次，由于pH改变了酶分子上一些基团的解离状态，酶的空间构象也会随之发生改变，酶活力也会相应地变大或变小，甚至使酶变性，完全丧失活性。

【实验材料】

1. **实验器材** 试管，漏斗，恒温水浴锅，温度计，移液管。

2. **实验试剂**

（1）1% 酪蛋白溶液 参照"碱性蛋白酶活力测定"。

（2）1/2000 碱性蛋白酶溶液 参照"碱性蛋白酶活力测定"。

（3）pH 10 硼砂 - 氢氧化钠缓冲液 参照"碱性蛋白酶活力测定"。

（4）0.1mol/L 盐酸溶液 参照"碱性蛋白酶活力测定"。

（5）0.2mol/L 氢氧化钠溶液 称取 8g 氢氧化钠溶解于 1L 蒸馏水中。

（6）0.4mol/L 碳酸钠溶液 参照"碱性蛋白酶活力测定"。

（7）0.4mol/L 三氯醋酸溶液 参照"碱性蛋白酶活力测定"。

（8）福林试剂 参照"碱性蛋白酶活力测定"。

【实验步骤】

取 3 支试管，按表 17 - 6 加入试剂。

表 17 - 6 pH 对酶活力的影响

试　剂	管　号		
	1	2	3
1% 酪蛋白溶液（ml）	1.0	1.0	1.0
pH 10 硼砂 - 氢氧化钠缓冲液（ml）	1.0		
0.1mol/L 盐酸溶液（ml）		1.0	
0.2mol/L NaOH 溶液（ml）			1.0
1/2000 碱性蛋白酶溶液（ml）	1.0	1.0	1.0

混合均匀后，于 40℃ 水浴中保温 15 分钟，各加入 0.4mol/L 三氯醋酸溶液 3.0ml，分别过滤，各吸取滤液 1.0ml，加入 0.4mol/L 碳酸钠溶液 5.0ml、福林试剂 1.0ml，摇匀，于 40℃ 水浴保温 15 分钟。观察现象，分析在不同 pH 情况下碱性蛋白酶活力的大小。

【注意事项】

1. 每个人的唾液淀粉酶活性并不相同，有时差别很大，因此稀释倍数可因个人情况而定。

2. 少量的激动剂或抑制剂就能影响酶的活性，但激动剂和抑制剂不是绝对的，有些物质在低浓度时为某种酶的激动剂，而在高浓度时则为该酶的抑制剂。甚至有些物质对一种酶是激动剂，对另一种酶则是抑制剂。

3. 酶促反应时间要准确，实验所用器皿必须干净、干燥，定量准确。

【思考题】

1. 什么是酶的最适温度、最适 pH？有何实际意义？

2. 影响酶活力的因素有哪些？简要说明作用原理。

3. 酶的性质研究实验必须注意控制哪些条件？为什么？

4. 什么是酶活力? 酶活力是怎样计算的?

5. 酶活力测定过程中应注意哪些问题?

Experiment 17　Measurement of Enzyme Activity and Properties

Purpose

1. To enhance the comprehension about enzyme properties.

2. To master the factors affecting enzyme properties and the principles.

3. To master the principle of alkaline protease activity measurement and the calculation method of enzyme activity.

4. To learn the method and the basic operations of enzymatic reaction rate measurement.

Ⅰ. Measurement of alkaline protease activity

Principle

Enzyme activity is the capability of catalyzing chemical reaction. The greater the enzyme activity is, the faster the enzymatic reaction rate is. On the contrary, the lower the enzyme activity is, the slower the enzymatic reaction rate is. So enzyme activity may be represented by the rate of enzymatic reaction under certain conditions. Measurement of enzyme activity is to measure the rate of enzymatic reaction.

The rate of enzymatic reaction may be represented by the decrease of substrates or the increase of products in unit time. Usually, the output of products in unit time is measured for sensitivity. During the initial stage of enzymatic reaction, the rate is in direct proportion to the enzyme activity. But as time goes on, the concentration of substrates decreases and the concentration of product increases which can inhibit the enzyme activity, so the enzymatic reaction rate will decrease. In order to measure enzyme activity correctly, it is necessary to measure the initial rate of enzymatic reaction.

Alkaline protease can hydrolyze casein to tyrosine under alkaline conditions. Tyrosine has phenolic hydroxyl group, which reacts with Folin reagent. Folin reagent is a mixture of phosphotungstic acid and phosphomolybdic acid. It is unstable in alkaline conditions and can be easily reduced by tyrosine in a qualitative way and generate tungsten blue and molybdenum blue. The depth of blue color is in direct proportion to the quantity of tyrosine. Therefore, the tyrosine quantity can be measured with colorimetric method. Alkaline protease activity is represented by tyrosine production in unit time.

Materials

1. Apparatus

Thermostatic water bath, analytical balance, volumetric flask, pipettes, glass funnels, 721 type spectrophotometer.

2. Reagents

(1) Folin reagent　Add 50g $Na_2WO_4 \cdot 2H_2O$, 125g $Na_2MoO_4 \cdot 2H_2O$, 350ml distilled

water, 25ml 85% H_3PO_4 and 50ml concentrated HCl into a 1L round-bottom stoppered flask, mix well and reflux for 10h. After refluxing, add 25g Li_2SO_4, 25ml distilled water, several drops of liquid Br_2, boil for 15min without cap to get rid of excessive Br_2. After cooling, dilute to 500ml and filtrate. Keep the filtrate in brown flask in darkroom. Add 4 times distilled water before using.

(2) 1% Casein solution Take 1g casein in a mortar, make it humid with a little distilled water, add 4ml 0.2mol/L NaOH slowly and grind. Wash it out into a volumetric flask, and keep in boiling water bath for 15min. Cool and dilute to 100ml with distilled water, store in a refrigerator.

(3) pH 10 Borax-NaOH buffer solution

Solution A (0.05mol/L borax solution): Dissolve 19g borax ($Na_2B_4O_7 \cdot 10H_2O$) into distilled water and dilute to 1000ml.

Solution B: 0.2mol/L sodium hydroxide solution.

Borax-NaOH solution pH 10: Mix 50ml solution A with 21ml Solution B, and dilute to 200ml with distilled water.

(4) Standard tyrosine solution Weigh 50mg tyrosine precisely and add 1ml 1mol/L hydrochloric acid. When it is dissolved, dilute to 50ml with distilled water.

(5) 1/2000 Alkaline protease solution Dissolve 2g enzyme powder in 10ml pH 10 buffer solution and stir with a glass rod. Keep for a moment, and pour the upper layer of solution into the volumetric flask carefully. Add a little buffer solution to the residue. Repeat the steps four times. Transfer all solution into a 200ml volumetric flask at last. Dilute it with buffer solution to 200ml. Filter it with 2-layer or 4-layer gauze. Transfer 5ml filtrate solution into 100ml volumetric flask. Dilute it with distilled water to 100ml.

(6) 0.4mol/L Sodium carbonate solution Dissolve 42.4g anhydrous sodium carbonate into 1L distilled water.

(7) 0.4mol/L Trichloroacetic acid solution Dissolve 65.4g trichloroacetic acid solid into 1L distilled water.

Procedures

1. Draw the standard curve of tyrosine

(1) Take 7 dry tubes, number them, and prepare tyrosine solution as Table 17-1.

Table 17-1 Preparation of standard tyrosine solution

Tube No.	Content of tyrosine (μg)	1mg/ml Standard tyrosine solution (ml)	Distilled water (ml)
0	0	0.0	2.0
1	100	0.1	1.9
2	200	0.2	1.8
3	300	0.3	1.7
4	400	0.4	1.6
5	500	0.5	1.5
6	600	0.6	1.4

(2) Add 1.0ml 1% casein solution into each tube. Keep them in 40℃ water bath for 15

min. Add 3. 0ml 0. 4mol/L trichloroacetic acid, mix up and filter.

(3) Take 1. 0ml filtrate from each tube into another 7 dry tubes. Add 5. 0ml 0. 4mol/L so-dium carbonate solution, 1. 0ml Folin reagent, and mix up. Keep them in 40℃ water bath for 15 min. Then add 3. 0ml distilled water in each tube and mix up.

(4) Adjust 721 type spectrophotometer with tube No. 0. Determine the optical density of each tube at 680nm and note them down.

(5) Draw the standard curve by taking the tyrosine content (μg) as abscissa and optical density as vertical ordinate.

2. Sample measurement

Take 3 dry tubes. Number them. Add reagents and operate as Table 17 – 2.

Table 17 – 2   Sample measurement

Reagents	Tube No.		
	0	1	2
Borax-NaOH buffer solution pH 10 (ml)	1. 0	1. 0	1. 0
1/2000 Alkaline protease solution (ml)	1. 0	1. 0	1. 0
0. 4mol/L Trichloroacetic acid solution (ml)	3. 0	0. 0	0. 0
1% Casein solution (ml)	1. 0	1. 0	1. 0
40℃ Water bath (min)	15. 0	15. 0	15. 0
0. 4mol/L Trichloroacetic acid solution (ml)	0. 0	3. 0	3. 0

Mix up and filtrate. Tabe 1. 0ml filtrate from each tube into another 3 dry tubes. Add 5. 0ml 0. 4mol/L sodium carbonate solution and 1. 0ml Folin reagent. Mix up and keep them in 40℃ water bath for 15 min. Add 3. 0ml distilled water into each tube and mix up. Adjust 721 type spectrophotometer with control tube No. 0. Measure the optical density of each tube at 680nm and note them down.

Results

1. The definition of alkaline protease activity in this experiment

Alkaline protease hydrolyzes casein to produce 1μg tyrosine in one minute under the conditions of pH 10, 40℃, which is defined to be 1 enzyme activity unit.

2. Calculation of alkaline protease activity

Alkaline protease Activity units = $(m/t) \times f$

In this equation:

m—The amount of tyrosine (μg) which is calculated by the standard curve according to the optical density.

t—Time for enzymatic reaction (min).

f—The dilution multiple of enzyme. In this experiment, $f = 2000$.

Ⅱ. Enzyme specificity

Principle

Enzymes are highly specific both in the reactions that they catalyze and in the selection of substrates' and products' structure. An enzyme acts on a kind of compound or a definite chemical bond only and catalyzes a specific chemical reaction to form definite products.

Most enzymes are protein. They have intricate three-dimensional structures. Catalysis takes place at a particular site on the enzyme called the active site . The specificity of an enzyme is due to the precise interaction of the substrate with the active site of the enzyme.

In this experiment, enzyme specificities will be verified by the effects of alkaline protease and amylase hydrolyzing different substrates including the casein and starch. Tyrosine, the hydrolysis product of casein, shows the color of blue when interacting with Folin reagent. If casein can't be hydrolyzed, there is no blue color. Starch shows blue when interacting with iodine. While starch is hydrolyzed by corresponding enzyme, there is no blue. Color reactions can be used to determine whether there is enzymatic reaction or not and then identify the enzyme specificity.

Materials

1. Apparatus

Test tubes, pipette, beaker, thermostatic water bath.

2. Reagents

(1) 1% Starch solution　Dissolve1g starch in 100ml distilled water.

(2) 1% Casein solution　See "Measurement of alkaline protease activity"

(3) 1/2000 Alkaline protease solution　See "Measurement of alkaline protease activity"

(4) pH 10 Borax-NaOH buffer solution　See "Measurement of alkaline protease activity"

(5) 0.4mol/L Na_2CO_3 solution　See "Measurement of alkaline protease activity"

(6) 0.4mol/L Trichloroacetic acid solution　See "Measurement of alkaline protease activity"

(7) Folin reagent　See "Measurement of alkaline protease activity"

(8) 1/2000 Amylase solution　The same method as 1/2000 alkaline protease solution except for replacing pH 10 buffer solution with distilled water.

(9) Iodine-potassium iodide solution　Dissolve 10g iodine and 20g potassium iodide in 100ml distilled water, and keep it in brown flask. Add 10 times diluted water before using.

Procedures

Take 5 test tubes, number them, and add reagents as Table 17 – 3.

Table 17 –3　Enzyme specificity

Reagents	Tube No.				
	0	1	2	3	4
1% Casein solution (ml)	1.0	1.0	1.0		
Borax-NaOH buffer solution pH 10 (ml)		1.0			
Distilled water (ml)	2.0		1.0	1.0	1.0
1% Starch solution (ml)				1.0	1.0
1/2000 Alkaline protease solution (ml)		1.0			1.0
1/2000 Amylase solution (ml)			1.0	1.0	

2. Mix up and keep them in 40℃ water bath for 15min.

3. Add two drops of iodide solution to No. 3 and No. 4 tubes and observe the phenomena.

4. Add 3. 0ml 0. 4mol/L trichloroacetic acid solution to No. 0 tube, No. 1 tube and No. 2 tube, then filtrate and collect 1. 0ml filtrate respectively. Add 5. 0ml 0. 4mol/L Na_2CO_3 solution and 1. 0ml Folin reagent. Keep them in 40℃ water bath for 15min. Observe the phenomena.

Ⅲ. Effects of Agonist and inhibitor on enzyme activity

Principle

Many substances can affect enzyme activity. Activator increases enzyme activity and accelerates the enzymatic reaction. On the contrary, inhibitor decreases enzyme activity and inhibits the enzymatic reaction. In this experiment, the inhibition of $MnCl_2$ and the activation of $HgCl_2$ to alkaline protease are identified.

Materials

1. Apparatus

Test tubes, funnel, thermostatic water bath, thermometer, pipette, 721 type spectrophotometer.

2. Reagents

(1) 1% Casein solution   See "Measurement of alkaline protease activity"

(2) 1/2000 Alkaline protease solution   See "Measurement of alkaline protease activity"

(3) pH 10 Borax-NaOH buffer solution   See "Measurement of alkaline protease activity"

(4) 8×10^{-3} mol/L $MnCl_2$ solution   Dissolve 1g $MnCl_2$ into 1L distilled water.

(5) 8×10^{-3} mol/L $HgCl_2$ solution   Dissolve 2. 17g $HgCl_2$ into 1L distilled water.

(6) 0. 4mol/L Na_2CO_3 solution   See "Measurement of alkaline protease activity"

(7) 0. 4mol/L Trichloroacetic acid solution   See "Measurement of alkaline protease activity"

(8) Folin reagent   See "Measurement of alkaline protease activity"

Procedures

Take 3 test tubes and add reagents as Table 17 - 4.

Table 17 - 4   Effects of agonist and inhibitor on enzyme activity

Reagents	Tubes No.		
	1	2	3
1% Casein solution (ml)	1. 0	1. 0	1. 0
Borax-NaOH buffer solution pH 10 (ml)	1. 0	1. 0	1. 0
8×10^{-3} mol/L $MnCl_2$ solution (ml)			1. 0
8×10^{-3} mol/L $HgCl_2$ solution (ml)		1. 0	
Distilled water (ml)	1. 0		
1/2000 Alkaline protease solution (ml)	1. 0	1. 0	1. 0

Mix up and put them in 40℃ water bath for 15min. Add 3. 0ml 0. 4mol/L trichloroacetic acid solution to each tube, then filtrate and collect 1.0ml filtrate respectively. Add 5.0ml 0.4mol/L Na_2CO_3 solution and 1.0ml Folin reagent. Mix up and put them in 40℃ water bath for 15min. Observe the phenomena. Determinethe activator and inhibi to according to based on the results.

Ⅳ. Effects of temperature on enzyme activity

Principle

Temperature affects enzyme activity remarkably. At low temperature, both enzyme activity and the rate of enzymatic reaction increase with increasing temperature. Generally most enzymatic reaction rates double for every 10°C increase in temperature till the rate reaches maximum. On the other hand, most enzymes are proteins. They will denature at high temperature and lose activity. So, when the rate of enzymatic reaction reaches a maximum, if the temperature continues to rise, reaction rate gradually decreases instead, or even stop. Each enzyme has an optimum temperature, at which enzymatic reaction reaches the maximum value. If the temperature is over or under the optimum temperature, the enzyme activity and the rate of enzymatic reaction will reduce.

In this experiment, the effects of temperature on enzyme activity will be verified by the effects of salivary amylase hydrolyzing starch. Salivary amylases with different activities hydrolyze starch to generate different products at the same time. The product, preliminary hydrolysate of starch, is amylodextrin which interacts with iodine to show blue. Amylodextrin is hydrolyzed to erythrodextrin which interacts with iodine to show red. When the erythrodextrin becomes achrodextrin, there is no color. Finally, achrodextrin is hydrolyzed to maltose and glucose. So, the colour reaction can be used to determine the activity of salivary amylase at different temperatures.

Materials

1. Apparatus

Test tubes, glass funnel, flask, thermostatic water bath, thermometer.

2. Reagents

(1) 1% Starch solution　See "Enzyme specificity"

(2) Iodine-potassium iodide solution　Dissolve 10g iodine and 20g potassium iodide in 100ml distilled water, and keep it in brown flask. Add 10 times distilled water before using.

(3) Diluted saliva.

Procedures

1. Collect saliva, dilute them to 5 ~ 10 times and mix up.

2. Take 2 test tubes, add 2.0ml diluted saliva in each of them. One is heated in boiling water for 5min and the other is placed in icy bath for 5min.

3. Take 4 test tubes, number them and operate as Table 17 - 5.

Table 17 −5　Effects of temperature on enzyme activity

Procedures	Tube No.			
	1	2	3	4
Step 1	Add 20 drops of 1% starch solution			
Step 2	Icy bath for 5min		37℃ water bath for 5min	
Step 3	Add 10 drops of precooled saliva		Add 10 drops of saliva	Add 10 drops of boiled saliva
Step 4	Mix up, icy bath for 10min	Icy bath for 5min, then transfer to 37℃ water bath for 5min	Mix up, 37℃ water bath for 10min	
Step 5	Add 3 drops of iodide solution			

4. Observe the phenomena and analyze the causes.

Ⅴ. Effects of pH on enzyme activity

Principle

Enzyme activity is remarkably affected by pH. Enzyme has activity only in a narrow range of pH. Enzyme has an optimum pH at which its activity is maximal. At higher or lower pH, its activity decreases.

The pH affects enzyme activity in two ways. First, changes in pH affect the dissociation of certain groups in active site of enzyme and substrates. So, it can affect the interaction of active site of enzyme and substrates. Catalytic activity of enzyme is also affected. Secondly, changes in ionizable groups may change the spatial conformation of the enzyme. Enzyme activity increases or decreases in different pH. Enzyme may denature and lose activity completely in drastic changes of pH.

Materials

1. Apparatus

Test tubes, funnel, thermostatic water bath, thermometer, pipettes.

2. Reagents

(1) 1% Casein solution　See "Measurement of alkaline protease activity"

(2) 1/2000 Alkaline protease solution　See "Measurement of alkaline protease activity"

(3) pH 10 Borax-NaOH buffer solution　See "Measurement of alkaline protease activity"

(4) 0. 1mol/L HCl solution　Dilute 8. 2ml concentrated hydrochloric acid to 1L with distilled water.

(5) 0. 2mol/L NaOH solution　Dissolve 8g NaOH in 1L distilled water.

(6) 0. 4mol/L Na_2CO_3 solution　See "Measurement of alkaline protease activity"

(7) 0. 4mol/L Trichloroacetic acid solution　See "Measurement of alkaline protease activity"

(8) Folin reagent　See "Measurement of alkaline protease activity"

Procedures

Take 3 test tubes and add reagents as Table 17 – 6.

Table 17 – 6　Effects of pH on enzyme activity

Reagents	Tube No.		
	1	2	3
1% Casein solution（ml）	1.0	1.0	1.0
Borax-NaOH buffer solution pH 10（ml）	1.0		
0.1mol/L HCl solution（ml）		1.0	
0.2mol/L NaOH solution（ml）			1.0
1/2000 Alkaline protease solution（ml）	1.0	1.0	1.0

Mix up and keep them in 40℃ water bath for 15min. Add 3.0ml 0.4mol/L trichloroacetic acid solution to each tube, then filtrate and collect 1.0ml filtrate respectively. Add 5.0ml 0.4mol/L Na_2CO_3 solution and 1.0ml Folin reagent. Mix up and keep them in 40℃ water bath for 15min. Observe the phenomena and analyze the alkaline protease activity under different pH.

Cautions

1. The salivary amylase activity varies from person to person, and sometimes the difference is great, so dilution times should be adjusted accordingly.

2. A small amount of inhibitors and activators can affect enzyme activity. Inhibitors and activators are not absolute. Some of them are certain enzyme activators in low concentration, but are inhibitors in high concentration. They are ever activators for some enzymes but are inhibitors for other enzymes.

3. The enzymatic reaction time must be controlled strictly. Experimental apparatus must be clean and dry.

Questions

1. What are the optimum temperature and optimum pH of enzyme? What practical meanings do they have?

2. What are the factors that affect enzyme activity? Explain the principle of each.

3. What conditions must be strictly controlled when doing the experiments about enzyme properties? Why?

4. What is the enzyme activity? How to measure the enzyme activity?

5. What are the cautions in measuring enzyme activity?

实验十八　细胞色素 C 的制备及鉴定

【实验目的】

1. 学习细胞色素 C 的理化性质及其生物学功能。

2. 掌握制备细胞色素 C 的原理。

3. 掌握制备细胞色素 C 的操作技术。

【实验原理】

细胞色素 C 是呼吸链的重要组成成分，是一种含铁卟啉基团的蛋白质。在线粒体呼吸链上位于细胞色素 b 和细胞色素 aa_3 之间，在生物氧化过程中起传递电子的作用。

细胞色素 C 分子中含赖氨酸较多，等电点为 pI 10.8，分子量为 12000~13000。它易溶于水及酸性溶液，且较稳定，不易变性。将样品组织破碎后，用酸性水溶液就可以将细胞色素 C 浸提出来。细胞色素 C 分为氧化型和还原型两种，因为还原型较稳定并易于保存，一般都将细胞色素 C 制成还原型。氧化型细胞色素 C 在 408nm、530nm 有最大吸收峰，还原型细胞色素 C 的最大吸收峰为 415nm、520nm 和 550nm，这一特性可用于细胞色素 C 的含量测定。

由于细胞色素 C 在心肌组织和酵母中含量丰富，常以此为材料进行分离制备。本实验以猪心为材料，经过酸溶液提取，人造沸石吸附，硫酸铵溶液洗脱，三氯醋酸沉淀等步骤制备细胞色素 C，并测定其含量。

【实验材料】

1. **实验器材** 绞肉机、电磁搅拌器、电动搅拌器、离心机、721 型分光光度计、玻璃柱（2.5cm×30cm）、下口瓶、烧杯（2000ml、1000ml、500ml）、量筒、移液管、玻璃漏斗和纱布、玻璃棒、透析袋。

2. **实验试剂**

（1）1mol/L H_2SO_4 溶液 取密度为 1.836g/ml 的浓硫酸（98% 硫酸）2.72ml 到蒸馏水中，定容到 50ml。

（2）2mol/L NH_4OH 溶液 量取 7.5ml 的 25% 氨水溶于水，稀释至 100ml 即可。

（3）25% 硫酸铵溶液 称取 25g 硫酸铵，定溶于 100ml 蒸馏水中，约相当于 25℃ 时 40% 的饱和度。

（4）0.2% 氯化钠溶液 称 0.2g 氯化钠，用蒸馏水溶解并定容至 100ml。

（5）$BaCl_2$ 试剂 称 12g $BaCl_2$ 溶于 100ml 蒸馏水中。

（6）20% 三氯醋酸溶液 称取无水三氯醋酸 20g，加入量杯中，加水适量，搅拌使溶解，加水定容至 100ml。

（7）人造沸石（60~80 目）。

（8）联二亚硫酸钠（$Na_2S_2O_4 \cdot 2H_2O$）。

（9）固体硫酸铵。

【实验步骤】

1. **细胞色素 C 的制备**

（1）材料处理 取新鲜或冰冻猪心，除去脂肪和韧带，将猪心切成小块，用水洗去积血，放入绞肉机绞碎。

（2）提取 称取绞碎猪心肌肉 500g，放入 2000ml 烧杯中，加蒸馏水 1000ml，在电动搅拌器搅拌下以 1mol/L H_2SO_4 调 pH 至 4.0（此时溶液呈暗紫色），在室温下搅拌提取 2 小时，在提取过程中，使溶液的 pH 值保持在 4.0 左右。在即将提取完毕，停止搅拌之前，以 2mol/L NH₄OH 调 pH 至 6.0，停止搅拌。用 4 层普通纱布压挤过滤，收集滤液。滤渣加入 750ml 蒸馏水，再按上述条件提取 1 小时，两次提取液合并。

（3）中和 用 2mol/L NH₄OH 调上述提取液至 pH 7.2（此时，等电点接近 7.2 的一些杂蛋白从溶液中沉淀析出），静置 30~40 分钟后过滤，所得滤液准备通过人造沸石柱进行吸附。

（4）吸附与洗脱 人造沸石容易吸附细胞色素 C，吸附后能被 25% 的硫酸铵洗脱下来，利用此特性将细胞色素 C 与其他不被沸石吸附的杂蛋白分开。具体操作如下。

①人造沸石的预处理 称取人造沸石 11g，放入 500ml 烧杯中，加水搅拌，用倾泻法除去 12 秒内不下沉的过细颗粒。

②装柱 选择一个底部带有滤膜的干净的玻璃柱（2.5cm×30cm），柱下端连接一根乳胶管，用夹子夹住，柱中加入蒸馏水至 1/3 体积，保持柱垂直，然后将已处理好的人造沸石带水装填入柱，注意一次装完，避免柱内出现气泡。

③上样 柱装好后，打开夹子放水（柱内沸石面上应保留一薄层水），将提取液装入下口瓶，使其流过人造沸石柱，随着细胞色素 C 的被吸附，柱内人造沸石逐渐由白色变为红色。调节柱下端流出液的速度，保证流出液为黄色或微红色。

④洗脱 吸附完毕，将红色人造沸石从柱内取出，放入 500ml 烧杯中，先用自来水，后用蒸馏水搅拌洗涤至水清，再用 100ml 0.2%NaCl 溶液分 3 次洗涤沸石，再用蒸馏水洗至水清，按第一次装柱方法将人造沸石重新装入柱内，用 25% 硫酸铵溶液（约 50ml）洗脱，流速 2ml/min，收集含有细胞色素 C 的红色洗脱液，当洗脱液红色开始消失时，即洗脱完毕。回收人造沸石，可再生使用。

⑤人造沸石再生 将使用过的沸石，先用自来水洗去硫酸铵，再用 0.25mol/L 氢氧化钠和 1mol/L 氯化钠混合液洗涤至沸石成白色，然后用蒸馏水反复洗至 pH 7~8，即可重新使用。

（5）盐析 在收集的洗脱液中加入固体硫酸铵（按每 100ml 洗脱液加入 20g 固体硫酸铵的比例，使溶液硫酸铵的饱和度为 45%），边加边搅拌，放置 30 分钟后，杂蛋白便从溶液中沉淀析出，而细胞色素 C 仍留在溶液中，用滤纸过滤除去杂蛋白，即得红色透亮细胞色素 C 溶液。

（6）三氯醋酸沉淀 向细胞色素 C 溶液中加入 20% 三氯醋酸（10ml 三氯醋酸/100ml 细胞色素 C 溶液），边加边搅拌，细胞色素 C 立即沉淀出来（沉淀出来的细胞色素 C 属可逆变性），立即于 3000r/min 离心 15 分钟，收集沉淀。

（7）透析 将沉淀的细胞色素 C 溶解于 5ml 蒸馏水中，装入透析袋，在 500ml 烧杯中用蒸馏水进行透析除盐（电磁搅拌器搅拌），15min 换水 1 次，换水 3~4 次后；检查透析外液 SO_4^{2-} 是否已被除净。检查方法是：取 2ml $BaCl_2$ 溶液于试管中，滴加 2~3 滴透析外液至试管中，若出现白色沉淀，表示 SO_4^{2-} 未除净；反之，说明透析完全。将透析液过滤，即得细胞色素 C 制品。

2. 含量测定 还原型细胞色素 C 在波长 520nm 处有最大吸收值，根据这一特性，用 721 型分光光度计，先作出一条标准细胞色素 C 浓度和对应的吸光度的标准曲线

（图 18 - 1），然后根据待测样品溶液的吸光度和标准曲线求出细胞色素 C 的含量。具体操作如下。

（1）标准曲线的绘制　取 1ml 细胞色素 C 标准品溶液（81mg/ml），稀释至 25ml，从中分别取 0.2ml、0.4ml、0.6ml、0.8ml、1.0ml 置于 5 支试管中，每管补加蒸馏水至 4ml，并加少许联二亚硫酸钠作还原剂，然后在 520nm 处测定各管的吸光度，分别为 0.179、0.330、0.520、0.700、0.870。以细胞色素 C 浓度为横坐标，吸光度为纵坐标，作出标准曲线，图 18 - 1，从图中求得斜率为 1/3.71。

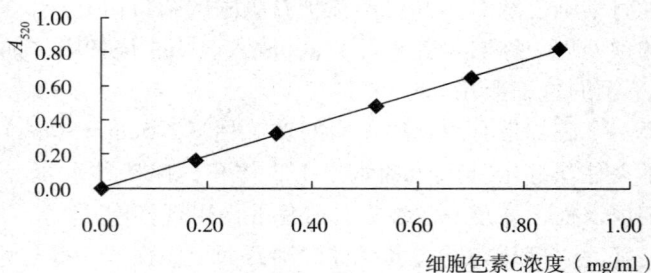

图 18 - 1　细胞色素 C 含量标准曲线

（2）样品测定　取 1ml 细胞色素 C 样品，稀释适当倍数，再加少许联二亚硫酸钠使其全部转变成还原型，在波长 520nm 处测定吸光度。根据标准曲线的斜率计算细胞色素 C 的含量。

3．等电点测定　方法和试剂参见实验七。

【实验结果】

计算公式：细胞色素 C 的含量 $= 3.71 \times A_{520} \times$ 稀释倍数 $\times 1/4 \times$ 终体积

在本实验中，500g 的猪心原料应获得 75mg 以上的细胞色素 C 制品。

说明：在细胞色素 C 制备的实际工作中，除了含量测定以外还要测定含铁量（纯度的鉴定）和活性，后两项测定，此处从略。

【注意事项】

1．尽可能除掉猪心中的韧带、脂肪和积血。

2．使用离心机之前，一定要配平。

3．透析之前要检查透析袋。

4．在 520nm 处测定各管的光密度时，要加少许联二亚硫酸钠作还原剂。

【思考题】

1．制备细胞色素 C 通常选取什么动物组织？为什么？

2．请说明细胞色素 C 制备相关步骤及其含量测定的基本原理。

3．请说出其他提取和纯化细胞色素 C 的方法，并写出相关的原理。

Experiment 18　Preparation and Identification
of Cytochrome C

Purpose

1. To learn physical and chemical properties and biology functions of cytochrome C.

2. To master the principle of cytochrome C purification.

3. To learn the experimental techniques of cytochrome C purification.

Principle

Cytochrome C, a key component in the respiratory chain, is a protein that contains heme prosthetic group. It is situated between cytochrome b and cytochrome aa_3 in the respiratory chain and functions as an electron transporter, which can both accept and donate electrons in the biological oxidation process.

The polypeptide chains of cytochrome C contain large amounts of lysine, which makes its pI alkaline (10.8). The molecular weight of cytochrome C is about $12000 \sim 13000$. It can be easily dissolved in water or acid solution and quite stable, so it is easily isolated and extracted from tissue using acid solution. Cytochrome C has the oxidized and reduced forms. The absorption peaks are at 415nm, 520nm, and 550nm in the reduced form, and at 408nm, 530nm in the oxidized form. In general, the reduced cytochrome C is more stable and easily conserved, so preparation of cytochrome C is in the reduced form. By this property, the content of cytochrome C can be determined.

Cytochrome C is relatively plentiful in tissues such as heart muscle and yeast, which can be the raw material for separating cytochrome C. In this experiment, a pig's heart is selected as the experimental material to obtain cytochrome C through the process of extracting at low pH, binding with man-made zeolite, eluting with ammonium sulfate, precipitating with trichloroacetic acid, and to measure its content.

Materials

1. Apparatus

Mincer, electromagnetic mixer, electromotive mixer, centrifuge, 721 type spectrophotometer, glass column (2.5cm × 30cm), flasks (2000ml, 1000ml, 500ml), cylinder, pipette, glass funnel, gauze, glass stick, dialytic bag.

2. Reagents

(1) 1mol/L H_2SO_4 solution　Add 98% H_2SO_4 ($\rho = 1.836g/ml$) 2.72ml in distilled water and set final volume to 50ml.

(2) 2mol/L NH_4OH　Dissolve 7.5ml 25% NH_4OH in water and dilute with water to 100ml.

(3) 25% $(NH_4)_2SO_4$ solution　100ml distilled water containing 25g ammonium sulfate,

which amounts to 40% saturation at 25℃.

（4）0.2% NaCl solution　Dissolve 0.2g NaCl in distilled water and dilute to 100ml.

（5）$BaCl_2$ solution　Dissolve 12g $BaCl_2$ in 100ml distilled water.

（6）20% Trichloroacetic acid solution　Add 20g anhydrous trichloroacetic acid to distilled water, stir and dissolve it and set final volume to 100ml.

（7）Man-made zeolite（60~80 screen）.

（8）Solid $Na_2S_2O_4 \cdot 2H_2O$.

（9）Solid $(NH_4)_2SO_4$.

Procedures

1. Preparation of cytochrome C

（1）Disposition of material　Take a fresh or frozen pig's heart, which is free from fat and ligaments, cut into small pieces and wash away blood with water. Turn on mincer at the highest speed to homogenize the tissue.

（2）Extraction　Weigh 500g samples and put into a 2000ml flask, then add 1000ml distilled water. Adjust the pH to 4.0 with 1mol/L H_2SO_4（till the color is about dark purple）. In the meantime, frequently stir with an electrical mixer. This step may take about 2h at room temperature. Be sure to keep the pH value at about 4.0 during the extracting process. Before stopping mixing, adjust pH to 6.0 with 2mol/L NH_4OH, and then stop swirling. Carefully squeeze the supernatant out with four-layer gauze and collect it. Add 750ml of distilled water to the residue to re-suspend the pellet, and re-extract for 1h. Combine the supernatant solutions. If the filtered solution is turbid, filter again.

（3）Neutralization　Adjust the pH of the extracted solvent to 7.2 with 2mol/L NH_4OH（during this process, some unwanted proteins will precipitate because of low solubility when the surrounding pH is equal to their pI）. After 30min to 40min of precipitation, the solution is filtrated and ready for next step.

（4）Binding and eluting　The man-made zeolite can easily bind with cytochrome C, which can be eluted by sulfate ammonium. According to this property, cytochrome C can be separated from other unwanted proteins. The detailed processes are listed below.

① Pretreatment of man-made zeolite　Weigh 11g man-made zeolite, put it into a 500ml flask, add water and stir, discard the small particles that can not precipitate in 12s with decantation method.

② Stuffing　Take a glass column（2.5cm×30cm）with filter membrane at the bottom, where a latex pipe is connected. Shut off the exit with a clip, add distilled water till it reaches 1/3 of the total volume, and keep the column upright. Suspend the pretreated man-made zeolite in water by swirling, and pour it into the column. Make sure that there is no bubble.

③ Loading samples　After stuffing the column, open the valve at the bottom of the column and allow the material in the column to settle（be sure to allow the water level to drop to just above the top of the material in the column）. Open the valve at the bottom of the column and pass the solution in Step（3）through the column. Allow all the solution to flow through the column, but do not let the solution level drop below the top of material in the column. The ingredient wanted can bind with the man-made zeolite in this step. Along with the binding of cytochrome C, the man-made zeolite in column gradually turns red from white, while the flow rate should be controlled in order to keep the solvent yellow or light red.

④ Elution　Take man-made zeolite out of the column after binding and put them into a 500ml flask. Wash it first with water, then with distilled water till the water is clear. Wash the man-made zeolite 3 times with 100ml 0.2% NaCl again. Finally wash it with water till the water is lucid. Re-stuff the man-made zeolite into the column and elute with 25% ammonium sulfate（about 50ml）at the flow rate of 2ml/min, then collect the red eluent, which contains cytochrome C. When the eluent turns from red to clear, it means the ending of elution. Do not discard the man-made zeolite because it can be regenerated.

⑤ Regeneration of man-made zeolite　Wash away the ammonium sulfate in the man-made zeolite with water, and then use the mixture of 0.25mol/L NaOH and 1mol/L NaCl to wash the zeolite till it becomes white, and wash it with water again and again until the pH is about 7 to 8, then the man-made zeolite can be reused.

（5）Salt precipitation　In order to further purify cytochrome C, add solid ammonium sulfate to the eluent（add 20g solid ammonium sulfate per 100ml to make the final saturation of ammonium sulfate 45%）and stir the eluent when adding, then place it statically. After 30 min, the impure proteins precipitate, while cytochrome C remains in the solution. Filtrate it with filter papers to collect the red clear filtrate that contains cytochrome C.

（6）Precipitation with trichloroacetic acid　Add 20% trichloroacetic acid to the clear liquid while swirling frequent（10ml trichloroacetic acid per 100ml liquid）, then the cytochrome C precipitates（this precipitation is reversible）. Put the sediment in a centrifugal tube immediately and centrifuge for 15min（3000r/min）, then collect the sediment.

（7）Dialysis　Make precipitates dissolve in 5ml distilled water. Transfer the suspension into a dialytic bag and dialyze with distilled water in a flask using electromagnetic mixer. Change the water every 15min, and after 3 to 4 times, check out whether SO_4^{2-} has been cleared away. The process is to put 2ml $BaCl_2$ into a test tube, and add 2 or 3 drops of water in the flask; if white precipitation appears, it means there is still some SO_4^{2-} in a dialysis bag, and vice versa.

2. Measurment of content

The cytochrome C in the solvent is in its reduced form, which has the maximum absorbance at the wavelength of 520nm. According to this property, draw absorbance-cytochrome C concentration calibration curve（Fig. 18 − 1）with 721 type spectrophotometer, then calculate the concentration of the sample from the slope of the curve and the absorbance. The process is listed below.

（1）Draw calibration curve　Take 1ml standard sample（81mg/ml）and dilute it to

25ml. Add different fraction of 0.2ml, 0.4ml, 0.6ml, 0.8ml and 1.0ml of sample to 5 test tubes marked respectively and distilled water till the final volume is 4ml in each test tube. Add little $Na_2S_2O_4 \cdot 2H_2O$ as reduced reagent, and measure absorbance at 520nm respectively. The OD Value is 0.179, 0.330, 0.520, 0.700, 0.870. Draw the calibration curve with the concentration on the x-axis, and the absorbance on the y-axis. From the calibration curve, the slope is 1/3.71.

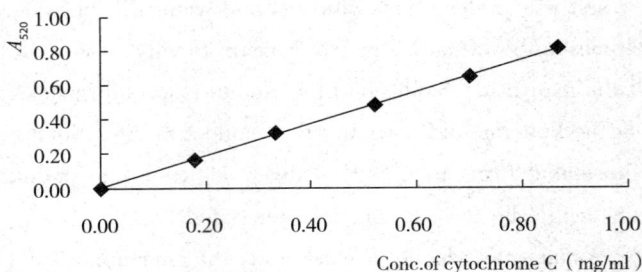

Fig. 18 − 1   Calibration curve of cytochrome C

(2) Sample assay   Take 1ml sample and dilute appropriate times. Add a little $Na_2S_2O_4 \cdot 2H_2O$ and measure absorbance at the wavelength of 520nm with 721 type spectrophotometer. Calculate the quantity of cytochrome C from the slope of calibration curve.

3. Determination of isoelectric point

See method and reagents of Experiment 7.

Results

Content of cytochrome C $= 3.71 \times A_{520} \times \mathrm{d}f \times V \times 1/4$

In this equation:

A—the absorbance of sample.

$\mathrm{d}f$—the dilution factor of sample.

V—the volume of sample.

In this experiment, with 500g pig's heart as the raw material, more than 75mg of final cytochrome C should be obtained.

Attention: In the actual extracting process of cytochrome C, both the amount of Fe^{2+} (the purity assay) and the activity of cytochrome C should also be analyzed. However, these procedures are not discussed here.

Cautions

1. Try your best to clear away fat, ligaments and blood in a pig's heart.

2. Keep balance when using centrifuge.

3. Check dialytic bag before dialysis.

4. Add a little $Na_2S_2O_4 \cdot 2H_2O$ to measure absorbance in 520nm wavelength.

Questions

1. What kind of animal tissue can be used to extract cytochrome C? and why?

2. Please describe in detail the principle of each step of cytochrome C preparation and quantification.

3. Can you use other separating method to extract and purify cytochrome C? Please describe the method and its principle.

实验十九　溶菌酶的制备及其性质

【实验目的】

1. 熟悉并进一步掌握酶的分离、纯化、检测及其生物学性质和理化性质研究等相关实验技能。

2. 初步培养从总体水平进行实验设计的能力，进一步加强并提高综合分析解决问题的能力。

3. 培养科研工作中的协作精神和勤俭而高效的科研作风。

【实验要求】

1. **实验内容**　本实验以蛋清为初始材料，制备高纯度溶菌酶，对溶菌酶生化性质进行检测。

2. **可行性报告**　通过相关文献资料的收集、分析，设计实验并撰写可行性报告。可行性报告包括实验目的、意义、国内外进展、实验方法和技术路线及可行性分析、实验预期结果。

3. **预实验报告**　在本实验开始前 1 个月，将实验报告草案提交指导教师，以审核和准备实验材料等；实验报告草案应提供最少 10 篇文献，其中至少有 2 篇是近 5 年内的文献，包括新技术、新方法在生物大分子研究中的应用；文献按学术期刊论文的格式要求，即作者、文章名、刊名、年、卷（期）、页码，参考书籍类同。

4. **实验报告**　包括采用实验的原理；实验所需试剂、仪器、设备；提取、分离、纯化的每步骤的蛋白质回收率、活性回收率，最终产率；按实验内容，提供实验结果及相关图表　完成实验后从整体上进行相关的讨论。

5. **操作要求**　本实验基本两人一组，在部分实验阶段中需几组合作进行。

【实验内容】

1. **溶菌酶活性检测**

（1）酶活力测定方法。

（2）酶活力单位定义。

（3）比活力定义。

（4）蛋白质含量测定方法 。

2. **蛋清溶菌酶的提取**

（1）每组 4～5 个新鲜鸡蛋。

（2）利用等电点沉淀及层析等方法进行溶菌酶提取。

3. **溶菌酶的分离、纯化**

（1）利用各种方法，从上述提取液中分离溶菌酶。

（2）每步纯化前需进行蛋白质纯度检测。

（3）分离纯化过程中跟踪检测活性组分的蛋白质含量和酶活性。

4. **溶菌酶理化性质**

（1）溶菌酶的分子量测定。

（2）溶菌酶的等电点测定。

5. **溶菌酶的酶学性质**

（1）在活力单位定义确定后，求出溶菌酶的 V_{max} 和 K_m。

（2）初步确定溶菌酶的最适 pH。

（3）初步确定溶菌酶的最适温度。

（4）提出最少两种溶菌酶的可逆抑制剂并验证抑制类型。

（5）提出溶菌酶的激活剂并验证。

（6）溶菌酶的热稳定性。

【实验原理】

溶菌酶（lysozyme）是由弗莱明在 1922 年发现，它是一种有效的抗菌剂，全称为 $1,4-\beta-N-$溶菌酶，又称作胞壁质酶。活性中心为天冬氨酸$_{52}$和谷氨酸$_{35}$，是一种糖苷水解酶，能催化水解黏多糖的 $N-$乙酰氨基葡萄糖（NAG）与 $N-$乙酰胞壁酸（NAM）间的 $\beta-1,4-$糖苷键，分子量 14700，由 129 个氨基酸残基构成，由于其中含有较多碱性氨基酸残基，所以其等电点高达 10.8 左右，最适温度为 50℃，最适 pH 为 6～7 左右。在 280nm 的消光系数 $[A_{1cm}^{1\%}]$ 为 13.0。该酶活性可被一些金属离子 Cu^{2+}、Fe^{2+}、Zn^{2+}（$10^{-5}～10^{-3}$mol/L）以及 $N-$乙酰葡糖胺所抑制，能被 Mg^{2+}、Ca^{2+}（$10^{-5}～10^{-3}$mol/L）、NaCl 所激活。

溶菌酶广泛存在于动、植物及微生物体内，鸡蛋（含量为 2%～4%）和哺乳动物的乳汁是溶菌酶的主要来源。溶菌酶具有抗感染、消炎、消肿、增强体内免疫反应等多种药理作用，目前广泛应用于医学临床。

溶菌酶常温下在中性盐溶液中具有较高天然活性，在中性条件下溶菌酶带正电荷，因此在分离制备时，先后采用等电点法，D152 型树脂柱层析法除杂蛋白，再经 Sephadex G-50 层析柱进一步纯化。最后用 SDS-PAGE 鉴定为一条带。采用福林酚法测蛋白质含量，分光光度法测定酶活性。

【实验材料】

1. **实验器材** 循环水式真空泵、蛋白质紫外检测仪、记录仪、紫外分光光度计、梯度混合器（500ml）、721 型分光光度计、冰冻离心机、冰箱、透析袋、酸度计、部分收集器、恒流泵、圆盘电泳装置、恒温水浴锅、层析柱（2.6cm×50cm）（1.6cm×30cm）、布氏漏斗（500ml）、吸滤瓶（1000ml）、G-3 砂芯漏斗（500ml）。

2. **实验试剂**

（1）鸡蛋清（鲜鸡蛋）。

（2）溶菌酶标准品，底物——微球菌粉。

（3）D152 大孔弱酸性阳离子交换树脂，Sephadex G – 50。

（4）固体氯化钠（NaCl），固体硫酸铵（NH₄）₂SO₄，固体磷酸氢二钠（Na₂HPO₄·12H₂O），固体磷酸二氢钠（NaH₂PO₄·2H₂O），固体磷酸钠（Na₃PO₄）。

（5）乙醇，蒸馏水，甲醇，考马斯亮蓝 G – 250，三氯乙酸，丙酮。

（6）N – 乙酰萄糖胺，硫酸铜，硫酸亚铁，硫酸锌，氯化镁，氯化钙，氢氧化钠，盐酸。

（7）SDS – 聚丙烯酰胺凝胶电泳试剂（见实验六），蛋白质含量测定（福林法）试剂（见实验二）。

（8）聚乙二醇 – 20000，两性电解质。

【实验步骤】

1. **蛋清的制备**　将 4～5 个新鲜的鸡蛋两端各敲一个小洞，使蛋清流出（鸡蛋清 pH 值不得小于 8），轻轻搅拌 5 分钟，使鸡蛋清的稠度均匀，用两层纱布过滤除去脐带块，量体积约为 100ml。

2. **鸡蛋清粗分离**　按过滤好的蛋清量边缓慢搅拌边加入等体积的去离子水，均匀后在不断搅拌下用 1mol/L HCl 调 pH 至 7 左右，用脱脂棉过滤并收滤液。

3. **D152 弱酸性阳离子交换层析**

（1）树脂处理　将 D152 树脂先用蒸馏水洗去杂物，滤出。用 1mol/L NaOH 搅拌浸泡并搅拌 4～8 小时，抽滤干 NaOH，用蒸馏水洗至近 pH 7.5，抽滤干。再用 1mol/L HCl 按上述方法处理树脂，直到全部转变成氢型，抽滤干 HCl。用蒸馏水洗至近 pH 5.5，保持过夜，如果 pH 不低于 5.0，抽滤干 HCl，用 2mol/L NaOH 处理树脂使之转变为钠型，pH 不小于 6.5。吸干溶液，加 pH 6.5 0.02mol/L 的磷酸盐缓冲液平衡树脂。

（2）装柱　取直径 1.6cm，长度为 30cm 的层析柱，自顶部注入经处理的上述树脂悬浮液，关闭层柱出口，待树脂沉降后，放出过量的溶液，再加入一些树脂，至树脂沉积至 15～20cm 高度即可。于柱子顶部继续加入 pH 6.5、0.02mol/L 磷酸盐缓冲液平衡树脂，使流出液 pH 为 6.5 为止，关闭柱子出口，保持液面高出树脂表面 1cm 左右。

（3）上柱吸附　将上述蛋清溶液仔细直接加到树脂顶部，打开出口使其缓慢流入柱内，流速为 1ml/min。

（4）洗脱　用柱平衡液洗脱杂蛋白，在收集洗脱液的过程中，逐管用紫外分光光度计检验杂蛋白的洗脱情况，当基线开始走平后，改用含 1.0mol/L NaCl 的 pH 6.5，浓度为 0.02mol/L 磷酸钠缓冲液洗脱，收集洗脱液。

（5）聚乙二醇浓缩　将上述洗脱液合并装入透析袋内，置容器中，外面覆以聚乙二醇，容器加盖，酶液中的水分很快被透析膜外的聚乙二醇所吸收。当浓缩到 5ml 左右时，用蒸馏水洗去透析膜外的聚乙二醇，小心取出浓缩液。

（6）透析除盐　蒸馏水透析除盐 24 小时。

4. Sephadex G-50 分子筛柱层析

（1）装柱 先将用 20% 乙醇保存的 Sephadex G-50 抽滤除去乙醇，用 6g/L NaCl 溶液搅拌 Sephadex G-50 数分钟，再抽滤，反复多次直至无醇味为止。如果 Sephadex G-50 是新的，则按实验五中的方法处理凝胶。加入胶体积 1/4 的 6g/L NaCl 溶液，充分搅拌，超声除去气泡，装入玻璃层析柱（1.6cm×50cm），柱床 45cm。

（2）上样 与实验五中的方法相同。

（3）洗脱 样品流完后，先分次加入少量 6g/L NaCl 洗脱液洗下柱壁上的样品，连接恒流泵，使流速为 0.5ml/min，用部分收集器收集，每 10 分钟收集一管。

（4）聚乙二醇浓缩 合并活性峰溶液，用聚乙二醇浓缩到 5ml 左右时，用蒸馏水洗去透析膜外的聚乙二醇，小心取出浓缩液。

（5）透析除盐 蒸馏水透析除盐 24 小时。收集透析液，量取体积。

5. 溶菌酶活力测定

（1）酶液配制 准确称取溶菌酶样品 5mg，用 0.1mol/L、pH 6.2 磷酸缓冲液配成 1mg/ml 的酶液，再将酶液稀释成 50μg/ml。

（2）底物配制 取干菌粉 5mg 加上述缓冲液少许，在乳钵中（或匀浆器中）研磨 2 分钟，倾出，稀释到 15~25ml，此时在光电比色上的吸光度最好在 0.5~0.7 范围内。

（3）活力测定 先将酶和底物分别放入 25℃ 恒温水浴预热 10 分钟，吸取底物悬浮液 4ml 放入比色杯中，在 450nm 波长读出吸光度，此为零时读数。然后吸取样品液 0.2ml（相当于 10μg 酶），每隔 30s 读 1 次吸光度，到 90s 时共记下 4 个读数。

活力单位的定义是：在 25℃，pH 6.2，波长为 450nm 时，酶蛋白每分钟引起吸光度下降 0.001 为 1 个活力单位。

$$酶的活力单位数 = \Delta A_{450}/t \times 0.001$$

$$比活力 = 酶的活力单位数/毫克蛋白质$$

6. 蛋白质含量的测定 采用 Folin-酚试剂法进行测定（参见实验二）。

7. 纯度检测 采用 SDS-PAGE 方法（参见实验六）。

8. 理化和酶学性质的测定 学生可根据酶纯化和活力测定的结果，运用已掌握的生化知识和实验技能自行设计方案进行探索研究。

【实验结果】

溶菌酶分离纯化和活性测定结果见表 19-1。

表 19-1 溶菌酶分离纯化和活性测定结果

步骤项目	体积（ml）	总蛋白质量（mg）	总活力单位	比活力（单位/毫克）	回收率（%）
1. 制备蛋清					
2. 溶菌酶分离					
3. D152 柱层析					
4. Sephadex G-50 层析					

【思考题】

1. 请说出其他提取和纯化溶菌酶的方法并说明相关原理。

2. 根据自身的实验体会，写出优化本实验的措施。

Experiment 19 Preparation of Lysozyme and Its Properties

Purpose

1. Be familiar with and further grasp experimental skills on the separation, purification, detection and the physical and chemical and biological properties of certain enzyme.

2. To train ability to design the experiment on the whole perspective level, and further improve the ability to analyze and solve problems.

3. To develop co-operative spirit and economical but efficient working style in the scientific research.

Requirements

1. Experiment content   Use albumen as the original material to extract and condense lysozyme, and assay its biochemical properties.

2. Feasibility report   By collecting relevant published papers, analyze and design the experiment and write the feasibility report. The report includes the purpose, the meaning, and the development on this experiment, methods and also technical route, while the analysis of possibility and the expected results of this experiment should be added.

3. Preliminary experiment report   One month before the beginning of this experiment, the draft of experiment report should be submitted to the teacher so that the teacher could look through and prepare for it. The draft of the report should be based on at least 10 published papers, among which at least 2 papers are published in recent 5 years, including new technology or new methods on the research of application of biomacromolecules. The quotation of published papers should follow the form which includes the author, article name, journal name, volume, page and reference books.

4. Experiment report   Experiment report should include principles, reagents, apparatus, equipment, protein product ratio, activity ratio and final product ratio in each step of extraction, separation and purification. According to the content of experiment, provide the results and related figures or charts and discuss the experiment on the whole perspective.

5. In this experiment, every group consists of two students. In part of the experiment, several groups need to cooperate.

Contents

1. Assay of lysozyme activity

（1）Method of enzyme activity assay.

（2）The definition of enzyme activity unit.

(3) The definition of specific activity.

(4) Quantification of protein.

2. Extraction of lysozyme from the egg white

(1) 4 ~ 5 eggs for every group.

(2) Extract lysozyme with some methods such as isoelectric point precipitation and chromatography.

3. Separation and purification of lysozyme

(1) Separation lysozyme from above-mentioned sample by various methods.

(2) Assay of protein purity before every step of purification.

(3) Assay of protein content and enzyme activity during every step of purification.

4. The physical and chemical properties of lysozyme

(1) Assay the molecular weight of lysozyme.

(2) Assay the isoelectric point of lysozyme.

5. The enzymatic properties of lysozyme

(1) Calculate V_{max} and K_m of lysozyme preliminarily.

(2) Determine the optimum pH of lysozyme preliminarily.

(3) Determine the optimum temperature of lysozyme.

(4) Propose at least two reversible inhibitors of lysozyme and prove the type of inhibition.

(5) Propose the activators of lysozyme and then prove them.

(6) Prove the thermal stability of lysozyme.

Principle

Lysozyme, discovered by Alexander Fleming in 1922, is an effective antimicrobial reagent, whose full name is 1,4-β-N-lysozyme, also called muramidase. The active site of this enzyme is Asp_{52} and Glu_{35}. It is a kind of glycoside hydrolase which hydrolyzes the β-1,4-glucosidic linkages between N-acetylmuramic acid and N-acetylglucosamine. The relative molecular weight of lysozyme is 14700, and is composed of 129 amino acid residues. As it contains more basic amino acids, the isoelectric point is about 10.8. The optimum temperature and pH are 50℃ and pH 6 ~ 7 respectively. At 280nm wavelength, the extinction coefficient $[A_{1cm}^{1\%}]$ is 13.0. The activity of lysozyme can be inhibited by some metal ions, such as Cu^{2+}, Fe^{2+}, Zn^{2+} (10^{-5} ~ 10^{-3} mol/L) and N-acetylglucosamine, while be activated by Mg^{2+}, Ca^{2+} (10^{-5} ~ 10^{-3} mol/L), NaCl.

Lysozyme extensively exists in the biosphere, including the animals, plants and microbes. The content of lysozyme in avian ovum (about 2% ~ 4%) and latex of mammalian is especially rich. It has many pharmacological effects, including anti-infection, anti-inflammation, detumescence, improving the immunity and so on. At present, lysozyme is widely used in clinical medicine.

As lysozyme has comparatively highly nature activity in neutral salt solution at room temperature, and has positive charge under this condition, it can be absorbed by cation-exchange-resin in the neutral environment. So in this experiment, the use of isoelectric point method can eliminate some of the unpurified proteins. D152 resin is used to remove most unpurified protein. In order to further purify lysozyme, we use sephadex G-50 to sieve out those unpurified protein. Identify to be a single band with SDS-PAGE. Protein content and enzyme activity are measured with Lowry method and spectrophotometric method respectively.

Materials

1. Apparatus

Vacuum pump of recycle water, ultraviolet detector, recorder, UV-visible spectrophotometer, gradient mixer (500ml), 721 type spectrophotometer (UV-9100), refrigerated centrifuge, refrigerator, dialysis bag, pH meter, automatic collector, constant speed pump, disc electrophoresis apparatus, constant temperature water bath, chromatography column (2.6cm × 50cm)(1.6cm × 30cm), buchner funnel, filter flask, G-3 core sand funnel (500ml).

2. Reagents

(1) Albumen (fresh egg).

(2) Standard sample of lysozyme, substrate – dried germ powder.

(3) D152 Acidic cation-exchange resin, Sephadex G-50.

(4) Solid NaCl, $(NH)_2SO_4$, $Na_2HPO_4 \cdot 12H_2O$, $NaH_2PO_4 \cdot 2H_2O$, Na_3PO_4.

(5) Ethanol, distilled water, methanol, Coomassie brilliant blue G-250, trichloroacetic acid, acetone.

(6) N-Acetylglucosamine, $CuSO_4$, $FeSO_4$, $ZnSO_4$, $MgCl_2$, $CaCl_2$, NaOH, HCl.

(7) Reagents of SDS-PAGE (the same as Experiment 6), Folin-phenol reagent of quantification of protein (the same as Experiment 2).

(8) Polyethylene glycol-20000, Ampholyte.

Procedures

1. Preparation of albumen

Choose 4~5 eggs and knock holes on each side to make the egg white flow out (the pH of egg white is no lower than 8), stir gently for 5min to get suitable viscosity, and then sieve with gauze, the total volume is about 100ml.

2. Preliminary separation of lysozyme

Stir the egg white gently while adding the same volume of deionized water, adjust the pH to 7 with 1mol/L HCl. Then filter with pledget and collect filtrate.

3. D152 weak acidic cation-exchange chromatography

(1) Disposal of Resin Wash D152 resin with clear water to eliminate the slight impurity. Add 1mol/L sodium hydroxide solution, keep for 4~8h and stir at intervals. Suck and filter the basic liquid, and wash it to pH 7.5 with distilled water. Soak the resin with 1mol/L hydrogen chloride solution as above. Add hydrogen chloride with stirring to assure that the resin changes to hydrogen mode totally. Then suck and filter the acid liquid, and wash it to pH 5.5

with distilled water, and keep over night. If the pH is not below 5. 0, suck and filter it, change the resin to sodium mode with 2mol/L sodium hydroxide solution, but keep the pH at no less than 6. 5. Suck and soak the resin with 0. 02mol/L phosphoric acid buffer pH 6. 5 over night.

(2) Packing   Take a chromatography column with the diameter of 1. 6cm and the length of 30cm; Pour the above prepared resin from the top. Close the exit of chromatography column. When the resin sediments, let out the excessive solution, add more resin until the height of the resin sediment is about 15 ~ 20cm. Add 0. 02mol/L phosphoric acid buffer pH 6. 5 from the top to wash it until the flowing liquor reaches pH 6. 5. Close the exit of the column, and keep the level of the liquor surface about 1cm higher than that of the resin.

(3) Loading   Add albumen solution to the top of resin directly and carefully, and open the exit to make it flow into the column slowly. The speed is about 1ml/min.

(4) Elution   Elute the inpurified protein with balanced solution; Collect the eluent and check with ultraviolet detector tube by tube. When base line goes flat, elute with 0. 02mol/L phosphate sodium buffer containing 1. 0mol/L NaCl, pH 6. 5. The eluent is collected.

(5) PEG condensation   Combine and move eluent into dialytic bag, put in flask and cover dialytic bag with PEG. Water in the enzyme solution will soon be absorbed by PEG outside the dialytic bag. When the final volume is about 5ml, wash away the PEG outside the dialytic bag with distilled water. Take out the condensed solution carefully.

(6) Desalting by dialysis   Dialyse above solution against distilled water for about 24h.

4. Sephadex G-50 gel filtration chromatography

(1) Stuffing   Suck the ethanol from the Sephadex G-50 storing solution which contains 20% ethanol, add 6g/L NaCl and stir for several minutes. Repeat suction till there is no ethanol in solution. (If the Sephadex G-50 is new, dispose the gel as described in Experiment 5). Add 6g/L NaCl about 1/4 of gel volume, eliminate the bubbles with ultrasonic, stuff the gel into the glass chromatography column (1. 6cm × 50cm), and the column bed height is 45cm.

(2) Loading sample   The same as Experiment 5.

(3) Elution   After all of the sample enters the gel, add 6g/L NaCl eluent to wash the sample on the inner wall of glass chromatography column. Connect with constant speed pump, the flowing speed being 0. 5ml/min, and collect the eluent into test tube every 10min with automatic collector.

(4) Condensing by PEG   Collect and combine the eluent. When it is condensed to 5ml with PEG wash away the PEG outside dialysis bag with distilled water. Take out condensed liquid carefully.

(5) Desalting by dialysis   Dialyse for 24h to desalt against distilled water, and then measure volume.

5. Assay of activity

(1) Preparation of enzyme solution   Accurately weigh 5mg of lysozyme, dissolve it with 0. 1mol/L pH 6. 2 phosphoric acid buffer to be 1mg/ml enzyme solution, and then dilute to

$50\mu g/ml$.

(2) Preparation of substrate　Take 5mg of dried germ powder, add a little above buffer, and triturate it in the mortar (or homogenizer) for 2min. Pour it out and dilute it to 15 ~ 25ml. It is the best that the optical density assayed by the photoelectric colorimeter is between 0.5 ~ 0.7.

(3) Activity determination　Preheat the enzyme and substrate respectively in constant temperature water bath of 25℃ for 10min. Suck 4ml of substrate suspension, and put it in cuvette. Then record the absorbance at 450nm, and this is the value at zero. Then draw 0.2ml of sample solution (equal to 10μg of enzyme), read the absorbance every 30s. Write down four readings after 90s.

One unit of activity is defined as the amount of enzyme that makes A_{450} decrease in absorbance of 0.001 every minute. When pH is 6.2, the temperature is 25℃, and the wavelength is 450nm.

Activity unit $= \Delta A_{450}/t \times 0.001$

Specific activity = Activity unit/1mg enzyme

6. Determination of protein content

Folin-phenol reagent method (the same as Experiment 2).

7. Identification of purity

SDS-PAGE method (the same as Experiment 6)

8. Determination of physical, chemical and enzymatic properties

According to the results of purification and activity assay and by applying the biochemistry knowledge and experiment techniques that students have grasped, students can design scheme by themselves to explore and research.

Results

The results of lysozyme purification and activity assay are shown in Table 19 – 1.

Table 19 – 1　The results of lysozyme purification and activity assay

Procedures	Volume (ml)	Total protein (mg)	Activity unit	Specific activity (U/mg)	Recovery ratio (%)
1. Preparation of Albumen					
2. Crude separation of lysozyme					
3. D152 resin chromatography					
4. Sephadex G-50 chromatography					

Questions

1. Can you use other separation method to extract and purify lysozyme? Please describe the method and its principle in detail.

2. Propose some feasible measures to optimize the experiment according to your experience in the experiment.

实验二十　碱性磷酸酶的分离纯化及其酶学研究

【实验目的】

1. 掌握酶分离纯化的相关原理。
2. 熟悉碱性磷酸酶分离纯化的方法步骤。
3. 掌握测定碱性磷酸酶比活力的原理和方法。
4. 培养综合运用各种方法从组织中分离纯化及鉴定特定蛋白质的技能。

一、碱性磷酸酶的分离纯化及比活力的测定

【实验原理】

碱性磷酸酶（alkaline phosphatase，AKP 或 ALP，EC 3.1.3.1）广泛存在于人体、动物、植物与微生物中，在生物体内直接参与磷酸基团的转移和代谢过程。AKP 是一种底物特异性较低，在碱性环境中能水解多种磷酸单酯化合物的酶，需要镁和锰离子作为激活剂。AKP 作用最适 pH 范围是 8.6～10。血清 AKP 主要来自肝，小部分来自骨骼。

大多数酶是蛋白质，其提取、分离与纯化的方法和蛋白质相似。常用蛋白质分离纯化的方法有中性盐盐析法（如硫酸铵盐析）、电泳法（如聚丙烯酰胺凝胶电泳）、层析法（如葡聚糖凝胶层析）以及有机溶剂法（如乙醇、丙酮、正丁醇等）。有机溶剂分级沉淀是分离蛋白质的常用方法之一。有机溶剂能使许多溶于水的生物大分子发生沉淀，其主要作用是降低水溶液的介电常数，从而使溶质的溶解度降低。同时有机溶剂溶于水，对大分子物质表面的水化膜具有破坏作用，最后使这些大分子脱水而互相聚集析出。沉淀不同物质所需有机溶剂的浓度不同，利用不同蛋白质在不同浓度的有机溶剂中发生沉淀作用而达到分离。用于生物大分子分级分离的溶剂主要是能与水互溶的有机溶剂，常用的有乙醇、甲醇和丙酮等。

本实验采用有机溶剂沉淀法从肝匀浆中提取分离 AKP。在制备肝匀浆时采用低浓度醋酸钠可以达到低渗破膜的作用，而醋酸镁则有保护和稳定 AKP 的作用。匀浆液中加入正丁醇能使部分杂蛋白变性，再通过过滤而除去。含有 AKP 的滤液可再进一步用冷丙酮和冷乙醇进行分离纯化。根据 AKP 在终浓度 33% 的丙酮或终浓度 30% 的乙醇中溶解，而在终浓度 50% 的丙酮或终浓度 60% 的乙醇中不溶解的性质，采用离心的方法重复分离提取，可从含有 AKP 的滤液中获得较为纯净的碱性磷酸酶。

以磷酸苯二钠为底物的苯基磷酸钠终点比色法是碱性磷酸酶活性检测方法中最常用的一种。它的基本原理是：在一定的 pH 和温度下，待测液中的碱性磷酸酶作用于底物液中的磷酸苯二钠，使之水解放出酚。酚在碱性溶液中与 4－氨基安替比林（AAP）作用并经铁氰化钾氧化，生成红色醌类化合物（反应原理如图 20－1）。以酚作标准液同样显色后在 510nm 波长处进行比色，根据红色深浅可以测定酶活力的高低，从而计算出酶的活力单位。本方法以每克组织蛋白在 37℃ 与底物作用 15 分钟产生 1mg 酚为一

个酶活力单位。这种方法操作简便，所需的设备简单，而且精度较高。其中，蛋白质含量测定采用考马斯亮蓝法。

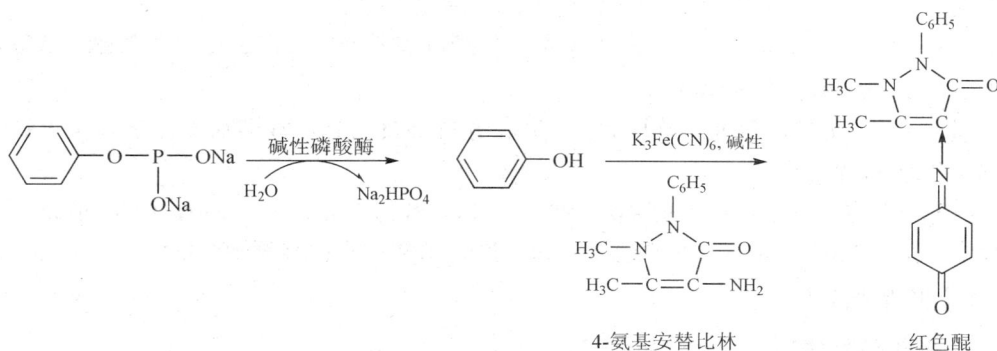

图 20 - 1 碱性磷酸酶活性测定反应原理

【实验材料】

1. 实验器材 分光光度计、离心机、恒温水浴锅、刻度离心管、量筒、移液管、电子天平、烧杯、剪刀、匀浆器。

2. 实验试剂

（1）0.1mol/L 醋酸钠溶液 称取醋酸钠 8.2g，溶于蒸馏水中，稀释至 1000ml。

（2）0.5mol/L 醋酸镁溶液 称取醋酸镁 107.25g，溶于蒸馏水中，稀释至 1000ml。

（3）0.01mol/L 醋酸镁 – 0.01mol/L 醋酸钠溶液 0.5mol/L 醋酸镁 20ml 及 0.1mol/L 醋酸钠 100ml，混合后加蒸馏水稀释至 1000ml。

（4）正丁醇（A. R.）。

（5）95% 乙醇（A. R.）。

（6）丙酮（A. R.）。

（7）0.01mol/L pH 8.8 Tris 缓冲液 称取三羟甲基氨基甲烷（Tris）12.1g，用蒸馏水溶解并定容至 1000ml，即为 0.1mol/L Tris 缓冲液。再取 0.1mol/L Tris 缓冲液 100ml，加蒸馏水约 700ml，再加 0.1mol/L 醋酸钠溶液 100ml，混匀后用 1% 醋酸溶液调节 pH 至 8.8，用蒸馏水稀释至 1000ml。

（8）酚标准液（0.1mg/ml） 称取重结晶酚 1.5g 溶于 0.1mol/L HCl 中，定容至 1000ml 即成贮备液。取上述酚液 25ml 于 250ml 碘量瓶中，加 50ml 0.1mol/L NaOH 并加热至 65℃，再加入 0.1mol/L 碘液 25ml，盖好碘量瓶塞，放置 30 分钟后，加浓盐酸 5.0ml，再加 0.1% 淀粉液作指示剂，用 0.1mol/L 标准硫代硫酸钠滴定。每毫升 0.1mol/L 碘溶液（含碘 12.7mg）所相当的酚毫克数为：$12.7 \times 94/(3 \times 254) = 1.567$。假设 0.1mol/L 碘溶液 25ml 与 25ml 酚液作用后剩余的碘用硫代硫酸钠滴定为 Xml，则 25ml 酚溶液中所含酚量为 $(25 - X) \times 1.567$mg，由此推算酚贮备液浓度。最后将贮备液稀释成 0.1mg/ml 作为标准液。

（9）复合底物液 称取磷酸苯二钠·$2H_2O$ 6g，4 – 氨基安替比林 3g，分别溶于煮沸冷却后的蒸馏水中，两液混合并稀释至 1000ml，加 4ml 三氯甲烷防腐，贮存于棕色瓶内，冰箱冷藏保存，可用1周。临用时将此液与等量0.1mol/L pH 10碳酸盐缓冲液混合。

（10）5g/L铁氰化钾　称取5g铁氰化钾和15g硼酸溶于400ml蒸馏水中，溶解后两液混合，再加蒸馏水至1000ml，置棕色瓶中暗处保存。

（11）0.1mol/L pH 10碳酸盐缓冲液　称取无水碳酸钠6.3g及碳酸氢钠3.36g溶解于蒸馏水中，稀释至1000ml。

（12）标准蛋白质溶液　称取50mg牛血清白蛋白，溶于蒸馏水中并定容至100ml，制成500μg/ml标准蛋白溶液。

（13）考马斯亮蓝G-250溶液　称取100mg考马斯亮蓝G-250，溶于50ml 95%乙醇中，加入85%（W/V）的磷酸100ml，最后用蒸馏水稀释至1000ml。

【实验步骤】

1. 碱性磷酸酶的提取和分离

（1）取新鲜兔肝脏2g，在烧杯中剪碎，加入2ml 0.01mol/L醋酸镁-0.01mol/L醋酸钠溶液，转入刻度离心管中进行匀浆（10000r/min大约30s），再用4ml上述溶液冲洗匀浆器并倒入离心管，混匀，此即为A液。记录体积，取A液0.1ml放入标记为A^E的试管中，再加入4.9ml 0.01mol/L pH 8.8 Tris缓冲液，待测酶活性，另取A液0.1ml放入标记为A^P的试管中，再加入4.9ml生理盐水（0.9%氯化钠溶液），待测蛋白质浓度。

（2）A液余液加入2ml正丁醇，用玻璃棒搅拌5分钟，室温静置10分钟，单层滤纸过滤，加入与滤液等体积的冷丙酮，立即搅拌混匀。2500r/min，离心5分钟，弃去上清，沉淀加入0.5mol/L醋酸镁4ml，搅拌使沉淀溶解，摇匀，此为B液。记录体积，取B液0.1ml放入标记为B^E的试管中，再加入2.9ml 0.01mol/L pH 8.8 Tris缓冲液，待测酶活性，另取B液0.1ml放入标记为B^P的试管中，再加入1.9ml加入生理盐水（0.9氯化钠溶液），待测蛋白质浓度。

（3）B液余液加入95%冷乙醇溶液至乙醇浓度达30%，迅速混匀，2500r/min，离心5分钟。弃去沉淀，上清液加入95%乙醇溶液至乙醇浓度为60%迅速混匀，2500r/min，离心5分钟。弃去上清，沉淀加0.01mol/L醋酸镁-0.01mol/L醋酸钠溶液2ml，搅拌沉淀使之溶解，此为C液。记录体积，取C液0.1ml放入标记为C^E的试管中，再加入1.9ml 0.01mol/L pH 8.8 Tris缓冲液，待测酶活性，另取C液0.1ml放入标记为C^P的试管中，再加入0.4ml 0.9%氯化钠溶液，待测蛋白质浓度。

（4）C液余液加入冷丙酮至丙酮浓度为33%，3000r/min，离心5分钟。弃去沉淀，上清液加入冷丙酮至浓度达50%，迅速混匀，3000r/min，离心5分钟。弃去上清液，沉淀加入0.01mol/L pH 8.8 Tris缓冲液5ml，3000r/min，离心5分钟。弃去沉淀，上清液即为D液。记录体积，取D液0.1ml放入标记为D^E的试管中，再加入0.9ml 0.01mol/L pH 8.8 Tris缓冲液，待测酶活性，另取D液0.1ml放入标记为D^P的试管中，待测蛋白质浓度。

2. 碱性磷酸酶比活力的测定

（1）碱性磷酸酶活力的测定　取干净干燥试管6支，分别编号，按表20-1操作。

表 20 -1　碱性磷酸酶活力测定反应体系

	O	S	A^E	B^E	C^E	D^E
不同提取阶段酶液（ml）			0.1	0.1	0.1	0.1
0.1mg/ml 酚标准液（ml）		0.1				
0.01mol/L pH 8.8 Tris 缓冲液（ml）	0.1					
预热至37℃复合底物液（ml）	3.0	3.0	3.0	3.0	3.0	3.0

加入复合底物液后立即混匀，置于37℃恒温水浴锅中准确保温15分钟。保温结束后各管立即加入5g/L铁氰化钾2ml并摇匀，以终止酶促反应，放置15分钟，显色后用721型分光光度计，以"O"号管作空白对照，在波长510nm处测定吸光度，计算每毫升酶液中的酶活力单位。

（2）蛋白质含量测定　用考马斯亮蓝法测定所提A、B、C、D液中的蛋白质含量。按表20-2操作。

表 20 -2　蛋白质含量测定反应体系

	O	S	A^P	B^P	C^P	D^P
不同蛋白质溶液（ml）			0.1	0.1	0.1	0.1
500μg/ml 标准蛋白质溶液（ml）		0.1				
0.9% 氯化钠溶液（ml）	0.1					
考马斯亮蓝 G -250（ml）	9.0	9.0	9.0	9.0	9.0	9.0

混匀静置5分钟后，以"O"号管作空白对照，在波长595nm处测定吸光度，计算样品中蛋白质含量。

【实验结果】

1. 活力单位的计算

$$P = A_E \times m_S \times n / (A_S \times V)$$

式中，P——每毫升样品中碱性磷酸酶的活力单位（U/ml）；

　　　A_E——测定管的吸光度；

　　　A_S——标准管的吸光度；

　　　m_S——标准管酚的质量（mg）；

　　　V——样品的体积（ml）；

　　　n——稀释倍数。

2. 比活力的计算

碱性磷酸酶的比活力 = 每毫升样品中碱性磷酸酶活力单位数/每毫升样品中蛋白质毫克数

3. 收率的计算

（1）各阶段碱性磷酸酶的总活力 = 每毫升样品中碱性磷酸酶活力单位数 × 样品体积数

（2）各阶段碱性磷酸酶得率 = 各阶段酶的总活力单位/匀浆 A 液中的酶总活力

单位 ×100%

4. 纯化倍数的计算

纯化倍数 = 各阶段所得比活力数 / 匀浆 A 液比活力数

按上述公式计算并将结果填入表 20 - 3。

表20 -3　碱性磷酸酶的分离纯化结果

分离阶段	总体积 (ml)	蛋白质浓度 (mg/ml)	总蛋白质 (mg)	每毫升酶活力单位 (U)	酶总活力单位 (U)	比活力 (U/mg)	纯化倍数	得率 (%)
匀浆（A液）								
第一次丙酮沉淀（B液）								
乙醇沉淀（C液）								
第二次丙酮沉淀（D液）								

【注意事项】

1. 加入有机溶剂的计算

进行有机溶剂沉淀时，欲使原溶液中有机溶剂达到一定浓度，需加入有机溶剂的浓度和体积可按下式计算：

$$V = V_0(S_2 - S_1)/(100 - S_2)$$

式中，V——需加入 100% 有机溶剂的体积；

V_0——原溶液的体积；

S_1——原溶液中有机溶剂的浓度；

S_2——要求达到的有机溶剂的浓度；

100——指加入的有机溶剂浓度为 100%。如所加入的有机溶剂的浓度为95%，则上式（$100 - S_2$）项应改为（$95 - S_2$）。

2. 用有机溶剂分离纯化酶（或蛋白质）时的注意事项

（1）有机溶剂沉淀是个放热过程，所以要在低温下进行，并在加入有机溶剂时溶剂应预冷并注意搅拌均匀，以避免局部浓度过大使酶蛋白变性并应立即离心，不宜放置过久。

（2）溶剂的 pH 值最好控制在被分离物质的等电点附近，以提高被分离物质的分离效果。蛋白质浓度应控制在 5～20mg/ml，以防止高浓度样品的共沉淀作用。

（3）分清实验过程中每次离心后保留的是上清液还是沉淀。

（4）有机溶剂中有中性盐存在时能增加蛋白质的溶解度，减少变性，提高分离效果。中性盐浓度一般在 0.05mol/L 左右为好，过高影响沉淀。

二、碱性磷酸酶米氏常数 K_m 的测定

【实验原理】

AKP 为通过上述实验获得的酶制品。AKP 作用于底物液中的磷酸苯二钠，使之水解释放出酚。酚在碱性溶液中与 AAP 作用，经过铁氰化钾氧化，可以生成红色醌类化合物。以酚作标准液同样处理显色并进行比色，测定酚的生成量，以此为基础计算酶

的活力单位。本法以37℃与底物作用15分钟产生1mg酚为一个酶活力单位。在酶的最适温度和最适pH的条件下，设置不同浓度的磷酸苯二钠为底物。每个底物浓度下的酶活力分别测定3次，然后按双倒数法作图，即可求出AKP的米氏常数K_m值。

【实验材料】

1. **实验器材** 试管、移液管、恒温水浴锅、分光光度计、坐标纸。

2. **实验试剂**

（1）0.04mol/L底物液 称取磷酸苯二钠·$2H_2O$ 10.16g，用煮沸冷却的蒸馏水溶解并稀释至1000ml，加4ml三氯甲烷防腐，贮于棕色瓶内，冰箱冷藏保存，可用1周。

（2）0.1mol/L pH 10碳酸盐缓冲液（含0.3% AAP） 称取AAP 3g，用0.1mol/L pH 10碳酸盐缓冲液溶解并稀释至1000ml，贮于棕色瓶内，冰箱冷藏保存。

（3）酶液 碱性磷酸酶液用0.01mol/L pH 8.8 Tris缓冲液稀释成每毫升含0.8～1.0单位的酶溶液。

【实验步骤】

取干净干燥试管8支，编号，按表20-4操作。

表20-4 碱性磷酸酶K_m的测定反应体系

	1	2	3	4	5	6	S	O
0.04mol/L底物液（ml）	0.1	0.2	0.3	0.4	0.8	1.0		
蒸馏水（ml）	1.4	1.3	1.2	1.1	0.7	0.5	1.5	1.5
含AAP的碳酸盐缓冲液（ml）	1.5	1.5	1.5	1.5	1.5	1.5	1.5	1.5
摇匀，37℃保温5分钟								
0.1mg/ml酚标准液（ml）							0.1	
酶液（ml）	0.1	0.1	0.1	0.1	0.1	0.1		0.1
充分摇匀，37℃准确保温15分钟								
5g/L铁氰化钾（ml）	2.0	2.0	2.0	2.0	2.0	2.0	2.0	2.0

混匀，室温放置15分钟后，以"O"号管调零作为对照，在510nm处测定各管光密度，并填入表20-5，计算有关数据并作图。

表20-5 底物浓度对酶促反应的影响结果

	1	2	3	4	5	6
吸光度						
V						
$1/V$						
$[S]$						
$1/[S]$						

【实验结果】

1. 计算各管的酶活力单位

即代表酶促反应速度 V:

$$(A_{1\sim6}/A_s) \times 0.01$$

2. 计算各管底物浓度 [S]

底物液浓度 × (加底物液体积/酶反应体系总体积) = 0.04 × (加底物液体积/3.1)

3. 计算各管的 1/V 和 1/[S] 值

按 Lineweaver – Burk 法作图，以 $1/[S]$ 为横坐标，$1/V$ 为纵坐标，在方格坐标纸上准确画出各坐标点，连接各点画出直线，向下延长此线与横轴交点即为 $-1/K_m$ 值。计算出该酶的 K_m 值。

【思考题】

1. 将本实验测得的 K_m 值与文献数据相比较，是否存在差异，分析可能的原因?

2. 酶的比活力在酶提取分离过程中的意义。

3. 碱性磷酸酶在科学研究及临床诊断中的应用。

Experiment 20　Separation，Purification of Alkaline Phosphatase and Its Enzymology Study

Purpose

1. To master the related principles of separation and purification of enzyme.

2. To be familiar with the method and procedure of purification of alkaline phosphatase.

3. To master the principle and method of measuring specific activity of alkaline phosphatase.

4. To train the ability of complex utilization of several methods for purifying and identifying specified proteins from tissues.

I. Separation，purification of alkaline phosphatase and measurement of specific activity

Principle

Alkaline phosphatase (alkaline phosphatase, AKP or ALP, EC 3. 1. 3. 1) widely exists in human bodies, animals, plants and microorganisms, and directly participates in the transfer and metabolic processes of phosphate group. AKP is an enzyme which has low substrate specificity, and can hydrolyse many kinds of phosphomonoester compounds, needing Mg^{2+} and Mn^{2+} as activators. The optimal pH range of AKP is 8. 6 ~ 10. Blood serum AKP mainly comes from the liver, and a few from the skeleton.

Most enzymes are proteins, therefore their extraction, separation and purification methods are similar to those of protein. The methods commonly used for protein separation and purification include salt fractionation with neutral salt (as $(NH_4)_2SO_4$ salt fractionation), electrophoresis method (as polyacrylamide gel electrophoresis), chromatography (as sephadex gel chromatography) and organic solvents precipitation (as ethanol, acetone, n-butyl alcohol, etc). Fractional precipitation with organic solvents is one of the methods commonly used for protein isolation. Organic solvents can precipitate most of the water soluble biomacromolecules, mainly through decreasing the dielectric constant of aqueous solution, consequently changing the dissolubility. At the same time, the organic solvents, when dissolving in water, can destroy hydration shell existing on the surface of the macromolecules, which finally assembles and separates the macromolecules through dehydration. For precipitating, different materials needs different concentrations of organic solvent. Different proteins can precipitate and separate in different concentrations of organic solvent. The solvents used for fractionation of biomacromolecules are mainly the organic solvents which can dissolve in water, such as ethanol, methanol and acetone, etc.

In this experiment, we apply organic solvents precipitation to extract and separate AKP from liver homogenate. In the procedure of preparing liver homogenate, using low concentration sodium acetate can ensure the rupture of membrane with hypotension, and magnesium acetate can protect and stabilize AKP. Adding the n-butyl alcohol to homogenate can denature part of the inpurity protein, which can then be removed through filtration. The filtrate including AKP can be further separated and purified by cold acetone and ethanol. According to the property that AKP is solvable in final concentraction of 33% acetone or 30% ethanol, but insolvable in final concentraction of 50% acetone or 60% ethanol, relatively pure AKP can be obtained by means of centrifugation and repeated separation and purification from the filtrate including AKP.

The end point colorimetric method of phenyl sodium phosphate with disodium phenyl phosphate as the substrate is the method mostly used for measuring AKP. Its basic principle is: in determining pH and temperature, the AKP existing in sample can interact with disodium phenyl phosphate, hydrolyse the substrate and produce phenol. The phenol can react with 4-aminoantipyrine (AAP) and be oxidized by $K_3Fe(CN)_6$, generating red quinone compound (for the principle, see the Fig. 20 – 1). Use phenol as the standard solution in the same color reaction and make color matching at 510nm. The enzyme activity can be determined according to the level of red shades, thus the enzyme activity unit can be calculated. This method defines one enzyme activity unit as 1mg phenol produced when tissue protein per gram reacts with substrate for 15min at 37℃. This method is easy to perform. The equipment is simple and has high precision. Hence it is one of the most commonly used in laboratory determination of alkaline phosphatase. The quantification of protein concentration is by Coomassie brilliant blue dye-binding method.

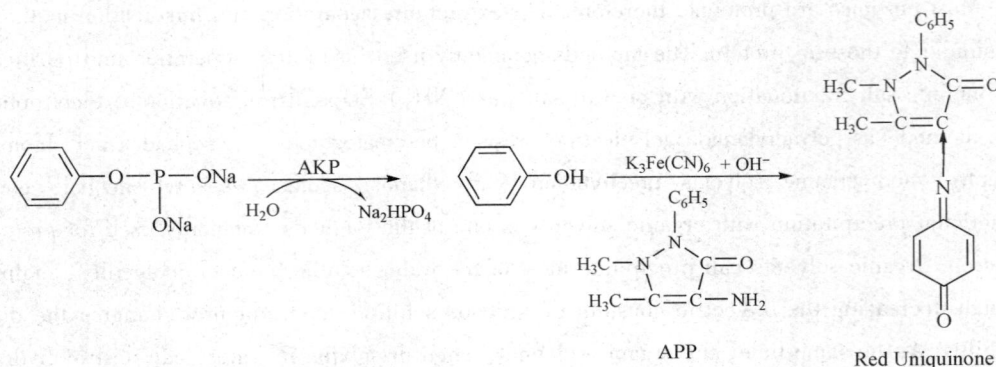

Fig. 20 - 1 The reaction principle of AKP activity measurement

Materials

1. Apparatus

Spectrophotometer, centrifuge, constant temperature water bath, cale centrifuge tube, cylinder, pipette, electronic balance, flask, scissors, homogenizer.

2. Reagents

(1) 0. 1mol/L Sodium acetate solution   Dissolve 8. 2g of sodium acetate in distilled water and dilute to 1000ml.

(2) 0. 5mol/L Magnesium acetate solution   Dissolve 107. 25g of magnesium acetate in distilled water and dilute to 1000ml.

(3) 0. 01mol/L Magnesium acetate – 0. 01mol/L sodium acetate solution   Mix 0. 5mol/L of magnesium acetate 20ml and 0. 1mol/L of sodium acetate 100ml, then dilute with distilled water to 1000ml.

(4) n-Butyl alcohol (A. R.) .

(5) 95% Ethanol (A. R.) .

(6) Acetone (A. R.) .

(7) 0. 01mol/L pH 8. 8 Tris buffer   Dissolve tris hydroxymethyl aminomethane (Tris) 12. 1g, in distilled water and dilute to of 1000ml. This is 0. 1mol/L Tris buffer. Take 0. 1mol/L Tris buffer 100ml, add distilled water (about 700ml), mix with 0. 1mol/L sodium acetate solution 100ml, then adjust pH value to 8. 8 with 1% acetic acid solution, dilute with distilled water to 1000ml.

(8) Standard phenol solution (0. 1mg/ml)   Weigh recrystallization phenol 1. 5g, Dissolve in 0. 1mol/L HCl and dilute to 1000ml as the stock solution. Drip 25ml of the above phenol solution in a 250ml iodometric flask, add 50ml 0. 1mol/L NaOH and heat it to 65℃, then add 0. 1mol/L of iodine solution 25ml, cork the iodometric flask, after 30min, add concentrated hydrochloric acid 5. 0ml, and add 0. 1% starch solution as the indicator. Titrate with 0. 1mol/L standard sodium thiosulfate. The number of phenol mg equivalent to 0. 1mol/L iodine solution per 1ml (iodine 12. 7mg) is: 12. 7 × 94/(3 × 354) = 1. 567. Assume that after the

reaction of 25ml iodine of 0. 1mol/L and 25ml phenol, the remaining iodine is titrated with sodium thiosulfate Xml, so 25ml phenol solution contains phenol $(25 - X) \times 1.567$mg. We can infer the concentration from the phenol stock solution. Finally, the stock solution is diluted to 0. 1mg/ml as the standard solution.

（9）Composite substrate solution　Dissolve 6g dihydrate disodium phenyl phosphate and 3g aminoantipyrine dissolved in cold boiled distilled water respectively, mix the two liquids and dilute to 1000ml, add 4ml chloroform for corrosion prevention. Store the solution in a brown flask in the refrigerator, and the solution is stable for one week. Mixing the solution with equal amounts of 0. 1mol/L pH 10 carbonate buffer solution before using.

（10）5g/L Potassium ferricyanide　Weigh 5g potassium ferricyanide and 15g boric acid , Dissolve in 400ml of distilled water, then mix two liquids, add distilled water to 1000ml, then keep in a brown flask in a darkroom.

（11）0. 1mol/L pH 10 Carbonate buffer　Weigh 6. 3g natrium carbonicum calcinatum and 3. 36g sodium bicarbonate, Dissolve in distilled water and dilute to 1000ml.

（12）Standard protein solution　Dissolve 50mg bovine serum albumin in distilled water, then dilute to 100ml to get the 500μg/ml protein standard solution.

（13）Coomassie brilliant blue G-250 solution　Dissolve 100mg Coomassie billiant blue G-250 in 50ml 95% ethanol, then add 85% (W/V) phosphate solution 100ml, finally dilute to 1000ml.

Procedures

1. Extraction and separation of alkaline phosphatase

（1）Cut 2g of fresh rabbit liver into pieces in a flask, add 2ml 0. 01mol/L magnesium acetate – 0. 01mol/L sodium acetate solution into the scale of centrifugal tube to homogenize （10000r/min for approximately 30s）, then wash the homogenizer with 4ml solution and pour into centrifugal tube. Blend it, and this is solution A. Record the volume. Put 0. 1ml solution A in tubes marked as A^E, then add 4. 9ml 0. 01mol/L pH 8. 8 Tris buffer for the determination of enzyme activity. Put 0. 1ml A solution into another test tube marked as A^P add 4. 9ml physiological saline （0. 9% sodium chloride solution）for the determination of protein concentration.

（2）Add 2ml n-butyl alcohol into the residue of solution A, mix with glass rod for 5min, keep at room temperature for 10min, filter with monolayer filter paper, add the same volume of cold acetone as the filtrate, stir immediately. Centrifuge at 2500r/min for 5min, then discard the supernatant, add 4ml 0. 5mol/L acetic acid magnesium to the precipitate, stir to dissolve the precipitate, shake well. This is solution B. Record the volume, and put 0. 1ml solution B in a test tube marked B^E, then add 2. 9ml 0. 01mol/L pH 8. 8 Tris buffer for the determination of enzyme activity. Put 0. 1ml solution B into another test tube marked B^P, add 1. 9ml physiological saline for the determination of protein concentration.

（3）Add 95% cold ethanol solution to the remaining solution B to the concentration of 30%, mix rapidly, centrifuge at 2500r/min for 5min. Discard the precipitate and add 95%

ethanol solution to the supernatant to the ethanol concentration of 60% , mix rapidly, then centrifuge at 2500r/min for 5min. Discard the supernatant, add 2ml 0.01mol/L magnesium acetate − 0.01mol/L sodium acetate solution to the precipitate, stir the precipitate to dissolve it, and this is solution C. Record the volume, put 0.1ml solution C in a test tube marked C^E, then add 1.9ml 0.01mol/L pH 8.8 Tris buffer for the determination of enzyme activity. Put 0.1ml solution C in another test tube marked C^P, add 0.4ml physiological saline, for the determination of protein concentration.

(4) Add cold acetone to the remaining solution C to the acetone concentration of 33% , centrifuge at 3000r/min for 5min. Discard the precipitate, add cold acetone to the supernatant to the acetone concentration of 50% , mix rapidly, then centrifuge at 3000r/min for 5min. Discard the supernatant, add 5ml 0.01mol/L pH 8.8 Tris buffer to dissolve precipitate, centrifuge at 3000r/min for 5min. Discard the precipitate, and the solution is solution D. Record the volume, put 0.1ml solution D in a test tube marked D^E, then add 0.9ml 0.01mol/L pH 8.8 Tris buffer for the determination of enzyme activity. Put 0.1ml D solution into another test tube marked D^P for the determination of protein concentration.

2. Specific activity assay of alkaline phosphatase

(1) Activity assay of alkaline phosphatase   Number 6 clean test tubes, and operate as Table 20 – 1.

Table 20 – 1   Activity assay of alkaline phosphatase

	O	S	A^E	B^E	C^E	D^E
Different extraction phase of enzyme solution (ml)			0.1	0.1	0.1	0.1
0.1mg/ml Standard phenol solution (ml)		0.1				
0.01mol/L pH 8.8 Tris buffer (ml)	0.1					
Preheat to 37℃ composite substrate solution (ml)	3.0	3.0	3.0	3.0	3.0	3.0

Mix the samples immediately after adding composite substrate solution, leave it at 37℃ in a constant temperature water bath for 15min. After that, add 2ml 5g/L potassium ferricyanide immediately and shake each tube to terminate the enzymatic reaction, leave it there for 15min. After coloring assay the absorbance at 510nm with 721 type spectrophotometer as control with tube "O" . Calculate the enzyme activity unit in each 1ml enzyme liquid.

(2) Quantitate protein concentration   Use the method of Coomassie brilliant blue dye-binding to quantitate protein concentration of the referred solution A, B, C and D. Operate as Table 20 – 2.

Table 20 −2 Quantitate protein concentration

	O	S	A^P	B^P	C^P	D^P
Different protein solution (ml)			0.1	0.1	0.1	0.1
500μg/ml Standard protein solution (ml)		0.1				
Physiological saline (ml)	0.1					
Coomassie brillant blue G-250 (ml)	9.0	9.0	9.0	9.0	9.0	9.0

Mix them up, leave it stand for 5min, measure the value of absorbance at 595nm, while the test tube numbered "O" is control. Calculate the concentration of protein in the sample solution.

Results

1. Calculate of activity unit

$$P = A_E \times m_S \times n / (A_S \times V)$$

In this equation:

P—Activity unit of each milliliter of alkaline phosphatase (U/ml).

A_E—The absorbance of determination tube.

A_S—The absorbance of standard tube.

m_S—Phenol quality of standard tube (mg).

V—The volume of the sample (ml).

n—Dilution multiple.

2. Calculate ratio of enzyme activity

Ratio of alkaline phosphatase activity = Alkaline phosphatase activity unit in each milliliter of sample / The number of milligrams of protein in each milliliter of sample.

3. Calculation of rate

Alkaline phosphatase activity of each stage = Alkaline phosphatase activity in each milliliter of sample unit × sample volume.

Alkaline phosphatase ratio of each stage = Each phase total enzyme activity unit / Enzyme activity unit in homogenate A solution × 100%.

4. Purification of multiples calculation

Multiple purification = Ratio of activity number in each stage / Ratio of activity number in homogenate A solution

Fill the results in Table 20 − 3 according to the above formula.

Table 20 −3 Separation and purification of alkaline phosphatase

Separation phase	Total volume (ml)	Protein concentration (mg/ml)	Total protein (mg)	Every milliliter enzyme unit (U)	Total enzyme activity unit (U)	Ratio of activity (U/mg)	Multiple purification	Rate (%)
Homogenate (A solution)								

(to be continued)

Separation phase	Total volume (ml)	Protein concentration (mg/ml)	Total protein (mg)	Every milliliter enzyme unit (U)	Total enzyme activity unit (U)	Ratio of activity (U/mg)	Multiple purification	Rate (%)
The first acetone precipitation (B solution)								
Ethanol precipitation (C solution)								
The second acetone precipitation (D solution)								

Cautions

1. Formula for adding organic solvent

In order to obtain certain concentration of organic solvent in the original solution during the precipitation, the concentration and volume of the organic solvent to be added can be calculated with the following equation: $V = V_0 (S_2 - S_1) / (100 - S_2)$

In this equation:

V—Volume of the 100% organic solvent to be added.

V_0—Volume of the original solution.

S_1—Concentration of organic solvent in the original solution.

S_2—The concentration of organic solvent to be obtained.

100—The concentration of organic solvent added is 100%. If the concentration of organic solvent is 95%, $(100 - S_2)$ in the equation should be replaced by $(95 - S_2)$.

2. Attention must be paid to the following while purifying enzyme or protein with organic solvents

(1) The organic solvent precipitation is an exothermic chemical process, so it should be conducted in the low temperature. The organic solvent added should be precooled. And stirred well in case local concentration is too great to cause the enzyme protein denaturation. It should be immediately centrifuged and should not be placed for too long.

(2) The solvent pH value should be perfectly controlled near the separated material's electricity point in order to improve the separation efficiency of the separated material. The protein concentration should be controlled at 5 ~ 20mg/ml in order to prevent the high concentration of samples of precipitation role.

(3) Distinguish between supernatant and precipitate from retentate after each centrifugation during the experiment.

(4) Organic solvents containing neutral salt can increase the solubility of protein, reduce degeneration and improve the separation effect. Because too much neutral salt affects precipitation, usually the neutral salt concentration is in 0.05mol/L or so.

II. Determination of AKP's Michaelis-Menton constant K_m

Principle

AKP are enzymatic products obtained by above-mentioned experiment. The AKP can interact with disodium phenyl phosphate, hydrolyse the substrate and produce phenol. The phenol can react with 4-aminoantipyrine (AAP) and be oxidized by $K_3Fe(CN)_6$, generate red quinone compound. Using phenol as the standard solution and treating with the same method, measure the quantity of phenol on this basis to calculate enzymatic activity unit. In this method, per mg of tissue protein reacts with substrate for 15min at 37℃, 1mg phenol has been produced, which is defined an enzyme activity unit. In the condition of optimal temperature and pH for enzyme, set different concentrations of disodium phenyl phosphate as the substrate. The enzyme activity of each substrate concentration is measured three times, then plotted in double reciprocal method and the AKP's Michaelis-Menton constant K_m values can be calculated.

Materials

1. Apparatus

Test tube, pipette, constant temperature water bath, spectrophotometer, coordinate paper.

2. Reagents

(1) 0.04mol/L Substrate solution　Add 10.16g dihydrate disodium phenyl phosphate to 1L cooled boiled distilled water, add 4ml chloroform for corrosion protection, store in a brown bottle, in refrigerator at 4℃ and the solution is stable for one week.

(2) 0.1mol/L Carbonate buffer (pH 10, including 0.3% AAP)　Add 3g AAP to 1L 0.1mol/L carbonate buffer (pH 10), store in a brown bottle in refrigerator at 4℃.

(3) Enzyme solution　Alkaline phosphatase solution is diluted with 0.01mol/L pH 8.8 Tris buffer to make it 0.8 to 1.0 units per 1ml of enzyme solution.

Procedures

Take 8 clean and dry test tubes, number them, and operate according to Table 20-4.

Table 20-4　Determination of AKP's K_m

	1	2	3	4	5	6	S	O
0.04mol/L Substrate solution (ml)	0.1	0.2	0.3	0.4	0.8	1.0		
Distilled water (ml)	1.4	1.3	1.2	1.1	0.7	0.5	1.5	1.5
Carbonate buffer including AAP (ml)	1.5	1.5	1.5	1.5	1.5	1.5	1.5	1.5
Shake up, incubate at 37℃ for 5min								
0.1mg/ml Phenol standard solution (ml)							0.1	
Enzyme solution (ml)	0.1	0.1	0.1	0.1	0.1	0.1		0.1
Shake up thoroughly, incubate at 37℃ for 5min accurately								
5g/L $K_3Fe(CN)_6$ (ml)	2.0	2.0	2.0	2.0	2.0	2.0	2.0	2.0

Mixing and standing for 15min at room temperature, then reset the "O" tube as control and determine the optical density of each tube at 510nm, filling in Table 20 – 5, calculating the data and plotting.

Table 20 – 5 Substrate concentration on enzymatic reaction

	1	2	3	4	5	6
Absorbance						
V						
$1/V$						
$[S]$						
$1/[S]$						

Results

1. Calculating the enzymatic activity of each tube

As that represents reaction rate V: $(A_{1\sim6}/A_s) \times 0.01$.

2. Calculating each substrate concentration $[S]$

Substrate solution concentration × (volume of added substrate solution / Total volume of enzyme reaction system) = 0.04 × (Volume of added substrate solution / 3.1)

3. Calculating the values of $1/V$ and $1/[S]$ of each tube

Setting $1/[S]$ as x-axis, $1/V$ as y-axis, drawing each coordinate point in the grid graph paper accurately, connecting every point to draw a straight line, downward extension of this line and the intersection with the horizontal axis is the value of $-1/K_m$. Calculating the K_m value of this enzyme.

Questions

1. Compare the K_m value of this experiment with literature data, and see whether there exists any difference. What is the possible reason?

2. Describe the significance of the specific activity of the enzyme in its extraction and separation process.

3. Describe the applications of alkaline phosphatase in scientific research and clinical diagnosis.

实验二十一　香菇多糖的制备及初步分析

【实验目的】

1. 掌握多糖含量测定及组成分析的一般方法。
2. 了解真菌多糖分离纯化的基本原理。

【实验原理】

香菇（*Lentinus edodes*）是中国及其他东亚国家广泛栽培的食用真菌之一，不但含有丰富的营养，而且含有多种有效药用组分。研究表明，香菇多糖具有抗氧化、抗肿瘤、抗衰老、免疫调制、抗病毒和抗动脉硬化等作用。香菇多糖是一种以 $\beta-D$（$1\rightarrow3$）- 葡萄糖残基为主链，侧链为 $\beta-D$（$1\rightarrow6$）- 葡萄糖残基的聚糖，其糖成分还包括甘露糖和木糖。香菇多糖对光和热稳定，在水中最大溶解度为 3mg/ml，不溶于甲醇、乙醇、乙醚、丙酮等有机溶剂。

热水浸提法是多糖提取常用的方法之一。苯酚 - 硫酸试剂与游离寡糖、多糖中的己糖、糖醛酸起显色反应，己糖在 490nm 处有最大吸收，吸收值与糖含量呈线性关系。多糖在浓硫酸中保温一定时间可完全水解为单糖，通过纸层析分离，特定试剂显色后与已知糖的标准混合物作对比，可以鉴定多糖水解产物中单糖的组成。

本实验采用热水浸提法从香菇子实体获取香菇多糖，三氯甲烷 - 正丁醇法脱蛋白质，乙醇沉淀，苯酚 - 硫酸法测定糖含量。酸水解香菇多糖，通过纸层析鉴定其单糖组成。

【实验材料】

1. 实验器材　烧杯、水浴锅、透析袋、磁力搅拌器、离心机、真空干燥器、分光光度计、容量瓶、移液管、水解管、滤纸、玻璃毛细管、层析缸、喷雾器。

2. 实验试剂

（1）香菇子实体。

（2）98% 的浓硫酸，95% 乙醇，无水乙醇，乙醚，过氧化氢，氢氧化钠，五氧化二磷，碳酸钡。

（3）80% 苯酚　80g 苯酚加 20ml 水使之溶解，置冰箱中避光贮存。

（4）6% 苯酚　临用前用 80% 苯酚配制。

（5）三氯甲烷 - 正丁醇溶液　4:1（V/V）。

（6）2mol/L 氢氧化钠　4g 氢氧化钠溶于蒸馏水中，定容到 50ml。

（7）标准葡萄糖溶液（0.1mg/ml）　精确称取 100mg 葡萄糖（预先在 105℃ 干燥至恒重），用蒸馏水溶解，定容至 1L。

（8）1mol/L 硫酸　1ml 98% 的浓硫酸加入到 17ml 蒸馏水中。

（9）展层剂　正丁醇 - 醋酸 - 水（4:1:5，V/V）（上层）。

（10）显色剂　苯胺 - 邻苯二甲酸 - 正丁醇饱和水溶液　将 1.6g 邻苯二甲酸溶于 100ml 水饱和的正丁醇溶液中，再向溶液中加入 0.93g（相当于 0.9ml）苯胺。

【实验步骤】

1. 香菇多糖的制备

（1）材料预处理　取干香菇 100g，用水浸泡 2h，剪碎。

（2）提取　将剪碎的香菇置烧杯中，加入 600ml 蒸馏水，沸水浴搅拌提取 3h，3000r/min 离心 20 分钟，以除去残渣。

（3）浓缩　上清液 80℃ 水浴浓缩至 120ml。

（4）脱蛋白　加入 1/4 体积的三氯甲烷 - 正丁醇溶液，剧烈振荡 30 分钟，3000r/min 离心 10 分钟，取上层液置于新的离心管中，重复脱蛋白质两次。

（5）脱色　上层液用 2mol/L NaOH 调节 pH 至 7.0，加入 H_2O_2 至体积分数为 7%，搅拌脱色 3 小时。

（6）透析　流水透析 12 小时，蒸馏水透析 24 小时。

（7）沉淀　透析液 80℃ 水浴浓缩至 120ml，边搅拌边加入 3 倍体积的 95% 乙醇，静置 12 小时，离心 3000r/min，20 分钟。

（8）干燥　沉淀用 95% 乙醇、无水乙醇、乙醚依次洗涤，置于盛有五氧化二磷及氢氧化钠的真空干燥器内干燥。

2. 香菇多糖含量测定

（1）标准曲线制作　取 9 支干燥试管，按表 21-1 操作。

表 21-1　标准曲线制作

管　号	0	1	2	3	4	5	6	7	8
标准葡萄糖溶液（ml）	0.0	0.4	0.6	0.8	1.0	1.2	1.4	1.6	1.8
蒸馏水（ml）	2.0	1.6	1.4	1.2	1.0	0.8	0.6	0.4	0.2
6% 苯酚（ml）	1.0	1.0	1.0	1.0	1.0	1.0	1.0	1.0	1.0
浓硫酸（ml）	5.0	5.0	5.0	5.0	5.0	5.0	5.0	5.0	5.0
静止 10 分钟，摇匀，室温放置 20 分钟									
A_{490}									

横坐标为糖微克数，纵坐标为 490nm 吸光度，绘制标准曲线。

（2）样品测定　精确称取香菇多糖干品 50mg，加少量热水溶解后定容至 500ml。取 1.0ml（相当于约 100μg 的多糖），按标准曲线制作的方法操作，测 490nm 光密度。计算多糖含量及香菇多糖制品的纯度。

（3）计算

$$糖含量（\%）= m/(c_0 V) \times 100\%$$

式中，m——由标准曲线查得的糖微克数（μg）；

c_0——样品溶液的浓度（0.1mg/ml）；

V——测定时用的样品溶液体积（1.0ml）。

3. 香菇多糖的单糖组分鉴定

（1）完全酸水解　称取 20mg 多糖样品，加入 1mol/L H_2SO_4 2ml；封管，100℃ 水解 8 小时，然后加入 $BaCO_3$ 中和，定量滤纸过滤，滤液留作分析。

（2）纸层析　将层析滤纸剪成 7cm×40cm 的纸条，距层析滤纸一端 2cm 处画一横线作为点样线，在点样线上画两个点分别作为标准糖溶液和多糖水解液的点样位置。用玻璃毛细管点样，斑点尽可能小，而且每点 1 滴，待点样点干燥后，在同一位置再点第二滴，然后将滤纸条悬挂于层析缸中进行层析，展层时间约为 36 小时。将滤纸取出，自然干燥，喷上苯胺 - 邻苯二甲酸 - 正丁醇饱和水溶液，100℃ 条件下 15 分钟即可显色。标准单糖混合物色斑在滤纸上由下而上的顺序是：半乳糖、葡萄糖、甘露糖、阿拉伯糖。与标准单糖混合物色斑比较，即可判断多糖样品的单糖组成。

【思考题】

1. 除苯酚 - 硫酸法外，还有哪些方法可以测定多糖的糖含量？

2. 设计一种实验方法，对所获得的香菇多糖进行精制。

Experiment 21   Preparation and Primary Analysis of Lentinan

Purpose

1. To master the general methods of content determination and composition identification of polysaccharide.

2. To understand the basic principle of seperation and purification of fungus polysaccharide.

Principle

Lentinus edodes, a valuable edible fungus, has been widely cultivated in China and other East Asian countries for centuries, and its importance is attributed to both its nutritional value and medical application. Studies have demonstrated that lentinan exhibits multiple bioactivities, including anti-oxidation, anti-tumor, anti-aging, immunoregulation, antiviral, reducing blood fat and resisting arteriosclerosis etc. The reported structure of lentinan comprises β-1,3-linked-D-glucose with β-1,6 branches. Mannose and xylose are also the monosaccharide compositions of lentinan. Lentinan is stable to light and heat, its solubility in water can be 3mg/ml, while the polysaccharide can not dissolve in organic solvents, such as methanol, alcohol, ether and acetone.

Usually, polysaccharides can be extracted by solvent extraction method using hot water. Phenol-sulfuric acid reagents can react with free oligosaccharide and alduronic acid or hexose in polysaccharide. After the reaction, the solution has the maximum absorption at 490nm (hexose), at which the relationship between absorbance and the content of polysaccharide takes on linearity in definite range. Polysaccharide can be completely hydrolyzed at definite temperature in concentrated sulfuric acid for enough time. Separate the hydrolysate with paper chromatography, and separated monosaccharide can form colored compound with definite chromogenic reagent. Compare with standard saccharide, the composition of monosaccharide in polysaccharide hydrolysate can be determined.

Here we will extract lentinan from the fruiting bodies of *Lentinus edodes* by using hot water. Chloroform-*n*-butanol method is used to remove the protein and ethanol is used to separate the precipitate. Phenol-sulfuric acid method is used to determine the content of saccharide. After acid hydrolysis, the monosaccharide composition of lentinan is identified with paper chromatography.

Materials

1. Apparatus

Flask, water bath, dialysis bag, magnetic stirring apparatus, centrifuge, vacuum desiccators, spectrophotometer, volumetric flask, pipette, ampoule, filter paper, glass capillaries, developing tank, vaporization.

2. Reagents

(1) Fruiting body of *Lentinus edodes*   100g.

（2）98% Concentrated sulfuric acid, 95% alcohol, absolute alcohol, ether, hydrogen peroxide, sodium hydroxide, phosphorus pentoxide, barium carbonate.

（3）80% Phenol Dissolve 80g of phenol into 20ml water, the solution can be stock-piled in the darkness in refrigerator for a long time.

（4）6% Phenol Dilute with 80% phenol on the day needed.

（5）Chloroform-n-butanol 4∶1（V/V）.

（6）2mol/L Sodium hydroxide Dissolve 4g sodium hydroxide in distilled water, and di-lute it to 50ml with distilled water.

（7）Standard glucose solution（0.1mg/ml） Dissolve 100mg of glucose in distilled wa-ter, and dilute it to 1L with distilled water.

（8）1mol/L Sulfuric acid Add 1ml 98% concentrated sulfuric acid into 17ml distilled water.

（9）Develop reagent n-Butanol∶acetic acid∶water =4∶1∶5（V/V）（upper phase）.

（10）Chromogenic reagent Water saturation solution of anilin-phthalic acid-n-buta-nol. Dissolve 1.6g phthalic acid in 100ml water with saturate n-butanol, then add 0.93g of（e-qual to 0.9ml）anilin to the solution.

Procedures

1. Preparation of lentinan

（1）Material preparation Cut up 100g *Lentinus edodes* into tiny pieces after soaking it in distilled water for 2h.

（2）Extraction Put the *Lentinus edodes* and 600ml distilled water in a flask, stir while heating in boiling water for 3h. Remove the residue by centrifugation at 3000r/min for 20min.

（3）Concentration Concentrate the supernatant in 80℃ water till its volume decreases to 120ml.

（4）Deprotein Add 1/4 volume chloroform-n-butanol to the concentrated solution, vi-brate it strongly for 30min, then centrifuge the mixture at 3000r/min for 10min and pipette the upper layer solution. Put the upper layer solution into another centrifuge tube and repeat the deprotein operation twice.

（5）Decolorize Adjust the pH of upper layer solution to 7.0 with 2mol/L NaOH. Add H_2O_2 to the solution till the volume fraction is 7% and stir the solution for 3h.

（6）Dialysis Dialyze the solution with running tap water for 12h and distilled water for 24h.

（7）Precipitation Concentrate the dialysate in 80℃ water till its volume decreases to 120ml. Stir the solution while adding triple volume of 95% alcohol. Let the mixture stand for 12h before the centrifugation（3000r/min, 20min）.

（8）Drying Wash the precipitate with 95% alcohol, absolute alcohol and ether succes-sively, then dry the precipitate in a vacuum desiccator with P_2O_5 and NaOH.

2. Quantitation of lentinan

(1) Drawing standard curve   Prepare 9 dry test tubes and operate as Table 21 – 1.

Table 21 –1   Drawing standard curve

Tube No.	0	1	2	3	4	5	6	7	8
Standard glucose solution（ml）	0.0	0.4	0.6	0.8	1.0	1.2	1.4	1.6	1.8
Distilled water（ml）	2.0	1.6	1.4	1.2	1.0	0.8	0.6	0.4	0.2
6% Phenol（ml）	1.0	1.0	1.0	1.0	1.0	1.0	1.0	1.0	1.0
Concentrated sulfuric acid（ml）	5.0	5.0	5.0	5.0	5.0	5.0	5.0	5.0	5.0
	Place Statically for 10min, shake evenly and place at room temperature for 20min.								
A_{490}									

Draw the calibration curve while the optical density is y-axis, the content of polysaccharide is x-axis.

(2) Quantitation of saccharide   Dissolve 50mg of lentinan in hot water and dilute with water to 500ml. Pipette 1.0ml sample (equal to 100μg polysaccharide), and perform as described above, determine the optical density at 490nm. Calculate the content of saccharide of the sample solution according to the optical density of sample solution and the calibration curve.

(3) Calculation   Saccharide content（%）$= m / (c_0 \times V) \times 100\%$

In this equation：

m—Saccharide content looked up from standard curve（μg）.

c_0—Sample concentration（0.1mg/ml）.

V—Sample volume（1.0ml）.

3. Identification of monosaccharide composition of lentinan

(1) Complete acid hydrolysis   Weight 20mg of the polysaccharide sample, add 2ml of 1mol/L H_2SO_4 in an ampoule and seal it, hydrolyze at 100℃ for 8h. Neutralize with $BaCO_3$, filter and collect the filtrate for sugar analysis.

(2) Paper chromatography   Cut chromatography filter paper into 7cm×40cm pieces. Draw a line as spotting end 2cm near the edge. Draw two spots on the line as spotting location of standard saccharide solution and hydrolysate respectively. Spot the solution on the filter paper with glass capillary; the spot should be as small as possible. Dry the spot in the air and then spot the same solution again at the same location. Hang the filter paper inside chromatography tank and develop for 36h, take out the paper and dry in the air. Spray water saturation solution of anilin-phthalic-n-butanol on the filter paper. Dry 15min at 100℃ till the color spot emerge. The upward sequence of standard monosaccharide sample spot is：galactose, glucose, mannose, arabinose. Compare with color spots of standard saccharide, sample composition can be determined.

Questions

1. What other ways can be used to determine the content of polysaccharide except for Phenol-sulfuric acid method?

2. Design an experiment about the further purification of the lentinan prepared in this work.

实验二十二　激素对血糖浓度的影响

【实验目的】

1. 掌握胰岛素和肾上腺素调节血糖水平的作用机制。

2. 熟悉邻甲苯胺法测定血糖浓度的原理与操作。

【实验原理】

正常人的血糖水平相对恒定，这种恒定是通过血糖的来源和去路的调节维持的。影响血糖水平的因素很多，最重要的因素是激素的调节。激素水平的变化主导着血糖水平。在调节血糖的激素中，胰岛素是体内唯一能降低血糖的激素。其他多种激素则具有升高血糖的作用，如肾上腺素、胰高血糖素、肾上腺皮质激素、生长素等，其中以肾上腺素作用较为迅速而明显。本实验给两只家兔分别注射胰岛素和肾上腺素，取注射前、后家兔的静脉血，测定血糖含量，比较注射前后血糖浓度变化，从而验证胰岛素和肾上腺素对血糖浓度的影响。本实验测定血糖的方法采用邻甲苯胺法。

【实验材料】

1. **实验器材**　注射器、微量移液器、移液管、台式磅秤、刀片、试管及试管架、烧杯、分光光度计、恒温水浴箱、离心机。

2. **实验试剂**

（1）胰岛素注射液（4U/ml）　取40U/ml胰岛素注射液1ml，用pH 2.5～3.5的酸性生理盐水（0.9%氯化钠溶液）配制成4U/ml。

（2）肾上腺素（1mg/ml）　纯药用pH 2.5～3.5的酸性生理盐水配制。

（3）抗凝剂（肝素或氟化钠）。

（4）标准葡萄糖贮存液（55.6mmol/L）　将葡萄糖置于硫酸干燥器内过夜，精确称取葡萄糖100.0mg，于100ml容量瓶内以0.02mol/L苯甲酸溶液稀释至刻度，置冰箱中可长期保存。

（5）标准葡萄糖应用液（8.3mmol/L）　取15.0ml标准葡萄糖储存液放于100ml容量瓶内，用0.02mol/L苯甲酸溶液稀释至刻度。

（6）0.02mol/L苯甲酸溶液　称取苯甲酸2.5g，加入蒸馏水1000ml中，加热溶解，冷却后盛于试剂瓶中。

（7）邻甲苯胺试剂　称取硫脲2.5g溶于冰醋酸700ml中，将此溶液转入1000ml容量瓶内，加邻甲苯胺150ml，2.4%硼酸溶液100ml，用冰醋酸定容至1000ml刻度，充分混匀后置棕色瓶中保存。

【实验步骤】

1. 动物及血样品处理

（1）取禁食 16 小时以上的健康家兔两只，称体重并记录。

（2）取空腹血 兔耳缘静脉靠近耳根部分周围去毛，用乙醇棉球擦拭，扩张血管，再用干棉球擦干，用刀片刺破或纵向划破耳缘静脉取血，将血液收集入抗凝瓶中，边收集边摇匀，以防血液凝固。每只家兔取血 2～3ml，分别标注为 "肾上腺素注射前" 和 "胰岛素注射前"。采血后用干棉球压迫血管止血。

（3）注射激素 取血后，分别向两只兔子臀部皮下或腹部皮下注射激素。一只注射胰岛素，剂量为 0.5ml/kg 体重；另一只注射肾上腺素，剂量为 0.4ml/kg 体重。分别记录注射时间。

（4）取注射激素后血样 注射激素 30 分钟后，再次取血 2～3ml 于另两只抗凝瓶中，分别标注为 "肾上腺素注射后" 和 "胰岛素注射后"。取血方法同上。也可采用心脏取血。

（5）血样品离心 取血后及时离心，3000r/min 离心 5 分钟，分离出血浆用于血糖测定。

2. 血糖测定

（1）测定 取洁净大试管 6 只，编号，按下表 22 - 1 加入试剂。

表 22 - 1 血糖含量的测定

试剂（ml）	肾上腺素注射前	肾上腺素注射后	胰岛素注射前	胰岛素注射后	标准管	空白管
血浆	0.1	0.1	0.1	0.1		
标准葡萄糖应用液					0.1	
蒸馏水						0.1
邻甲苯胺试剂	5.0	5.0	5.0	5.0	5.0	5.0

混匀各管后，置沸水浴加热 15 分钟后取出，流水冷却，以空白管调零，630nm 波长下，分别测各测定管和标准管的吸光度（A 值）。

（2）结果计算 分别计算肾上腺素注射前、肾上腺素注射后，胰岛素注射前、胰岛素注射后的血糖值。

计算出注射胰岛素后血糖降低和注射肾上腺素后血糖增高的百分率。

$$血糖改变百分率（\%）= \frac{\Delta BS}{注射前 BS} \times 100\%$$

【注意事项】

（1）尽量选取个头较大、耳静脉血管较粗的家兔，取血前让兔子充分活动，双手充分揉搓兔子耳朵，以加速血液循环，便于取血。

（2）取血及注射激素时，应尽可能使家兔保持安静状态。

（3）用刀片垂直于血管流向，割或挑破血管，不要用力过猛，否则易割断耳朵，一只手按住耳缘根部血管的回流方向，让血液滴到抗凝瓶中，接血的过程中要经常轻晃小瓶，以防血液凝固，取血过程尽量迅速，操作时间过长也容易造成溶血。

（4）注射胰岛素时务必严格按家兔体重计算所需激素的量，否则可能因血糖过低引起痉挛，发生胰岛素性休克，直至死亡。

（5）离心后取血浆时要缓慢仔细，勿吸取下层红细胞。

【思考题】

1. 简述血糖的来源与去路。
2. 正常人如何维持血糖水平的恒定？
3. 简述肾上腺素和胰岛素调节血糖浓度的作用机制。

Experiment 22　Effects of Hormone on Blood Sugar Concentration

Purpose

1. To master the mechanism of regulation of insulin and epinephrine on blood glucose level.

2. Be familliar with the principle and operation of measurement of blood glucose concentration with *o*-Toluidine method.

Principle

Normal blood glucose level is relatively constant, which is regulate by the source and the way of blood glucose. Many factors affect the blood glucose level, the most important of which is hormone, the changes of hormone levels dominate blood sugar levels. Of all the hormones to regulate blood sugar, insulin is the only one in the body that can decrease the blood sugar hormone. Many other hormones can elevate blood sugar, such as epinephrine, glucagon, adrenal cortical hormone, growth hormone etc. , among which the effect of adrenaline is more rapid and significant.

In this experiment, two rabbits are injected with insulin or epinephrine, and their venous blood will be taken before and after the injection to determine the blood sugar levels and compare blood glucose concentration changes, so as to verify the effects of insulin and epinephrine on blood sugar concentration. The *o*-Toluidine method will be used to determine the concentration of glucose in this experiment.

Materials

1. Apparatus

Injector, micropipette, pipette, bench scale, blade, test tubes and test tube shelf, flask, spectrophotometer, constant temperature water bath, centrifuge.

2. Reagents

（1）Insulin solution for injection （4U/ml）　Take 40U/ml insulin solution and dilute it with acidic physiological saline pH 2. 5 ~ 3. 5.

（2）Epinephrine （1mg/ml）　Make with acidic physiological saline pH 2. 5 ~ 3. 5.

（3）Anticoagulantion solution （heparin or sodium fluoride）.

（4）Standard glucose stock solution （55. 6mmol/L）　Place the glucose in the sulfuric acid dryer overnight. Then weigh accurately 100. 0mg glucose and dilute with 0. 02mol/L benzoic acid solution to 100ml. The solution can be stored in refrigerator for a long time.

（5）Standard glucose application solution（8. 3mmol/L）　Put 15. 0ml standard glucose storage solution to a 100ml volumetric flask, and dilute it to the scale with 0. 02mol/L benzoic acid solution.

（6）0. 02mol/L Benzoic acid solution　Weigh 2. 5g benzoic acid into 1000ml distilled water. After heated, dissolved and cooled, the solution is placed in a reagent bottle.

（7）*o*-Toluidine reagent　Weigh 2. 5g thiourea into 700ml glacial acetic acid. Transfer into a 1000ml volumetric flask , the solution is added with 150ml *o*-toluidine, 100ml 2. 4% boric acid solution and dilute with acetic acid to the scale. After fully mixed, the solution is stored in amber bottle.

Procedures

1. Treatment of animals and blood samples

（1）Take two healthy rabbits which have fasted for over 16h, weigh them and record.

（2）Fasting blood　Cut the hair around the vein of rabbit ear, wipe with alcohol cotton, dilate blood vessels and wipe with cotton again. Use a blade to perforate or cut longitudinally the vein of the ear to take blood, collect the blood into anticoagulant bottle and shake to prevent blood coagulation. 2 ~ 3ml blood are collected form each rabbit and labled labeled as "before adrenaline injection" and "before insulin injection" respectively. After blood collection, vessels are oppressed with dry cotton to stop bleeding.

（3）The hormone injection　After taking blood, the two rabbits are injected hormone through gluteal subcutaneous or abdominal subcutaneous. One with insulin（0. 5ml/kg）, the other with epinephrine（0. 4ml/kg）. Record the injection time.

（4）Blood sample after the injection of hormone　Through 30min after injection of the hormone, take 2 ~ 3ml blood again in the other two anticoagulant bottles labeled as "after adrenaline injection" and "after insulin injection". Blood as above. Heart blood may also be used.

（5）Centrifugation of blood samples　Blood is centrifuged promptly for 5min at 3000r/min, and then plasma is separated for the determination of glucose.

2. Measurement of blood glucose

（1）Measurement　Number six clean dry tubes, and add reagents as Table 21 – 1.

Table 22 – 1　The content of blood glucose measurement

Reagent（ml）	Before epinephrine injection	After epinephrine injection	Before insulin injection	After insulin injection	Standard tube	Blank tube
Blood plasma	0. 1	0. 1	0. 1	0. 1		
Standard glucose solution					0. 1	

(to be continued)

Reagent (ml)	Before epinephrine injection	After epinephrine injection	Before insulin injection	After insulin injection	Standard tube	Blank tube
Distilled water						0.1
o-Toluidine reagent	5.0	5.0	5.0	5.0	5.0	5.0

After mixing the tube, heating in boiling water bath and water cooling. After setting zero with blank tube, the measuring tube and standard tube are measured at a wavelength of 630nm (A value).

(2) The results of calculation   Calculate blood sugar levels before and after the injection of epinephrine and insulin respectively.

Calculate the percentage of blood glucose decrease after epinephrine injection and blood glucose increase after insulin injection.

$$\text{Percentage of blood glucose change (\%)} = \frac{\Delta BS}{BS \text{ before injection}} \times 100\%$$

Cautions

1. Try to choose the larger size rabbit having thicker ear vein. Before taking blood, let rabbits make full activity. Rubbing rabbit's ear to accelerate blood circulation in order to take blood easily.

2. When takeing blood and injecting hormone, keep rabbits quiet as far as possible.

3. When using a blade to perforate or cut longitudinally the vein of the ear to take blood, don't put too much force so as not to cut off ear. One hand holds the reflux direction of vein to let blood drip into the anticoagulant bottle. Shake the bottle in the process of collecting blood in case of blood clotting. Taking blood should be quick as soon as possible in case of hemolysis.

4. Insulin injection must be in strict calculation on the required amount of hormone accordance with the rabbit body weight, otherwise spasm may caused by low blood sugar, insulin shock, until death.

5. After centrifugation, the plasma must be collected slowly and carefully, and do not absorb the lower red cell.

Questions

1. Describe the source and the way of blood glucose.

2. How to maintain a constant normal blood glucose level?

3. Describe the mechanism of epinephrine and insulin regulating blood glucose concentration.

实验二十三　降钙素基因在大肠埃希菌中的重组表达

【实验目的】

1. 掌握大肠埃希菌感受态细胞的制备及重组质粒转化。
2. 掌握碱变性法提取质粒 DNA 的原理和相关技术。
3. 学习外源基因在原核细胞中表达的过程及特点。

一、细菌感受态的制备及重组表达载体的转化

【实验原理】

基因工程的主要操作过程如下：寻找目的基因→目的基因与载体的酶切→酶切产物连接→重组载体转化宿主细胞→筛选并验证阳性转化子→诱导表达并验证目的产物。

本实验以载有人降钙素基因的 pET－32a－c（＋）的重组载体为材料，转化大肠埃希菌 BL21（DE3）。

感受态是指菌体生长到一定时期所出现的一种能够接受外源目的基因的状态。自然状态下转化率极低，因此在生物技术操作中经常需人工诱导，以使转化效率大大提高。细菌在 4℃和低渗溶液中膨胀成球形，转化的 DNA 与溶液中的 Ca^{2+} 形成羟基磷酸钙复合物黏附于细胞表面，经 42℃短时间热冲击处理，促进细胞吸收 DNA 复合物，在培养基上培养数小时后，球形细胞复原并进行增殖。$CaCl_2$ 处理的感受态细胞，一般每微克 DNA 能获得 $10^5 \sim 10^6$ 个转化子（即转化率），重组子越小，转化率越高。环状 DNA 分子比线性 DNA 转化率高 1000 倍。加二价阳离子（如 Mn^{2+}，Co^{2+}）、DMSO 或还原剂，可提高转化率。

【实验材料】

1. **实验菌株与载体**　pET－32a－hCT 重组质粒，大肠埃希菌 BL21（DE3），质粒 pET－32a－c（＋）。

2. **实验器材**　恒温水浴锅，微量移液器，离心机，恒温震荡培养箱，超净台。

灭菌材料见表 23－1。

表 23－1　灭菌材料

仪器名称	规格	数量
培养皿	直径 10cm	4
锥形瓶	250ml	2
枪头	10μl、200μl、1000μl	若干
Eppendorf 管	1.5ml	若干
T_1 buffer	1×	10ml
T_2 buffer	1×	10ml
三角耙		4
接种环		2

3. 实验试剂

（1）常规试剂 见表23-2。

表23-2 常规试剂

试剂	T_1缓冲液（mmol/L）	T_2缓冲液（mmol/L）
NaCl	10	
$MnCl_2$	50	100
NaAc - HCl pH 5.6	10	10
$CaCl_2$		75

（2）LB 培养基配方（100ml） 见表23-3。

表23-3 LB 培养基配方

试剂	用量（g）
胰蛋白胨	1.0
酵母提取物	0.5
NaCl	1.0

用2mol/L NaOH 调 pH 至7.2~7.4，121℃高压蒸汽灭菌20分钟，LB 液体培养基中加入1.5%琼脂粉即为LB 固体培养基。

【实验步骤】

（1）取保存的菌种 BL21（DE3）进行菌落画线，待长出后（12~16h）挑取单菌落接入20ml LB 培养基，于37℃下220r/min 培养过夜（12~16h）。

（2）按1∶100的比例将过夜培养菌液接种至20ml LB 培养基中，37℃下220r/min 培养至 OD_{650} 为0.4~0.5（大约3小时）。

（3）取上述菌液1.5ml 于 Eppendorf 管中，共4管，将其置于冰浴冷却，然后于3500r/min 离心3分钟，弃去上清液。

（4）向 Eppendorf 管中加入 T_1 缓冲液300μl，用枪头冲匀菌体后，置于冰浴20分钟，然后于3500r/min 离心3分钟，将上清弃去。

（5）向 Eppendorf 管中加入 T_2 缓冲液30μl，用枪头混匀菌体后，按表23-4加入各溶液，分散均匀后置于冰浴30分钟，42℃水浴（静置）90s，转置冰浴1~2分钟。

（6）向 Eppendorf 管中加入1.0ml LB 液体培养基置于37℃静置培养45分钟，于3000r/min 离心2分钟，取出上清液850μl，用枪头混匀余下的菌体后，涂于 LB + 抗生素（氨苄西林100μg/ml）琼脂固体平板培养基，于37℃下倒置培养过夜（最多不超过16 小时）。

【实验结果】

取出培养皿观察菌落生长情况，将每皿菌落数记录于表23-4。

表 23 – 4　实验结果记录

培养皿编号	菌落数
阴性对照（1μl 水）	
阳性对照 [1μl pET – 32a – c（+）]	
1μl 重组载体	
2μl 重组载体	

【注意事项】

（1）感受态细胞制备过程中应密切观察细菌的生长状态和密度，尽量使用对数生长期的细胞。

（2）所有操作均应在无菌条件和冰浴中进行。

二、PCR 方法验证重组克隆

具体内容见实验十四 PCR 扩增 DNA 及实验十二琼脂糖凝胶电泳。

【实验结果】

PCR 反应样品经琼脂糖凝胶电泳，溴化乙锭（EB）染色，观察 DNA 条带。

三、碱变性法提取质粒 DNA

【实验原理】

碱变性法提取质粒 DNA 是基于染色体 DNA 与质粒 DNA 的变性与复性的差异而达到分离目的的。在 pH 高达 12.6 的碱性条件下，染色体 DNA 的氢键断裂，双螺旋结构解开而变性。质粒 DNA 的大部分氢键也断裂，但超螺旋共价闭合环状的两条互补链不会完全分离，当以 NaAc 高盐缓冲液去调节其 pH 至中性时，变性的质粒 DNA 又恢复原来的构象，而染色体 DNA 不能复性而形成不溶性的网状结构。因此，通过离心，可将质粒 DNA 与染色体 DNA 及细胞破碎物分开。

【实验材料】

1. **实验菌株与载体**　含 pET – 32a – hCT 的重组菌。

2. **实验器材**　超净台，离心机，微量移液器，旋涡混合器，恒温培养箱。

3. **实验试剂**　裂解溶液 I，溶液 II，溶液 III，LB 液体培养基，100mg/ml 氨苄西林（Ampicillin，Amp）。

（1）溶液 I 配方　见表 23 – 5。

表 23 – 5　溶液 I 配方

试剂	浓度
葡萄糖	50mmol/L
EDTA	10mmol/L
Tris（pH 8.0）	25mmol/L

121℃灭菌 20 分钟，4℃保存。

（2）溶液Ⅱ配方　见表 23 - 6。

表 23 - 6　溶液Ⅱ配方

试剂	浓度
NaOH	0.2mol/L
SDS	1%

（3）溶液Ⅲ配方　见表 23 - 7。

表 23 - 7　溶液Ⅲ配方

试剂	组成
醋酸钾（5mol/L）	60.0ml
冰醋酸	11.5ml
蒸馏水	28.5ml

【实验步骤】

（1）将验证过的阳性转化菌落接入 20ml 含有 100μg/ml 氨苄西林的 LB 液体培养基中，37℃ 220r/min 过夜培养。

（2）将 1.5ml 培养物转入 EP 管中，以 14000r/min 离心 30 秒，弃上清。

（3）将沉淀悬于 100μl 溶液Ⅰ中，混匀，冰浴 10 分钟。

（4）加入 200μl 新配制的溶液Ⅱ，快速颠倒 5 次，并在 5 分钟中内加入 150μl 溶液Ⅲ。

（5）温和振荡 10s，冰浴 5 分钟，14000r/min 离心 5 分钟，将上清转移到另一 Eppendorf 管中约 400μl。

（6）加入 200μl 酚，200μl 三氯甲烷/异戊醇，振荡混匀，14000r/min 离心 2 分钟，转移上清到另一 Eppendorf 管中。

（7）重复步骤（6）1 次。

（8）加入 800μl 无水乙醇，振荡均匀，-20℃冰箱中放置 1 小时，14000r/min 离心 5 分钟，去上清。

（9）加入 1ml 70% 乙醇，用移液器吹洗沉淀，14000r/min 离心 5 分钟，去上清，37℃干燥。

（10）加入 20μl 含有 20μg/ml RNA 酶的 TE 缓冲液溶解核酸，37℃水浴 30 分钟。

（11）电泳 20μl 上样量检测所提质粒质量。

【注意事项】

（1）沉淀细菌后，菌液一定要弃干净。未移尽的菌液将导致质粒 DNA 抵抗限制性内切酶消化反应，因为细菌菌株的细胞壁成分会散落在培养基中，而这些有效成分有抑制许多内切酶反应的作用。

（2）裂解和中和时，手法要轻柔，加完试剂要立即混匀。

（3）溶解质粒时，可在 37 ℃放置几分钟，确保质粒完全溶解。

四、外源基因在大肠埃希菌中的诱导表达

【实验原理】

如图 23 -1 所示，pET - 32a - c（+）为一个融合表达载体，其使用的启动子为 T7 启动子，含 *Lac* 操纵基因，并可自身表达 Lac I 阻遏蛋白，此阻遏蛋白既可与 *Lac* 操纵基因结合，也可与乳糖结合，当其与乳糖结合后构象改变，随即失去与 *Lac* 操纵基因结合的能力。在无诱导物存在的条件下，阻遏蛋白结合于操纵基因区，阻止 T7 启动子下游基因的转录和表达。IPTG 为乳糖类似物，可与 Lac I 阻遏蛋白结合使其构象改变，从而失去与 *Lac* 操纵基因结合的能力。当加入 IPTG 诱导时，IPTG 与阻遏蛋白结合使其从操纵基因上脱落，T7 启动子下游基因转录并表达，从而菌体内合成大量基因产物。

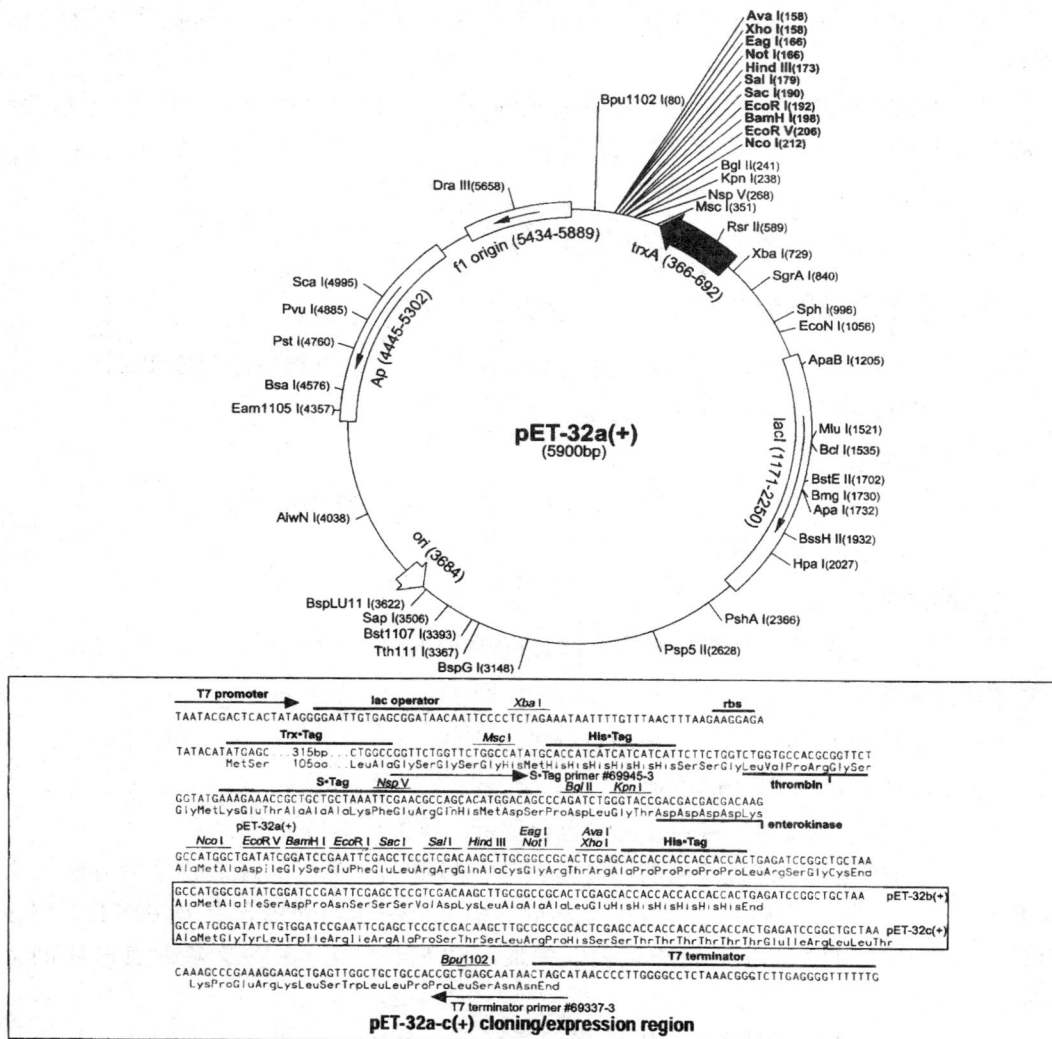

图 23 -1　pET - 32a（+）质粒

【实验材料】

1. **实验菌株与载体**　实验一阳性转化子保藏菌种以及含有 pET – 32a – c（＋）空载体的 BL21 保藏菌种。

2. **实验器材**　恒温培养摇床，超净台，微量移液器，离心机。

3. **实验试剂**　0.2mol/L IPTG，LB 液体培养基。

【实验步骤】

（1）取实验一阳性转化子以及含有 pET – 32a – c（＋）空载体的 BL21 甘油管保藏菌种按 1∶100 接种至 20ml 含 100μg/ml 氨苄西林 LB 液体培养基中，37℃ 220r/min 过夜培养。

（2）取出培养物按 1∶100 分别接种至另外两瓶含 100μg/ml 氨苄西林的 20ml LB 液体培养基中，37℃ 220r/min 培养 3 小时。

（3）培养物内分别加入 IPTG，使其终浓度为 0.2mmol/L，放回摇床内继续培养 4h。

（4）取出锥形瓶，将菌液转至 1.5ml Eppendorf 管中，5000r/min 离心 5 分钟，弃上清，收集菌体，–20℃ 冷冻保存待用。

【注意事项】

注意无菌操作，接种过程中防止杂菌污染。

五、基因产物的分析验证

具体内容见实验六 SDS – 聚丙烯酰胺凝胶电泳法、实验九蛋白质免疫印迹法。

（一）SDS – 聚丙烯酰胺凝胶电泳法

【实验结果】

根据凝胶中标准品与待测样品的相对迁移率判断样品所在的位置。

（二）蛋白质免疫印迹法

【实验结果】

检查膜上显色结果，色带所对应的即是目标蛋白。

【注意事项】

（1）丙烯酰胺有神经毒，应用时需戴手套。

（2）加样时尽量选择中间泳道。

（3）脱色时注意观察，避免过度脱色导致蛋白质条带不易观察。

（4）蛋白质免疫印迹最常见的问题是背景信号过高。最好的降低背景的方法（大多数情况下）是进一步稀释一抗浓度。其他的解决方法包括使用含有去污剂的封闭缓冲液，使用其他封闭试剂（如酪蛋白、牛血清蛋白、血清），以及减少蛋白质的上样量。

（5）如果无带或弱带发生，则可增加蛋白质上样量，或增加一抗和（或）二抗的量。

【思考题】

1. 制备感受态细菌的原理是什么？
2. 如果实验中对照组本不该长出菌落的平板长出了菌落，分析原因。
3. 为什么感受态制备时要在冰浴中操作？
4. 碱变性法提取质粒过程中，加入Ⅱ号液后，为什么溶液会出现黏丝状物质？
5. 如果实验未能得到质粒 DNA，可能有哪些原因？
6. 质粒 DNA 电泳结果可为 3 条带，各代表何种构型？
7. IPTG 诱导基因表达的原理是什么？

Experiment 23　Recombinant Expression of Calcitonin Gene in *Escherichia coli*

Purpose

1. To master the methods of the preparation of competent bacteria and the transformation of the recombinant plasmid.

2. To master the principle and related technique of the extraction of plasmid DNA by alkaline lysis.

3. To learn the process and the characteristics of the foreign genes expressed in prokaryotic cells.

｜ Preparation of competent bacteria and transformation of the recombinant expression vector

Principle

The procedures of genetic engineering are as follows: find the target gene → restriction digestion of target gene and vector → connection of the enzyme-digested products → transformation of recombinant vector to host cell → screen and verify the positive transformant → inducible expression and verify the target products. This experiment chose the recombinant vector which contained the human calcitonin gene as the material, and transformed it into *E. coli* BL21 (DE3).

Competence is a state that a cell grows to a certain period to accept the exogenous target gene. Transformation efficiency in natural state is very low, therefore artificial induction in the biotechnology operations is often used to increase the transformation efficiency. Bacteria expand into spheres within hypotonic solution at 4℃, the Ca^{2+} destabilizes the cell membrane, and a calcium phosphate-DNA complex is formed, which adheres to the cell surface, the DNA is absorbed during a heat-shock step when the cells are exposed briefly at 42℃. Culture the cells in the medium for a few hours, the spherical cell recover and start to proliferate. The competence induced by the calcium chloride yields up to $10^5 \sim 10^6$ transformed colonies per microgram of supercoiled plasmid DNA. The smaller the recombinants, the higher the conversion rate. The transformation efficiency of circular DNA molecule is 1000 times higher than that of linear DNA. Adding divalent cations (Mn^{2+}, Co^{2+}), DMSO or reducing agents will increase the transformation efficiency.

Materials

1. Strain and vector

Recombinant plasmid pET-32a-hCT, *E. coli* BL21 (DE3), plasmid pET-32a-c (+).

2. Apparatus

Water bath, micropipette, centrifuger, constant temperature incubator shaker, clean bench. Sterilizing materials: see Table 23 – 1.

Table 23 – 1   Sterilizing materials

Materials	Specification	Amount
Petri dishes	diameter 10cm	4
Triangular flask	250ml	2
Pipette tip	10μl、200μl、1000μl	Several
Eppendorf tube	1.5ml	Several
T_1 buffer	1 ×	10ml
T_2 buffer	1 ×	10ml
Triangular harrow		4
Transferring loop		2

3. Reagents

(1) Common reagents　See Table 23 – 2.

Table 23 – 2   Common reagents

Reagent	T_1 buffer	T_2 buffer
NaCl	10mmol/L	
MnCl₂	50mmol/L	100mmol/L
NaAc-HCl pH 5.6	10mmol/L	10mmol/L
CaCl₂		75mmol/L

(2) LB medium recipe (100ml)　See Table 23 – 3.

Table 23 – 3   LB medium recipe

Reagent	Dose (g)
Tryptone	1.0
Yeast extract	0.5
NaCl	1.0

Adjust pH to 7.2 ~ 7.4 with 2mol/L NaOH, sterilizing at 121℃ for 20min. LB solid medium: Add 15g agar per liter LB medium.

Procedures

1. Streak the strain BL21 (DE3) onto a plate, pick a single bacterial colony from the plate that has been incubated for 12 ~ 16h at 37℃. Transfer the colony into 20ml LB medium. Incubate the culture for 12 ~ 16h at 37℃ with vigorous agitation (approximately 220r/min).

2. Transfer 200μl of the overnight culture to 20ml LB medium. Incubate at 37℃ for 3h with continuous shaking. Check the OD_{650}, you should have an OD between 0.4 ~ 0.5.

3. Transfer 1.5ml of the bacterial cells to Eppendorf tubes, four tubes in total. Cool the cultures by storing the tubes on ice. Recover the cells by centrifugation at 3500r/min for 3min.

4. Add 300μl T_1 buffer in each of the Eppendorf tubes, resuspend each pellet by swirling or gentle vortexing, and then store the tubes on ice for 20min, recover the cells by centrifugation at 3500r/min for 3min, discard the supernant.

5. Add 30μl T_2 buffer in each of the Eppendorf tubes, resuspend each pellet by swirling or gentle vortexing, add the solution according to Table 23 - 4. After being well-distributed, store the tubes on ice for 30min. Transfer the tubes into 42℃ circulating water bath. , keep for exactly 90s. Rapidly transfer the tubes to an ice bath. Allow the cells to chill for 1 ~ 2min.

6. Add 1.0ml LB of LB medium to each tube. Incubate the cultures for 45min at 37℃. Recover the cells by centrifugation at 3000r/min for 2min, take out 850μl supernatant, resuspend each pellet by swirling or gentle vortexing, transfer the competent cells onto agar LB medium containing 100μg/ml Ampicillin. Invert the plates and incubate at 37℃ for less than 16h.

Results

Observe the phenomenon, note the mumber of colonies in the Table 23 - 4.

Table 23 - 4 Records of the results

Petri dishes No.	Bacterial colony No.
Negative control (1μl water)	
Positive control [1μl pET-32a-c (+)]	
1μl Recombination vector	
2μl Recombination vector	

Cautions

1. Monitor the state of bacterial growth and density closely, and use the cells from the logarithmic phase of growth as far as possible .

2. All operations should be in the aseptic and icy conditions.

Ⅱ. Verify the recombinant clone by PCR

Content see Experiment 14 PCR amplify DNA and Experiment 13 agarose gel electrophoresis.

Results

Recycle the samples and analyze them by an agarose electrophoresis. Stain the gel with ethidium bromide to visualize the DNA.

III. Extraction of plasmid DNA by alkaline lysis

Principle

This method exploits the difference in denaturation and renaturation characteristics of covalently closed circular plasmid DNA and chromosomal DNA. In the condition of alkali (pH = 12.6), hydrogen bond in chromosomal DNA break, which results in the uncouple of double helix structure and denaturation. Most hydrogen bond of plasmid DNA also break, but two strands of the covalently closed circular plasmid DNA remain in close proximity. When adding potassium acetate and in the condition of neutrality, denatured plasmid DNA restore its conformation rapidly, but chromosome DNA could not renature and aggregates to form an insoluble network. When centrifuged, the plasmid DNA still stays in the supernatant while the chromosome DNA sediments together with cellular fragments.

Materials

1. Strain and vector

Recombinant bacteria containing plasmid pET-32a-hCT.

2. Apparatus

Clean bench, centrifuger, micropipette, vortex mixer, constant temperature incubator shaker.

3. Reagents

Alkaline lysis solution I, II, III, LB liquid medium, Ampicillin (Amp) 100mg/ml.

(1) Solution I See Table 23 – 5.

Table 23 – 5 Solution I recipe

Reagents	Concentration
Glucose	50mmol/L
EDTA	10mmol/L
Tris (pH 8.0)	25mmol/L

Sterilize at 121℃ for 20min, store at 0℃.

(2) Solution II See Table 23 – 6.

Table 23 – 6 Solution II recipe

Reagents	Concentration
NaOH	0.2mol/L
SDS	1%

(3) Solution III See Table 23 – 7.

Table 23 – 7 Solution III recipe

Reagents	Concentration
Potassium acetate (5mol/L)	60.0ml
Ice acetic acid	11.5ml
Distilled water	28.5ml

Procedures

1. A single colony of transformed bacteria is inoculated in 20ml of LB medium containing Ampicillin (100mg/ml). Incubate the culture at 37℃ overnight with 200r/min agitation.

2. Pour 1.5ml of the culture into a microfuge tube. Centrifuge at 14000r/min for 30s, and remove the supernatant.

3. Resuspend the bacterial pellet in 100μl of solution I by vigorously vortexing. Place the tube in ice bath for 10min.

4. Add 200μl of freshly prepared solution II to each bacterial suspension. Mix the contents by inverting the tube rapidly five times. And add 150μl of solution III.

5. Gently invert the tube for 10min, store the tube on ice for 5min. Centrifuge the bacterial lysate at 14000r/min for 5min. Transfer the supernatant to a fresh tube (approximately 400μl).

6. Add 200μl phenol, 200μl chloroform or isoamylol. Mix the organic and aqueous phases by vortexing and then centrifuge the emulsion at 14000r/min for 2min. Transfer the aqueous upper layer to a fresh tube.

7. Repeat Step 6 one time.

8. Add 800μl 100% ethanol. Mix the solution by vortexing and keep at -20℃ for 1h. Centrifuge at 14000r/min for 5min, pour off the supernatant.

9. Add 1ml of 70% ethanol to the pellet and purge with pipette. Centrifuge at 14000r/min for 5min. Pure off the supernatant and dry the pellet at 37℃.

10. Dissolve the nucleic acids in 20μl of TE (pH 8.0) containing 20μg/ml DNase-free RNase A. Incubate at 37℃ for 5min.

11. Load 20ml sample for electrophoresis to identify the quality of the plasmid.

Cautions

1. After the bacterium are precipitated, the supernatant should be removed completely. The penalty for failing to remove all traces of medium from the bacterial pellet is that plasmid DNA will be resistant to cleavage by restriction enzymes. This is because the cell-wall components in the medium inhibit the action of many restriction enzymes.

2. The lysed step and neutralized step are characterized by gentle operation, and the reagents added to the system should be mixed immediately.

3. When the plasmids are dissolved, we should place them at 37℃ for few minutes to ensure the plasmids are completely dissolved.

IV. Expression of exogenous genes in *E. coli*

Principle

As shown in Fig. 23-1, the pET-32a-c (+) is a fusion expression vector, using the T7 promoter, containing Lac operator gene, and can express the Lac I repressor protein. This repressor protein can combined with both Lac operator gene and lactose. The conformational change will occur after its combination with lactose, and then lose the ability to bind with Lac operator gene. Without inducer, the repressor protein binds with operator gene, and prevents

transcription and expression of the gene downstream of the T7 promoter. IPTG is lactose ana-
logue, and the combination with the Lac I repressor protein causes its conformational changes,
and thus loses the ability to combine with Lac operator gene. When the inducer IPTG is added,
it combines with repressor protein so that it detaches from the operator gene, then starts the
transcription and expression of the gene downstream of the T7 promoter, and the bacteria syn-
thesizes a large number of gene products in *vivo*.

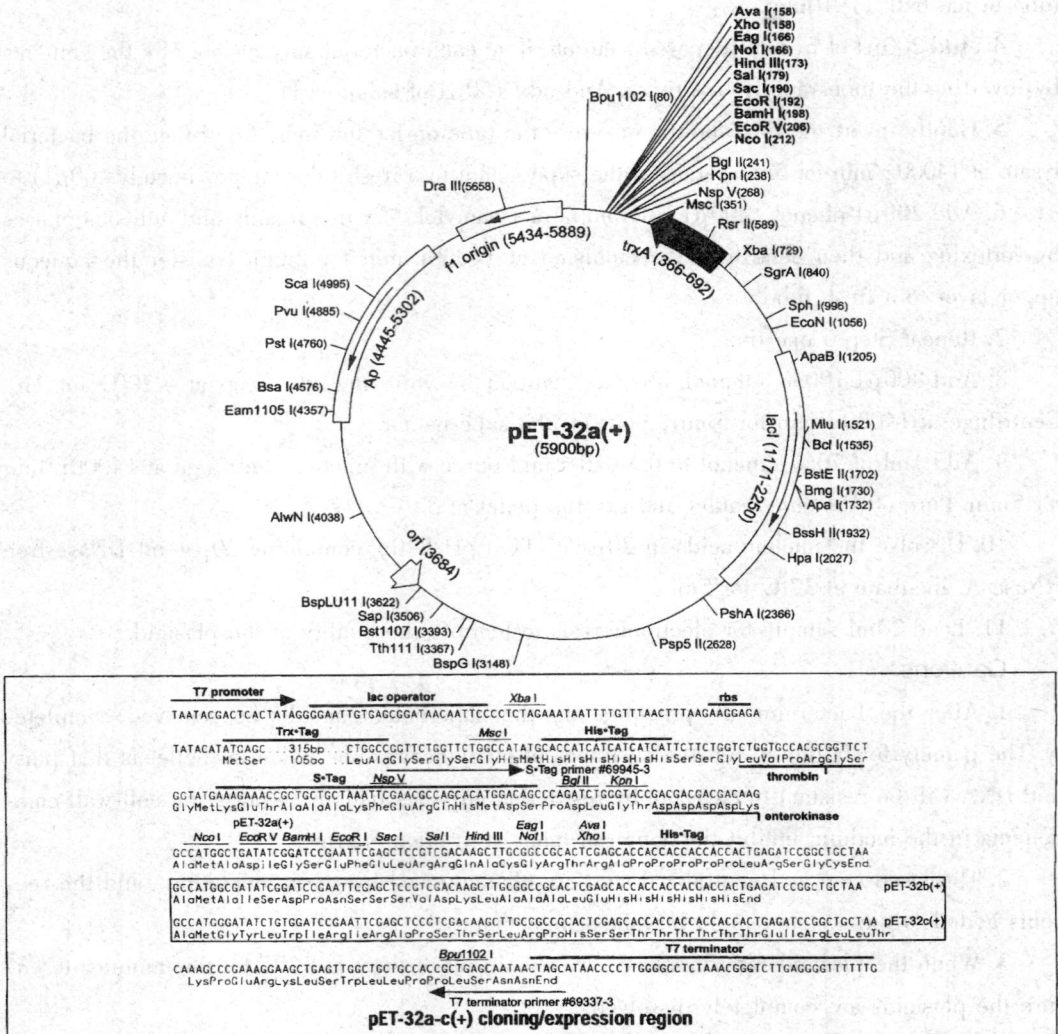

Fig. 23 – 1　pET-32a-c（+）

Materials

1. Strain and vector

Positive transformant strains, strains BL21 containing empty vector of pET-32a-c（+）.

2. Apparatus

Constant temerature incubator, clean bench, micropipette, centrifuge.

3. Reagents

0.2mol/L IPTG，LB liquid medium.

Procedures

1. Inoculate positive transformant strain and strains BL21 containing empty vector of pET-32a-c（+）to 20ml LB medium containing 100μg/ml Ampicillin with 1∶100 dilution. Incubate the culture overnight at 37℃ with vigorous agitation（approximately 220r/min）.

2. Inoculate culture to 20ml LB medium containing 100μg/ml ampicillin with 1∶100 dilution. Incubate the cultures at 37℃ for 3h with vigorous agitation（approximately 220r/min）.

3. Induce each culture by adding IPTG to a final concentration of 0.2mmol/L in the clean bench and continue to incubate at 37℃ for another 4h.

4. Take out the triangular flask, transfer each culture to a 1.5ml Eppendorf tube, centrifuge at 5000r/min for 5min. Remove the supernatants and collect the bacterial pellet, store at −20℃.

Caution

Prevent bacterial from contamination in the inoculation process.

V. Analysis and validation of the gene product

Content see Experiment 6 SDS-Polyacrylamide Gel Electrophoresis, and Experiment 9 Western Blot Analysis.

（Ⅰ）SDS-polyacrylamide gel electrophoresis

Results

Identification of the position of the target protein according to the relatively electrophoretic mobility of the standard protein and the sample to be tested.

（Ⅱ）Western blot analysis

Results

Check the bands on membrane, the band with color corresponding to the target protein.

Cautions

1. Acrylamide is a toxic substance, so use carefully and wears gloves while handling solutions that contain it.

2. Try to choose the middle lane when add samples.

3. Avoiding excessive decolorization so that we could observe protein bands clearly.

4. The most common problem in Western blotting is the occurrence of background staining. The best remedy for high background (in many cases) is simply to dilute the primary antibody further. Other solutions include ensuring that detergent is used in blocking reagent, using an alternate blocking reagent (casamino acids, BSA, serum), and decreasing the amount of protein applied to the electrophoresis gel.

5. No or low signal can be remedied by loading more protein in the gel or increasing the amount of primary and/or secondary antibody applied to the blot.

Questions

1. What is the principle of the preparation of competent bacteria?

2. If the control group grows colonies in the experiment, what are the possible causes?

3. Why should we prepare for the competent bacteria in an ice bath?

4. Why the solution will appear sticky filaments after solution Ⅱ was added in the process of alkaline lysis?

5. What are the reasons if the experiment fails to obtain the plasmid DNA?

6. If there are three bands in the electrophoresis result of the plasmid DNA, what configuration do they represent?

7. What is the principle of gene expression induced by IPTG?

实验二十四 动物基因组多态性分析

【实验目的】

1. 掌握基因组多态性分析的原理。

2. 熟悉动物基因 PCR – RFLP 分析方法的操作过程。

3. 熟悉 PCR、胶回收、酶切和琼脂糖电泳等技术在基因多态性分析中的应用。

【实验原理】

多态性（polymorphism）是指在一个生物群体中，同时和经常存在两种或多种不连续的变异型或基因型（genotype）或等位基因（allele），亦称遗传多态性（genetic polymorphism）或基因多态性。从本质上来讲，多态性的产生在于基因水平上的变异，一般发生在基因序列中不编码蛋白的区域和没有重要调节功能的区域。基因多态性现象十分普遍，按引起关注和研究的先后，通常分为 3 大类：DNA 片段长度多态性、DNA 重复序列多态性、单核苷酸多态性。其中 DNA 片段长度多态性是指 DNA 限制性内切酶酶切片段长度的多态性（restriction fragment length polymorphism）。由于碱基顺序的差异，在不同的种或同一个种的不同个体之间，它们的基因组 DNA 限制性内切酶位点的种类和数目不同，经特定的限制性内切酶切割后，所产生的限制性酶切片段在大小（长度）和数目方面自然也存在着差异。通过琼脂糖凝胶电泳分离和核酸染料染色，在紫外检测仪下观察，即可直接看到这种差异。电泳分离后，再经过 Southern 杂交也可显示出已知 DNA 片段的差异。

CAPs（cleaved amplification polymorphism sequence-tagged sites）技术又称为聚合酶链式反应——限制性片段长度多态（PCR – RFLP）分析技术，是在 PCR 技术和 DNA 序列分析技术的基础上发展起来的。DNA 碱基置换正好发生在某种限制性内切酶识别位点上，使酶切位点增加或者消失。利用这一酶切性质的改变，PCR 特异扩增包含碱基置换的这段 DNA，经某一限制酶切割，再利用琼脂糖凝胶电泳分离酶切产物，与正常比较来确定是否变异，或进行不同物种基因型分析。

【实验材料】

1. **实验样品** 不同种动物或同种动物不同个体提取出的基因组 DNA。

2. **实验器材** 微量移液器、灭菌微量移液器吸头、灭菌 Eppendorf 管、PCR 扩增仪、台式高速离心机、恒温水浴锅、电泳仪、水平式电泳槽、凝胶成像系统。

3. **实验试剂**

（1）*Taq* DNA 聚合酶（5U/μl），10×*Taq* PCR 缓冲液，引物 F（10μmol/L），引物 R（10μmol/L），dNTP（2.5mmol/L），灭菌双蒸水。

（2）Silver Beads DNA 胶回收试剂盒，限制性内切酶，10×限制性内切酶缓冲液。

（3）λDNA/*Hind*Ⅲ 标准分子量标记物，DL 2000 标准分子量标记物，6×样品缓冲液，0.5×TBE 电泳缓冲液，Golden view 核酸染色液，琼脂糖。

【实验步骤】

1. **PCR 反应**

（1）依据实验材料基因组 DNA 来源选取待分析基因，输入基因名称在 Genbank 查询序列，使用 Primer Premier 5.0 软件设计引物。

（2）取 2μl −20℃保存的动物基因组 DNA 为模板，在灭菌 0.2ml Eppendorf 管中按表 24 −1 和表 24 −2 组成和条件进行 PCR 反应。反应完毕取出后放入 4℃冰箱保存备用。

表 24 −1　PCR 反应体系

组　　成	体积（μl）
模板	2.0
10×*Taq* PCR 缓冲液	2.0
引物 F	0.4
引物 R	0.4
dNTP	0.4
蒸馏水	14.6
Taq DNA 聚合酶	0.2
终体积	20.0

表 24 −2　PCR 反应扩增过程

步　　骤	温　　度	时　　间
步骤 1	95℃	5min
步骤 2	94℃	30s
步骤 3	50~60℃	40s
步骤 4	72℃	30s
步骤 5	多于 29 次循环到步骤 2	
步骤 6	72℃	5min
步骤 7	4℃	24h
步骤 8	结束	

（3）配制 1% 琼脂糖凝胶溶液，待溶液冷至 50～60℃按每 100ml 凝胶溶液加 5μl Golden View 核酸染色液，而后制胶。取 PCR 产物样品 10μl 与 6×样品缓冲液按照比例混合后，用微量移液器缓慢加入样品池中，确保电泳正负极正确，100V 恒压电泳至距离前沿 4cm 左右，切断电源，于凝胶成像系统观察电泳结果。

2. PCR 产物的胶回收

（1）取干净手术刀从琼脂糖凝胶中分割下含有 PCR 扩增产物条带的胶块，放入灭菌 1.5ml Eppendorf 管中。

（2）按每 100mg 琼脂糖凝胶加入 400μl 溶胶溶液和 10μl 玻璃珠，50～60℃水浴中 10min，使胶彻底融化，溶胶过程每两分钟混匀 1 次。10000r/min 高速离心 1 分钟。

（3）小心吸掉上清，用 500μl 洗涤溶液将玻璃珠悬浮起来，10000r/min 离心 1 分钟。重复本次操作 1 次。

（4）小心吸掉上清，Eppendorf 管倒置，室温干燥 10 分钟。用 20μl 灭菌双蒸水将玻璃珠悬浮起来，室温或 37℃放置 5～10 分钟，中途混匀若干次。

（5）10000 r/min 离心 1 分钟，小心将上清液移到另一个灭菌的 Eppendorf 管中，不要吸取玻璃珠。10000 r/min 离心 1 分钟，除去溶液中的微量 Beads。

3. 限制性酶切及电泳检测

（1）取 PCR 胶回收产物 10μl 于另一个 1.5ml 灭菌 Eppendorf 管，按表 24-3 组成进行酶切反应。

表 24-3　限制性内切酶反应体系

组　成	体积（μl）
蒸馏水	5
10×限制性内切酶缓冲液	4
PCR 产物	10
用移液器混匀	
限制性内切酶	1
终体积	20

（2）用手指轻弹管壁，使各种试剂混合，快速离心集中溶液。于 37℃水浴中 60～180 分钟。80℃水浴灭活 20 分钟，备用。

（3）配制 1% 琼脂糖凝胶溶液，并制胶。取酶切产物样品 10μl 与 6×样品缓冲液按照比例混合，上样进行琼脂糖凝胶电泳，于凝胶成像系统观察并记录电泳结果。根据片段大小和条数判断基因型。

【思考题】

基因组多态性分析的原理是什么？

Experiment 24　Analysis of the Animal Gene Polymorphism

Purpose

1. To master the principle of gene polymorphism analysis.

2. To learn about the operative procedures of PCR-RFLP analysis of the animal gene polymorphism.

3. Be familliar with the application of PCR, gel recovery, restrict enzyme digestion and agarose gel electrophoresis in gene polymorphism analysis.

Principle

Polymorphism means that there are two or multiple discontinuous genotypes or allele in a group of organisms, and it is also named genetic polymorphism. In fact, polymorphism is produced by the gene mutation and it occurs in the area of gene sequences which don't encode the protein and don't have important regulating function. Genetic polymorphism is widespread and can be classified into 3 categories: DNA fragment length polymorphism, DNA repeat sequences polymorphism and single-nucleotide polymorphism by the sequences of research. DNA fragment length polymorphism means DNA restriction fragment length polymorphism (RFLP). In the different species or the different individual organisms of a species, the variety and quantity of gene restriction enzyme digestion sites are diverse, and the restriction fragments are diverse in length and quantity by specific restriction enzyme digestion. The difference can be observed through agarose gel electrophoresis, nucleic acid stain coloration and UV detection. After electrophoresis, the distinction of known DNA can be also shown by southern blotting.

Cleaved amplification polymorphism sequence-tagged sites (CAPs) analysis, or PCR-RFLP analysis, is developed by the foundation of PCR and DNA sequence analysis. DNA base substitution occurs on some restriction enzyme digestion sites and makes the restriction enzyme digestion sites increase or disappear. Using the change of enzyme digestion properties, the DNA containing base substitution is specifically amplified and digested by the restriction enzyme, and then the enzyme digestion products are separated to ensure variation or not, and analyze the genotype of different species.

Materials

1. Sample

Animal DNA from different species or different individual organisms.

2. Apparatus

Micropipette, sterilized micropipette tips, sterilized eppendorf tubes, PCR thermal cycler, table high-speed centrifuge, constant temperature water bath, electrophoresis apparatus, horizontal electrophoresis bath, gel imaging system.

3. Reagents

(1) *Taq* DNA polymerase (5U/μl), 10 × *Taq* PCR amplification buffer, primer F

（10μmol/L），primer R （10μmol/L），dNTPs solution containing all the four dNTPs （2.5mmol/L），sterilized double distilled water.

（2）Silver Beads DNA gel recovery kit, restriction enzyme, 10×restriction enzyme buffer.

（3）λDNA/HindⅢ marker, DL 2000 marker, 6×loading buffer, 0.5×TBE buffer, Golden view nucleic acid stain, agarose.

Procedures

1. The process of PCR

（1）Choose the gene to be analyzed according to the species origin of DNA, input the gene name on Genbank to inquire about the gene sequences and design the primers with Primer Premier 5.0 software.

（2）Take 2μl animal DNA stored at −20℃ as template, mix the components in a 0.2ml sterilized Eppendorf tube as Table 24 − 1 and amplify the process as Table 24 − 2. Store the PCR products at −4℃.

Table 24 −1　Reaction mixture for PCR

Component	Volume （μl）
Template	2.0
10 × Taq PCR buffer	2.0
Primer F	0.4
Primer R	0.4
dNTP	0.4
Distilled water	14.6
Taq DNA polymerase	0.2
Final volume	20.0

Table 24 −2　Cycles of PCR

Step	Temperature	Time during
Step 1	95℃	5min
Step 2	94℃	30s
Step 3	50~60℃	40s
Step 4	72℃	30s
Step 5	29 more cycles to step 2	
Step 6	72℃	5min
Step 7	4℃	24h
Step 8	End	

（3）Prepare 1% （W/V） agarose solution in electrophoresis buffer, and add 5μl Golden View nucleic acid stain when the agarose buffer is cooled to 50~60℃. Make agarose gel. Mix 10μl PCR products and 6×loading buffer in proportion, and load the sample mixture into the slots with a micropipette. Correct the direction of electrophoresis, and apply a voltage of 100V. Run the gel until the bromophenol blue has migrated to the position which is about 4cm away from the edge of the gel. Turn off the electric current and examine the results with gel imaging system.

2. Gel recovery of PCR products

(1) Cut the agarose gel containing PCR amplifying bands with a clean knife, and then put the gel into a 1.5ml sterilized Eppendorf tube.

(2) Mix 400μl solubization solution and 10μl silver beads in every 100mg agarose gel, and then keep the tube in 50 ~ 60℃ constant temperature bath for 10min. Melt the gel absolutely and mix it every 2 min. Centrifuge the tube at 10000r/min for 1min.

(3) Remove the supernatant liquid carefully and suspend the silver beads with 500μl wash solution, centrifuge the tube at 10000r/min for 1min. Repeat this step.

(4) Remove the supernatant liquid carefully, reverse the tube and dry it for 10min. Suspend the silver beads with 20μl sterilized double distilled water, keep the tube at room temperature or 37℃ for 5 ~ 10min and mix it several times.

(5) Centrifuge the tube at 10000r/min for 1min, remove the supernatant liquid carefully to another sterilized tube without beads. Centrifuge the tube at 10000r/min for 1min to remove the trace of beads from liquid.

3. Restriction enzyme digestion and gel electrophoresis analysis

(1) In a 1.5ml sterilized Eppendorf tube, mix the components as Table 24 − 3 and enzyme digestion.

Table 24 −3   Reaction mixture of restriction enzyme digestion

Component	Volume (μl)
Distilled water	5
10 × Restriction enzyme buffer	4
PCR products	10
Mix by pipetting	
Restriction enzyme	1
Final volume	20

(2) Flip the tube gently to mix the components and centrifuge quickly. Keep the tube in a 37℃ constant temperature bath for 60 ~ 180min. Then finish the reaction at 80℃ for 20min.

(3) Prepare 1% (W/V) agarose solution, and make agarose gel. Mix 10μl restriction enzyme digestion products and 6 × loading buffer in proportion, load the sample mixture into the slots and run the electrophoresis. Examine the gel by gel imaging system and record the results. Determine the genotype according to the length and quantity of fragments.

What is the principle of gene polymorphism analysis?

实验二十五　多克隆抗体的制备、纯化及鉴定

【实验目的】

1. 加深了解抗体基本知识。
2. 掌握多克隆抗体制备、纯化和鉴定的基本方法及其原理。

一、多克隆抗体的制备

【实验原理】

当将抗原注射入实验动物体内时，一系列抗体生成细胞会不同程度地与抗原结合，受抗原刺激后在血液中产生不同类型的抗体，这种由一种抗原刺激产生的抗体称为多克隆抗体。多克隆抗体中不同的抗体分子可以以不同的亲和能力与抗原分子表面不同抗原决定簇相结合。

将抗原导入敏感动物体内后，可刺激网状内皮细胞系统，尤其是淋巴结和脾脏中的淋巴细胞大量增殖。如图 25 – 1 所示，实验动物对初次免疫和二次免疫的应答有明显的不同。通常初次免疫应答往往比较弱，尤其是针对于易代谢、可溶性的抗原。首次注射后大约 7 天，在血清中可以观察到抗体，但抗体的浓度维持在一个较低的水平，在大约 10 天左右抗体的滴度会达到最大值。但同种抗原注射而产生的二次免疫应答的结果明显不同，和初次免疫应答相比，抗体的合成速度明显增加，并且保留时间也长。

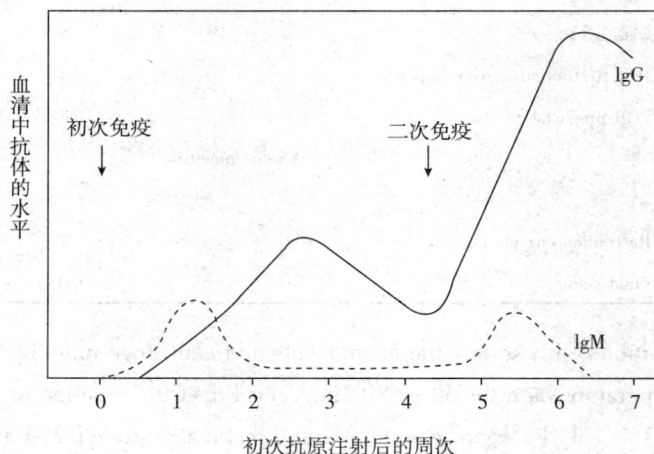

图 25 – 1　抗体产生的基本特点

免疫应答的动力学结果取决于抗原和免疫动物的种类，但初次和二次免疫应答之间的关系是免疫应答的一个重要特点。3 次或以后的抗原注射所产生的应答和二次应答

结果相似：抗体的滴度明显增加并且血清中抗体的种类和性质发生了改变，这种改变被称为免疫应答的成熟，具有重要的实际意义。通常在抗原注射 4~6 周后会产生具有高亲和力的抗体。

【实验材料】

1. **实验动物**　成年兔。

2. **实验器材**　特制兔盒、刀片、针头、注射器、20ml 血液收集管、药铲、离心机以及塑料离心管、加样器、烧杯。

3. **实验试剂**

（1）抗原，乙醇，20mmol/L 磷酸缓冲溶液 pH 7.2

（2）福氏完全佐剂和福氏不完全佐剂　见表 25 – 1。

表 25 – 1　福氏完全佐剂和福氏不完全佐剂的成分

成　分		完全佐剂	不完全佐剂
石蜡油	6 份	+	+
无水羊毛脂	4 份	+	+
杀死的分枝杆菌	3~5mg	+	–
磷酸缓冲溶液	10 份	+	+

福氏完全佐剂的制备：使用前在福氏不完全佐剂中加入适量杀死的分枝杆菌。

【实验步骤】

1. **抗原的制备**　抗原制备的主要目的在于在免疫动物体内产生最强、最适当的抗体。由于纯化的抗原适合产生抗体，因此在注射前通常采用一些经典的方法，比如柱层析、分级萃取、亚细胞分离等进行抗原的分离和纯化。如果多肽抗原在 SDS – PAGE 中为可见的单一带，抗原从凝胶中的抽提可作为纯化的最后一个步骤。

2. **预放血**　轻轻地将兔子放在特制兔盒中，按压兔子耳根部直至血管突出，然后将针头插入耳部血管的中上部，观察到进针后小心推出活塞收集血液 1~5ml。结束收集后，退出针头并按压伤处，以制止血流，再用乙醇消毒。取收集的血液在 37℃ 恒温箱中放置 30 分钟，以防止激活补体系统，再将试管在 4℃ 放置过夜使血液凝固。用药铲将血凝块从管壁上拨落，将血液转移至塑料离心管中，4℃，10000r/min 离心 10 分钟，收集上清液在 4℃ 保存。

3. **注射抗原**

（1）准备两只成年兔，将 100μg 抗原/兔溶入 1ml 磷酸缓冲溶液中待用。在 1ml 福氏不完全佐剂中加入分枝杆菌制成完全佐剂，并加入 1ml 抗原溶液，剧烈振荡使之充分乳化，用 3ml 注射器抽取该乳化液，接上 25G 针头，排除注射器中的气泡。从笼中取出兔子，抚去注射处的兔毛并用乙醇消毒暴露的皮肤。捏出皮肤，将针头以相对皮肤 15°的角度进针，进针深度为 1~2cm，小心不要刺入肌肉中，在 4 个不同部位（两处后背，两处大腿）分别各注射约 500μl 抗原溶液。注射结束后，将针在注射处放置几秒钟后轻轻拔出，并用乙醇消毒。用相同方法免疫另一只家兔。

（2）每4~6周注射抗原，并在注射后的7~10天按照步骤2收集血液。将收集的血液与注射前收集的血液进行比较，检查是否有抗体产生。待确定产生抗体后可大量收集血液，但每只兔子收集血液通常不多于40ml，以防止休克。

4. 放血和收集抗血清

（1）将家兔放入固定架上固定，二甲苯涂于耳部血管的上中部，用刀片倾斜45°在该处切出0.23~0.3cm的切口，使血液能自由地流出。用消毒后的管收集血液，若在结束之前出现凝固，可用温水轻擦切口处，再继续收集。收集适量血液后可用消毒后的纱布轻擦患处，轻按患处10~20s确定血流停止后方可结束。

（2）将血液在37℃恒温箱中放置30分钟，再在4℃放置过夜。用药铲将血凝块从管壁上拨落，将血液转移至塑料离心管中，4℃，10000r/min离心10分钟，收集上清液即为抗血清，可在-20℃保存数年。

【实验结果】

利用蛋白质免疫印迹法或免疫电泳方法检查抗体产生情况。

二、亲和层析法纯化抗体

【实验原理】

如图25-2所示，亲和层析的高度选择性使得从某一初始材料中纯化，富集某一含量较低的目的蛋白成为可能，因此亲和层析是蛋白质分离纯化过程中最有效的方法之一。另外，如果配基与蛋白质的亲和能力很强，也可同时进行样品的浓缩。

虽然多数情况下不需要将抗体与其他血清蛋白分开，但如果一旦需要，蛋白A亲和层析是一种非常有效的分离方法。蛋白A从 *Staphylococcus aureus* 中获得，可与抗体重链的Fc片段相结合。现在已知蛋白A可与多种哺乳动物的IgG相结合，也可与某些IgM和IgA相结合。如果将蛋白A与固相载体相连，例如Sepharose CL-4B，这种填料可以成为分离和纯化不同类型、不同亚类抗体或抗体片段的重要工具。

【实验材料】

1. 实验仪器 蛋白A柱（含10ml或5ml填料）、蠕动泵、离心管、离心机、pH试纸、过滤器、玻璃柱。

2. 实验试剂

（1）TBS缓冲溶液 6.06g Tris（50mmol/L），8.78g NaCl（150mmol/L）以及0.5g叠氮化钠（0.05%）溶于1L蒸馏水中，HCl调节pH至7.4。

（2）中和缓冲溶液 121.2g Tris（1mol/L），87.8g NaCl（1.5mol/L），0.37g EDTA（1mmol/L）及5g叠氮化钠（0.5%）溶于1L蒸馏水中，HCl调节pH至8.0。

（3）洗脱缓冲溶液（pH 2.7） 将3.75g甘氨酸（50mmol/L）溶解于1L蒸馏水中，HCl调节pH至2.7。

（4）洗脱缓冲溶液（pH 1.9） 将3.75g甘氨酸（50mmol/L）溶解于1L蒸馏水中，HCl调节pH至1.9。

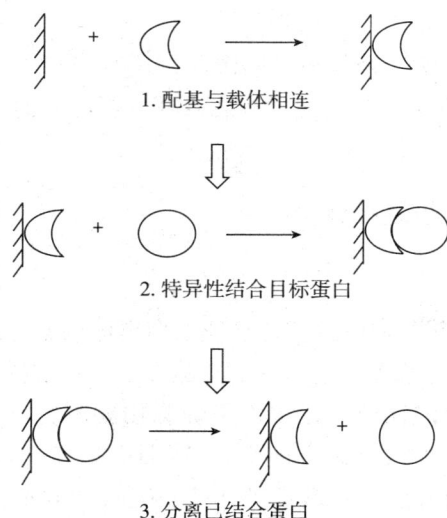

1. 配基与载体相连

2. 特异性结合目标蛋白

3. 分离已结合蛋白

图 25 – 2 亲和层析的基本过程

【实验步骤】

1. **准备蛋白 A Sepharose CL – 4B 亲和柱**　通常准备 5ml 或 10ml 蛋白 A Sepharose CL – 4B 填料，在真空瓶中将等体积的填料和 TBS 缓冲溶液混合，搅拌。抽真空约 15min，以除去填料中的气泡，否则在柱中形成的气泡影响柱子的容量和分离效果。将蛋白 A Sepharose CL – 4B 填料缓慢加入玻璃柱中，利用蠕动泵控制填充速度为 1 ~ 2ml/min，避免柱干，利用 10 倍于床体积并经过预冷的 TBS 缓冲溶液平衡柱子。

2. **制备抗血清**　将抗血清放入冰水或冰箱中过夜解冻，以避免蛋白质的聚集。在蛋白质解冻过程中出现的聚集可通过 37℃ 预热而溶解。加入固体叠氮化钠至浓度为 0.05%，4℃、15000g 离心 5 分钟，移出澄清的抗血清再经过滤器过滤除去多余的脂。

3. **亲和层析**　将抗体用 TBS 缓冲溶液以 1∶5 的比例进行稀释，再用过滤器进行过滤。以 0.5ml/min 的速度将抗血清上到柱上，为保证抗血清与填料的结合，需连续上柱 2 次，并保留上样流出液。用 TBS 缓冲溶液清洗柱子至 $A_{280} < 0.008$ 后加 pH 2.7 洗脱缓冲溶液，以 0.5ml/min 的速度洗脱至所有蛋白质均流下来。用已经加入 100μl 中和缓冲溶液的 1.5ml EP 管分管收集洗脱液，混匀后用 pH 试纸检查洗脱液的 pH，如果 pH 低于 7，可利用中和缓冲液调至约 pH 7.4，以防止抗体的变性。

在柱中加入 10ml、pH 1.9 洗脱缓冲溶液，按上述方法收集洗脱液至 $A_{280} < 0.008$。

利用分光光度计测定各管中蛋白质的含量。若蛋白质浓度低于 0.5mg/ml 可加入 10% 的甘油以便保存，将纯化的抗体分装后在 2 ~ 8℃ 保存。

用含 0.05% 叠氮化钠的 TBS 缓冲溶液清洗柱子后 2 ~ 8℃ 储存。

【实验结果】

利用 SDS – PAGE 检查洗脱获得的蛋白质纯度，利用免疫电泳技术检查纯化后抗体的滴度。

【注意事项】

1. 叠氮化钠有毒，应戴手套并小心操作。

2. 在纯化过程中，预冷的 TBS 缓冲溶液可减少蛋白质的非特异性结合和微生物的代谢。

三、免疫电泳技术鉴定抗体

【实验原理】

免疫电泳又称为 γ - 球蛋白电泳或免疫球蛋白电泳技术，这是一种能够判断血液中三种免疫球蛋白 IgM、IgG、IgA 含量水平的实验方法。在这项实验技术中，首先利用蛋白质的分子量和所带电荷的比值，运用水平琼脂糖凝胶电泳技术将蛋白质进行分离，然后将特异性的抗体引入到与电泳方向平行的凹槽中，在抗原和抗体的扩散过程中，抗原和抗体适当比例的结合会导致沉淀的产生。0.85％ 盐不仅可以终止扩散过程，也可用于洗去未结合的蛋白质，抗原和抗体结合所形成的沉淀线即可以肉眼观察，也可利用染色方法观察。

免疫电泳技术不仅可用于血清或尿样中单克隆抗体的鉴定，也可用于免疫复合物的筛选、各种异常丙种球蛋白血症的识别和鉴定等。同时，免疫电泳技术也是进行蛋白质常规评价的一种可靠、精确的实验方法，可观察蛋白质结构的变化和浓度的改变。

【实验材料】

1. 实验器材 水平电泳仪、打孔器、刀片、电源、恒温水浴、烧杯、微量移液器。

2. 实验试剂

（1）纯化的抗体，蛋白质混合物，1％琼脂。

（2）Tris - 巴比妥缓冲溶液 2.24g 巴比妥酸，4.43g Tris，0.053g 乳酸钙及 0.065g 叠氮化钠溶于 100ml 蒸馏水中。

（3）电泳缓冲溶液 将 Tris - 巴比妥缓冲溶液与蒸馏水按 1∶4 的比例混合。

【实验步骤】

1. 准备琼脂糖凝胶 将琼脂和电泳缓冲溶液混合放入 90℃ 水浴加热至溶化，制成 1％琼脂，将琼脂在冷却前铺在水平玻璃板上，待冷却至室温后，按图用内径 4mm 的打孔器打孔及制作凹槽。

2. 电泳 将用电泳缓冲溶液稀释的 4％ ~5％ 的抗原用滴管小心放入小孔中，将胶板放入电泳槽中，并用润湿的滤纸将胶板和电泳槽中的缓冲溶液相连。盖上电泳槽盖，接通电源，6V/cm 通电至前沿移动约 35mm，时间约为 1 小时，利用示踪染料判断移动距离。

3. 扩散 将胶板移出电泳槽并放在水平位置上，用滤纸润干胶板凹槽中的缓冲溶液，在凹槽中加入适量的抗体（0.2～0.25ml），注意抗体不能溢出凹槽，以避免污染。将胶板移至含有叠氮化钠且有一定湿度的盒内，加盖密封后在30℃水浴扩散至少10h后，移至0.85%盐水中，以终止扩散并洗去未结合的蛋白质。

【实验结果】

观察抗原和抗体之间所形成的沉淀线，并进行记录。

【思考题】

1. 什么是抗原和抗体，并解释抗原抗体结合的特点。

2. 免疫电泳的基本原理是什么。

Experiment 25　Preparation，Purification and Identification of Polyclonal Antibody

Purpose

1. To deepen understanding of the basic knowledge of antibody.

2. To master the basic methods of preparation, purification and identification of polyclonal antibody.

I. Preparation of polyclonal antibody

Principle

If an antigen is injected into an animal, a number of antibody-producing cells will bind that antigen, albeit with varying degrees of affinity, and so the antibody which appears in the bloodstream will arise from several clones of cells, which will be a polyclonal antibody. Different antibody molecules in polyclonal antibody will bind to different epitopes and will do so with different binding affinities.

The introduction of an antigen into a susceptible animal results initially in increasing proliferation of lymphocytes in the tissues of the reticule-endothelial system, particularly the lymph nodes and the spleen. An animal will show different responses to a primary response and a secondary response as is shown in the Fig. 25 – 1. Primary responses are often very weak, particularly for readily catabolized, soluble antigens. Antibody is usually detected in the serum from around 7 days after the first injection and persists at a low level for a few days, typically reaching peak titer around the 10th day. The response to the second injection of the same antigen is dramatically different, and it shows a considerably increased rate of antibody synthesis compared with the primary response and the antibody persists for a longer period.

The kinetics of the response varies depending upon the antigen and the animal but the relationship between the primary response and the secondary responses is an important characteristic. The response to third and subsequent injections broadly mirrors that of the second injection. Higher titers of antibody are reached, but more importantly the nature and the quality of the antibodies present in the serum change. These changes are known as the maturation of the

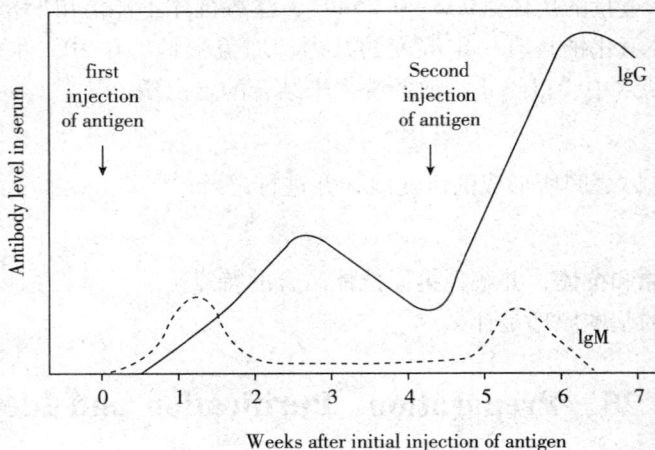

Fig. 25 – 1　The character of antibody production

immune response and have considerable practical importance because they yield high-affinity antibody preparations. The antibody with high affinity can be produced in 4 ~ 6 weeks after injection.

Materials

1. Animal

Adult rabbits.

2. Apparatus

Strainer, razor blade, needle, syringe, 20ml evacuated blood collection tube, spatula, centrifuge and plastic centrifuge tube, pipette, flask.

3. Reagents

(1) Antigen, ethanol, 20mmol/L phosphate buffered saline (PBS) pH 7.2.

(2) Freund's complete and incomplete adjuvant.

Table 25 – 1　The component of Freund's complete and incomplete adjuvant

Component		Complete adjuvant	Incomplete adjuvant
Paraffin	6 share	+	+
Dehydrated lanolin	4 share	+	+
Dead mycobacteria	3 ~ 5mg	+	−
PBS buffer	10 share	+	+

The complete adjuvant must be prepared by adding dead mycobacteria in incomplete adjuvant just before you need it.

Procedure

1. Preparation of antigen

The objective of preparing the antigen is to present it to the animal in a form that will induce the strongest and most appropriate response. Usually, pure antigens provide the best case for the production of antibodies, so the purification of antigens is necessary before antigen injection. The standard techniques, including column chromatography, differential extraction, and subcellular fractionation, are the most useful. If the polypeptide of interest can be seen as a unique band on a SDS-PAGE, then the gel extraction can be used as a final purification step.

2. Pre-bleeding

Calmly and gently place a rabbit in a restrainer. Press lightly on the base of the ear and the vein will stand out straight. Insert the needle into the top middle of the ear vein, and when the needle appears to be in the vein, gently withdraw the needle and collect blood. When you get the required amount of blood (1 ~ 5ml is sufficient for a pre-bleed), remove the needle and apply pressure to the wound. When the bleeding has stopped, sterilize the ear with ethanol. Take the collected blood and place at 37℃ for 30min to inactivate complement, and then place the tube at 4℃ overnight to clot. Loosen the clot from the tube wall with a spatula and decant the blood into a plastic centrifuge tube. Centrifuge at 4℃ 10000r/min for 10min. Collect the supernatant and keep at 4℃.

3. Antigen injection

(1) For injection of two rabbits, antigen should be in 1ml PBS and 100μg/rabbit of antigen is best. Prepare Freund's adjuvant by warming in a flask of warm water, inject 1ml of antigen solution into the adjuvant, and vortex vigorously for 2min to get a good suspension. Draw antigen/adjuvant solution in a 3ml syringe. Calmly take the rabbit out of its cage and place it on a flat surface for the injection. Four subcutaneous injections are done, two on the lower back and two on the thigh. To inject, rub the hair away from the injection site and sterilize with a squirt of ethanol. Pinch the skin and pull up slightly to pull the skin away from the muscle, insert the needle 1 ~ 2cm at a 15°angle so as not to hit the muscle, and inject 500μl. After the required volume has been injected, let the needle remain in place for a few seconds, then pull it out and gently rub the injection site so nothing leaks out. Repeat for all four sites and repeat the process for the other rabbit.

(2) Injections will be done every 4 ~ 6weeks, with bleeding 7 ~ 10days after each injection according to Step 2. Bleeding are performed identically to the pre-bleed, but obtain at least 20ml per rabbit, with 40ml being the upper limit for an adult rabbit to prevent anemia.

4. Bleed and collection of antiserum

(1) Calmly and gently place rabbit in a restrainer. Rub xylene on the top middle of the ear to dilate the vein. Shave this position with a razor blade at a 45°angle to form a notch with 0.23 ~ 0.3cm length and check if the blood can effuse freely. Collect the blood by allowing it to drop into a sterilized tube. If the blood clot on the cut appears before the desired amount is collected, wipe the ear with warm clean water and continue to collect. The blood flow can be stopped by gently pressing to the cut with a sterilized piece of gauze. Press for 10 ~ 20s and then check to make sure the flow has stopped.

（2）Take the collected blood and place at 37℃ for 30min, then 4℃ overnight to contract. Remove the clot from the tube wall with a spatula and decant the blood into a plastic centrifuge tube. Centrifuge at 4℃ 10000r/min for 10 min, decant or pipet off the supernatant. This is the antiserum, which can be stored for many years at −20℃.

Result

Check the result of this experiment by using Western-blotting or immuno-precitpitation method.

Ⅱ. Purification of antibody with affinity chromatography

Principle

As is shown in Fig. 25 − 2, the affinity chromatography is the most powerful technique for protein purification since its high selectivity can, in principle, allow purification of a single protein of low abundance from a crude mixture of proteins at higher concentration. Secondly, if the affinity of the ligand for the protein is sufficiently high, this technique offers simultaneous concentration from a large volume.

Although for many purposes, it is not necessary to purify the antibodies away from other serum proteins, if desired this is best accomplished by protein A affinity chromatography. Protein A found from *Staphylococcus aureus* can bind to the Fc fragment of immunoglobulins through interactions with the heavy chain. The binding of protein A has been documented for IgG from a variety of mammalian species and for some IgM and IgA as well. So, if protein A is coupled with a matrix, such as Sepharose CL-4B, this kind of resin can be a powerful tool to isolate and purify classes, subclasses and fragments of immunoglobulins from biological fluids and serum.

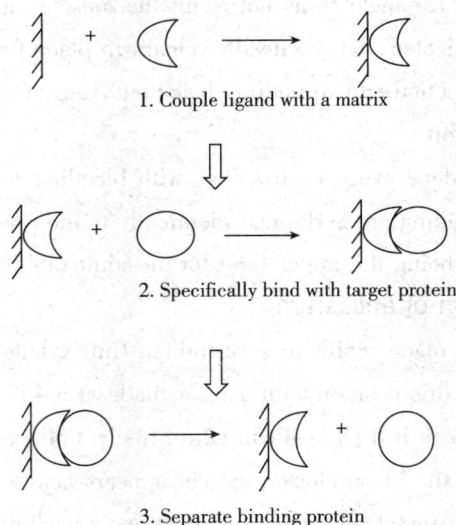

1. Couple ligand with a matrix

2. Specifically bind with target protein

3. Separate binding protein

Fig. 25 − 2 The procedure of affinity chromatography

Materials

1. Apparatus

Protein A column (10ml or 5ml of packed beads), pump, centrifuge, centrifuge tubes, pH strips, filter, glass columns.

2. Reagents

(1) Tris-buffered saline (TBS)　Add 6.06g Tris (50mmol/L), 8.78g NaCl (150mmol/L) and 0.5gNaN$_3$ (0.05%) to 1L distilled water and adjust pH to 7.4 with HCl.

(2) Neutralization buffer (NB)　Add 121.2g Tris (1mol/L), 87.8g NaCl (1.5mol/L), 0.37g EDTA (1mmol/L) and 5g NaN$_3$ (0.5%) to 1L distilled water and adjust pH to 8.0 with HCl..

(3) Elution buffer (pH 2.7)　Add 3.75g Glycine (50mmol/L) to 1L distilled water and adjust pH to 2.7 with HCl.

(4) Elution buffer (pH 1.9)　Add 3.75g Glycine (50mmol/L) to 1L distilled water and adjust pH to 1.9 with HCl.

Procedure

1. Preparation of a protein A Sepharose CL-4B Affinity column

Typically, columns containing 5ml or 10ml of packed protein A Sepharose CL-4B are prepared. After mixing equal volum of resin and TBS buffer, application of vacuum for at least 15min at room temperature is necessary to prevent bubble formation in the column that would reduce the column's capacity and resolution. Slowly add the degassed protein A Sepharose CL-4B to a glass column, and pack the column at a flow rate of about 1~2ml per min. Do not let the column run dry. Flow rate may be controlled by using a pump. Wash the column with 10 bed volumes of ice-cold TBS.

2. Preparation of antiserum

Thaw the antiserum in ice water or refrigerator overnight to prevent aggregation of proteins. Any protein aggregation that forms during thawing may be dissolved by briefly warming the thawed antiserum to 37℃. Add sodium azide to a final concentration of 0.05%. Clarify the antiserum by centrifugation at 15000 r/min for 5 min at 4℃ and remove it. Additional filtration may be required to remove residual lipid.

3. Affinity chromatography

Dilute antibody 1∶5 with binding buffer and filter through a 0.22 filter. Then, add the diluted antiserum to the column at a flow rate of 0.5ml per minute. Pass the antiserum through the column twice and save the effluent in case the antibody does not bind to the column. Wash column with TBS until $A_{280} < 0.008$ and add Elution Buffer pH 2.7 to column at a rate of 0.5ml/min until all protein has been eluted from the column, checking with spectrometer. Collect eluted antibody with 1.5ml microcentrifuge tubes which have been added 100μl of neutralization buffer (NB) and mix each tube, check its pH with pH test paper. If pH is lower than 7, neutralize with neutralization buffer to pH 7.4 which can prevent denaturation of the IgG.

Add 10ml of Elution Buffer pH 1.9 to the column. Collect, mix, and save fractions as described in the steps above. Continue to collect protein until $A_{280} < 0.008$.

Use spectrophotometer to determine the concentration of the antibody in the combined fractions. Add 10% glycerol if the antibody concentration of the combined fractions is less than 0.5mg/ml. Aliquot and store the purified antibody at 2℃ ~ 8℃.

Wash the column with 200ml of TBS with 0.05% sodium azide and store the column at 2℃ ~ 8℃.

Results

Check the purity of eluted protein with SDS-PAGE and identify the titer of purified antibody with immune electrophoresis.

Cautions

1. Since sodium azide is toxic, wear gloves and handle the stock solution with care.

2. During purification, pre-cooled TBS is used to reduce nonspecific binding of proteins and slow the metabolism of any remaining viable microbes.

III. Identification of antibodry with immunoelectrophoresis

Principle

Immunoelectrophoresis (IEP), also called gamma globulin electrophoresis, or immunoglobulin electrophoresis, is a method of determining the blood levels of three major immunoglobulins-immunoglobulin M (IgM), immunoglobulin G (IgG), and immunoglobulin A (IgA). In this method, the proteins are first separated by horizontal agarose gel electrophoresis on the basis of their different charge-to-mass ratios. The antibodies to the proteins are introduced into narrow troughs parallel to the separated antigens. Diffusion of both antigen and antibody takes place and, if solution of antigen and antibody are mixed in different ratios, it is found that at a specific ration, the binding is maximized and a precipitate of antigen-antibody complex is formed. Diffusion can be halted by rinsing the plate in 0.85% saline. Unbound protein is washed from the plate by the saline and the antigen/antibody precipitate line can be stained with a protein sensitive stain.

IEP is used for the identification of monoclonal antibody in serum or urine specimens. This method is also used for a number of other purposes, including screening for circulating immune complexes, recognition and characterization of the various forms of dysgammaglobuline-mias. IEP is a reliable and accurate method for routine protein evaluation, detecting both structural abnormalities and concentration changes.

Materials

1. Apparatus

Horizontal electrophoresis apparatus, drilling equipment, razor blade, power supply, constant temperature water bath, flask, micropipette.

2. Reagents

(1) Purified antibody, protein mixture, 1% agarose.

（2）Tris-barbitol buffer   Dissolve 2.24g barbituric acid, 4.43g Tris, 0.053g Calcium lactate and 0.065g sodium azide in 100ml distilled water.

（3）Electrophoresis buffer   1:4 dilute Tris-barbitol buffer with distilled water.

Procedure

1. Preparation of agarose gel

Mix agarose powder with electrophoresis buffer and heat in 90℃ water bath until it dissolves to make 1% agarose gel. Spread gel on a horizontal glass plate before freezing. After the gel cools to room temperature, puncture pores with 4mm internal diameter drilling equipment and make the trough with razor according to the figure.

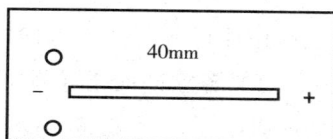

2. Electrophoresis

Add 4% ~5% antigen, which is diluted with electrophoresis buffer, into the small holes with glass pipette and put the agar plate in the electrophoresis chamber. Communicate two ends of plate to the buffer in the camber with wetted filter paper and put the cover on the chamber. Connect power supply, electrophorese at the 6V/cm for 1h with a migration distance of 35mm and the distance can be verified by observing the position of the marker.

3. Diffusion

Remove the agar plate from the chamber and put it on a flat surface. Get rid of the buffer in trough with filter paper and apply appropriate amount of antibody (0.2 ~0.25ml) in the trough. Severe overfilling may cause contamination. Stack the plate in a humidity chamber containing sodium azide, and incubate the plate at 30℃ water bath for at least 10h. Transfer the plate to 0.85% saline, which can stop the diffusion and wash out unbound proteins.

Results

Observe the precipitation line which is formed by combining antigen with antibody and make notes.

Questions

1. What is antigen and antibody? What is the characteristic of their combination with each other?

2. What is the basic principle of immunoelectrophoresis?

附 录

一、实验须知

（1）进入实验室须按实验指导教师要求，寻找自己的位置，清点自己的实验仪器，发现仪器丢失或破损，及时报告指导教师，做好记录登记，不得到实验室其他位置逗留。

（2）实验室公用物品用完之后按原样放回，不得擅自带出。必须严格按照仪器设备规范操作，发现仪器有故障者，有义务立即向指导教师报告，严禁擅自处理、拆卸、调整仪器，凡自行拆卸者一经发现将给予严重处罚。仪器用后切断电源，各种按钮调回到原位，并做好清洁工作。

（3）实验室放置的其他药品、试剂、仪器、设备等物品，进入人员不得翻动接触，以免出现丢失、破损或意外。学生应注意消防设施位置。如发生意外事故，应立即采取必要措施，并及时报告指导教师。

（4）实验室内禁止喧哗、吸烟、用餐和与本次实验内容无关的一切活动，保证通风洁净，闲杂人员不得入内；实验完毕后，值日同学要认真做好整理工作，打扫室内及分担区卫生，及时清理实验垃圾，关闭电源、水源、气源和门窗。

（5）学生实验结束后要清点好自己的仪器，并收拾好实验台面、试药架及搞好水槽卫生，经指导教师检查合格在学生实验登记表签字后，方可离去；否则按缺课处理。

（6）在实验期间指导教师是实验的主导，学生要听从指导教师指导，认真完成指导教师安排的工作。

二、常用仪器的使用方法

（一）移液管的使用

移液管（又称吸管）是生物化学与分子生物学实验中常用的取量容器。量取液体应选用与取液量最接近的吸管。用吸管移取溶液时，一般用右手的中指和拇指拿住管颈刻度线上方，把管尖插入溶液内大约 1cm 处，不得过深与过浅。用洗耳球吸液体至所需刻度上，立即用右手示指（食指）按住管口，提升吸管离开液面，左手拿起盛溶液器皿，保持吸管垂直，将吸管末端靠在盛溶液器皿的内壁上约 45° 夹角，略微放松示指，使液面平稳下降，直至溶液的弯月面与刻度标线相切（注意，此时溶液凹面、刻度和视线应在一个水平位置），立即用右手示指压紧管，取出吸管，插入接受容器中，吸管垂直，管尖靠在接受器内壁上约 45° 夹角，接受器保持垂直，松开示指，使液体自然流出，移液管靠在受器内壁 15s，不必吹出尖端残留液体；若标有"吹"字的刻度吸管以及奥氏吸管应吹出尖端残留液体。

（二）分光光度计测定 *A* 值的使用方法

分光光度计能在紫外、可见光谱区域内对样品物质作定性和定量的分析。该仪器可广泛应用于医药卫生、临床检验、生物化学、石油化工、环境保护、质量控制等部门，是实验室常用分析仪器之一。

（1）使用仪器前，使用者应该首先了解本仪器的结构和工作原理以及各个操作旋钮之功能。在未接通电源前，应该对仪器进行检查，电源线接线应牢固，通地要良好，各个调节旋钮的起始位置应正确，然后再接通电源开关。

（2）开启电源，指示灯亮，选择开关置于"T"，波长调置测试用波长。仪器预热 20min。

（3）将遮挡块放入光路位置管好试样室盖（若为 721 型此步操作为打开试样室盖，使光门自动关闭），调节"0"旋钮，使数字显示为"00.0"；将比色皿架处于对照溶液校正位置，将存有对照溶液的比色杯（液面高度在比色杯 2/3 以上）放入光路，使光电管受光，调节透过率"100%"旋钮，使数字显示为"100.0"。

（4）将选择开关置于"A"，调节吸光度调零旋钮，使得数字显示为"00.0"，然后将被测样品的比色杯移入光路，显示值即为被测样品的吸光度值。

（5）实验所用的比色皿，使用前应清洗干净，尽量消除干扰；否则，测量前要测定记录比色杯间差异，减去空白读数值，以做校正。

（三）移液器的使用

移液器（又称移液枪）是生化与分子生物学实验常用的精密仪器，按量程有 0.1~2.5μl、0.5~10μl、2.0~20μl、10~100μl、20~200μl、100~1000μl、500~5000μl 等不同规格，能否正确使用关系到实验的准确性与重复性，也关系到移液枪的使用寿命。

1. 移液枪的正确使用步骤

（1）根据需要选择所需量程的移液枪。左手拿移液枪，右手旋转刻度轮，顺时针方向旋转刻度变小，至所需刻度。调整过程动作要轻缓，切勿超过最大或最小量程。

（2）选择与移液器匹配的吸头，将吸头套在移液枪的吸杆上，按吸量按钮至第一档，将洗头垂直插入待取液体中，深度在液面下 2~3mm，以刚浸没吸头尖端为宜，慢慢放开吸量按钮吸取液体；释放所取液体时，先将吸头尖端垂直接触在受液容器壁上，慢慢按下吸量按钮至第一档，稍微停顿 2~3 秒后，再按至第二档，将液体全部排出。移液完成后，可除去或更换吸头时，轻按卸载按钮，吸头自动脱落。使用过程中带有残余液体吸头的移液枪，应将移液枪挂在移液器架上。

（3）移液枪使用完毕后，应将刻度调至其最大量程存放，以免影响移液枪使用寿命。

2. 移液枪常见的错误操作

（1）直接按到第二档吸液。

（2）吸液时，应该垂直吸液，慢吸慢放，移液器本身倾斜，导致移液不准确。

（3）装配吸头时，用力过猛，导致吸头难以脱卸。

（4）平放或倾斜放置带有残余液体吸头的移液枪。

（5）不按所需量程使用移液枪，例如用大量程的移液器移取小体积样品。

（6）使用丙酮或强腐蚀性的液体清洗移液器。

三、常用洗涤液的种类和用途

附表1　常用洗涤液的种类与用途

种类	配制与用途
铬酸洗液	（1）5g 重铬酸钾 +100ml 浓硫酸 （2）5g 重铬酸钾 +5ml 水 +100ml 浓硫酸 （3）80g 重铬酸钾 +1000ml 水 +100ml 浓硫酸 （4）200g 重铬酸钾 +500ml 水 +500ml 浓硫酸 广泛用于玻璃仪器的洗涤
5% 草酸溶液	用数滴硫酸酸化，可洗去高锰酸钾痕迹
45% 尿素洗涤液	为蛋白质的良好溶剂，可洗涤蛋白质及血样的容器
5%～10% EDTANa$_2$溶液	加热煮沸可洗玻璃仪器内壁的白色沉淀物
有机溶剂	丙酮、乙醇、乙醚等可脱油脂、脂溶性染料等痕迹，二甲苯可洗油漆的污垢
30% 硝酸溶液	洗涤微量滴管及 CO_2 测定仪器
乙醇与浓硝酸的混合液	滴定管中加3ml 乙醇，然后沿管壁慢慢加入 4ml 浓硝酸盖住管口，利用所产生的氧化氮洗净滴定管
强碱性洗涤液	氢氧化钾的乙醇溶液和含高锰酸钾的氢氧化钠溶液，可清除容器内壁的污垢，但对玻璃仪器的腐蚀性较强，使用时时间不宜过长
浓盐酸	可除去容器上的水垢或无机盐沉淀

四、常用缓冲溶液浓度及 pH 范围

附表2　常用缓冲溶液浓度及 pH 范围

缓冲液名称及常用浓度	配制 pH 范围	主要物质分子量 M_r
甘氨酸 – 盐酸缓冲液（0.05mol/L）	2.2～5.0	甘氨酸 $M_r = 75.07$
邻苯二甲酸 – 盐酸缓冲液（0.05mol/L）	2.2～3.8	邻苯二甲酸氢钾 $M_r = 204.23$
磷酸氢二钠 – 枸橼酸缓冲液	2.2～8.0	磷酸氢二钠 $M_r = 141.98$
枸橼酸 – 氢氧化钠 – 盐酸缓冲液	2.2～6.5	枸橼酸 $M_r = 192.06$

续表

缓冲液名称及常用浓度	配制 pH 范围	主要物质分子量 M_r
枸橼酸 – 枸橼酸钠缓冲液（0.1mol/L）	3.0 ~ 6.6	枸橼酸 $Mr = 192.06$；枸橼酸钠 $Mr = 257.96$
醋酸 – 醋酸钠缓冲液（0.2mol/L）	3.6 ~ 5.8	醋酸钠 $Mr = 81.76$；醋酸 $Mr = 60.05$
邻苯二甲酸氢钾 – 氢氧化钠缓冲液	4.1 ~ 5.9	邻苯二甲酸氢钾 $Mr = 204.23$
磷酸氢二钠 – 磷酸二氢钠缓冲液（0.2mol/L）	5.8 ~ 8.0	$Na_2HPO_4 \cdot 2H_2O$ $Mr = 178.05$；$Na_2HPO_4 \cdot 12H_2O$ $Mr = 358.22$ $NaH_2PO_4 \cdot H_2O$ $Mr = 138.01$；$NaH_2PO_4 \cdot 2H_2O$ $Mr = 156.03$
磷酸氢二钠 – 磷酸二氢钾缓冲液（1/15 molL）	4.92 ~ 8.18	$Na_2HPO_4 \cdot 2H_2O$ $Mr = 178.05$；KH_2PO_4 $Mr = 136.09$
磷酸二氢钾 – 氢氧化钠缓冲液（0.05mol/L）	5.8 ~ 8.0	KH_2PO_4 $Mr = 136.09$
巴比妥钠 – 盐酸缓冲液（18℃）	6.8 ~ 9.6	巴比妥钠 $Mr = 206.18$
Tris – 盐酸缓冲液（0.05mol/L 25℃）	7.10 ~ 9.00	三羟甲基氨基甲烷（Tris）$Mr = 121.14$
硼砂 – 盐酸缓冲液（0.05mol/L）	8.0 ~ 9.1	硼砂 $Na_2B_4O_7 \cdot 10H_2O$ $Mr = 381.43$
硼酸 – 硼砂缓冲液（0.2mol/L）	7.4 ~ 8.0	硼砂 $Na_2B_4O_7 \cdot 10H_2O$ $Mr = 381.4$；H_3BO_3 $Mr = 61.84$
甘氨酸 – 氢氧化钠缓冲液（0.05mol/L）	8.6 ~ 10.6	甘氨酸 $Mr = 75.07$
硼砂 – 氢氧化钠缓冲液（0.05mol/L）	9.3 ~ 10.1	硼砂 $Na_2B_4O_7 \cdot 10H_2O$ $Mr = 381.43$
碳酸钠 – 碳酸氢钠缓冲液（0.1mol/L）	9.16 ~ 10.83	碳酸钠 $Mr = 286.2$；碳酸氢钠 $Mr = 84.0$
碳酸钠 – 氢氧化钠缓冲液（0.025mol/L）	9.6 ~ 11.0	碳酸钠 $Mr = 286.2$
磷酸氢二钠 – 氢氧化钠缓冲液	10.9 ~ 12.0	$Na_2HPO_4 \cdot 2H_2O$ $Mr = 178.05$；$Na_2HPO_4 \cdot 12H_2O$ $Mr = 358.22$
氯化钾 – 盐酸缓冲液（0.2mol/L）	1.0 ~ 2.2	氯化钾 $Mr = 74.55$
氯化钾 – 氢氧化钠缓冲液（0.2mol/L）	12.0 ~ 13.0	氯化钾 $Mr = 74.55$

五、硫酸铵饱和度的常用表

（一）硫酸铵溶液饱和度的计算（0℃）

附表3　硫酸铵溶液饱和度计算表（0℃）

		在0℃硫酸铵终浓度,%饱和度															
	20	25	30	35	40	45	50	55	60	65	70	75	80	85	90	95	100
	每100ml溶液加固体硫酸铵的克数																
0	10.6	13.4	16.4	19.4	22.6	25.8	29.1	32.6	36.1	39.8	43.6	47.6	51.6	55.9	60.3	65.0	69.7
5	7.9	10.8	13.7	16.6	19.7	22.9	26.2	29.6	33.1	36.8	40.5	44.4	48.4	52.6	57.0	61.5	66.2
10	5.3	8.1	10.9	13.9	16.9	20.0	23.2	26.6	30.1	33.7	37.4	41.2	45.2	49.3	53.6	58.1	62.7
15	2.6	5.4	8.2	11.1	14.1	17.2	20.4	23.7	27.1	30.6	34.3	38.1	42.0	46.0	50.3	54.7	59.2
20	0	2.7	5.5	8.3	11.3	14.3	17.5	20.7	24.1	27.6	31.2	34.9	38.7	42.7	46.9	51.2	55.7
25		0	2.7	5.6	8.4	11.5	14.6	17.9	21.1	24.5	28.0	31.7	35.5	39.5	43.6	47.8	52.2
30			0	2.8	5.6	8.6	11.7	14.8	18.1	21.4	24.9	28.5	32.3	36.2	40.2	44.5	48.8
35				0	2.8	5.7	8.7	11.8	15.1	18.4	21.8	25.4	29.1	32.9	36.9	41.0	45.3
40					0	2.9	5.8	8.9	12.0	15.3	18.7	22.2	25.8	29.6	33.5	37.6	41.8
45						0	2.9	5.9	9.0	12.3	15.6	19.0	22.6	26.3	30.2	34.2	38.3
50							0	3.0	6.0	9.2	12.5	15.9	19.4	23.0	26.8	30.8	34.8
55								0	3.0	6.1	9.3	12.7	16.1	19.7	23.5	27.3	31.3
60									0	3.1	6.2	9.5	12.9	16.4	20.1	23.1	27.9
65										0	3.1	6.3	9.7	13.2	16.8	20.5	24.4
70											0	3.2	6.5	9.9	13.4	17.1	20.9
75												0	3/2	6.6	10.1	13.7	17.4
80													0	3.3	6.7	10.3	13.9
85														0	3.4	6.8	10.5
90															0	3.4	7.0
95																0	3.5
100																	0

左侧纵向标注：硫酸铵初浓度,%饱和度

（二）不同温度下饱和硫酸铵溶液的制备

附表4　不同温度下饱和硫酸铵溶液的数据表

温度（℃）	0	10	20	25	30
重量百分数	41.42	42.22	43.09	43.47	43.85
摩尔浓度	3.9	3.97	4.06	4.10	4.13
每1000g水中含硫酸铵摩尔数	5.35	5.53	5.73	5.82	5.91
1000ml水中用硫酸铵克数	706.8	730.5	755.8	766.8	777.5
每1000ml溶液中含硫酸铵克数	514.8	525.2	536.5	541.2	545.9

（三）调整硫酸铵溶液饱和度的计算（25℃）

附表5　调整硫酸铵溶液饱和度计算表（25℃）

在25℃硫酸铵终浓度, %饱和度

	10	20	25	30	33	35	40	45	50	55	60	65	70	75	80	90	100
	每1000ml溶液加固体硫酸铵的克数																
0	56	114	144	176	196	209	243	277	313	351	390	430	472	516	561	662	767
10		57	86	118	137	150	183	216	251	288	326	365	406	449	494	592	694
20			29	59	78	91	123	155	189	225	262	300	340	382	424	520	619
25				30	49	61	93	125	158	193	230	267	307	348	390	485	583
30					19	30	62	94	127	162	198	235	273	314	356	449	546
33						12	43	74	107	142	177	214	252	292	333	426	522
35							31	63	94	129	164	200	238	278	319	411	506
40								31	63	97	132	168	205	245	285	375	469
45									32	65	99	134	171	210	250	339	431
50										33	66	101	137	176	214	302	392
55											33	67	103	141	179	264	353
60												34	69	105	143	227	314
65													34	70	107	190	275
70														35	72	153	237
75															36	115	198
80																77	157
90																	79

硫酸铵初浓度, %饱和度

六、离心机转数和相对离心力换算

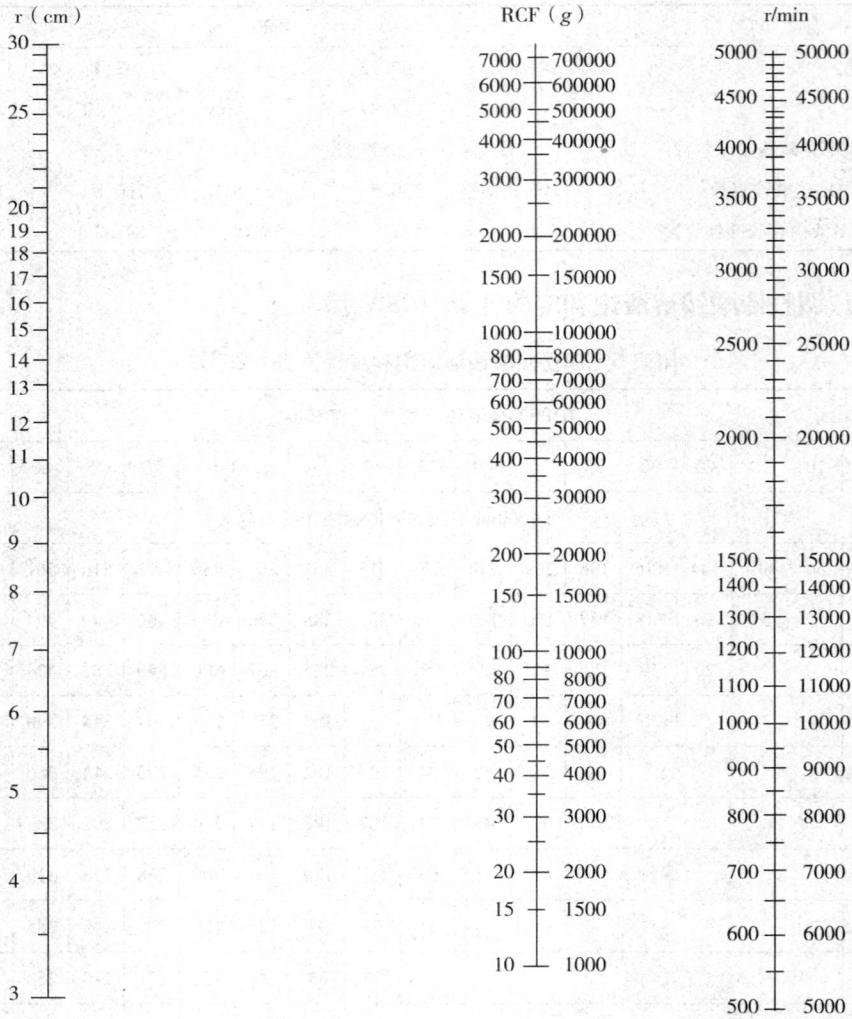

附图1　离心机转数和相对离心力换算

七、生物大分子常用分离纯化柱料使用及处理

层析柱常用于分离纯化蛋白质（包括酶类）核酸、多糖、激素、病毒、氨基酸和抗生素等生物大分子，也可用于样品的浓缩和脱盐及测定生物大分子的分子质量等方面，具有设备简单、操作方便、重现性好、产品收率高等特点。生化常用的有以下几类。

（一）DEAE 阴离子交换纤维素

1. DEAE 阴离子纤维素的处理　取纤维素干品用蒸馏水浸泡，充分溶胀并搅拌均匀，过夜。次日再搅匀，静止30分钟留下沉集部分（重复3次），用真空泵抽干，然后用适量的 0.5mol/L 的氢氧化钠溶液浸泡 30 分钟，抽干，蒸馏水洗至中性；再用适量的 0.5mol/L 的盐酸溶液浸泡 30 分钟，抽干，蒸馏水洗至中性；重复用 0.5mol/L 的氢氧化钠溶液浸泡 30 分钟，抽干，蒸馏水洗至中性。最后用 0.005mol/L pH 6.0 的磷酸缓冲液浸泡待用。

2. DEAE 阴离子纤维素的重生　回收的纤维素先用 0.5mol/L 氯化钠－0.5mol/L 氢氧化钠溶液浸泡，再按上述（1）操作处理，即可再次投入使用。

3. DEAE 阴离子纤维素的保存　回收后，用 0.5mol/L 氢氧化钠溶液浸泡 30 分钟后，蒸馏水洗至中性，抽干，于鼓风干燥箱中 60℃ 烘干后，保存。

（二）Sephadex G 型葡聚糖凝胶

1. 凝胶的特性　葡聚糖 G 后面的数字代表不同的交联度，数值越大交联度越小，吸水量越大，其数值为吸水量的 10 倍。Sephadex 对碱和弱酸稳定。在中性时可以高压灭菌。不同型号中又有颗粒粗细之分。颗粒粗的分离效果差，流速快。颗粒越细，分离效果越好，但流速也越慢。交联葡聚糖工作时的 pH 稳定在 2～11 的范围内使用。葡聚糖 G 型凝胶分离的分子量分级范围为 $700 \times 10^5 \sim 8 \times 10^5$。可根据所需分离样品选择凝胶型号，Sephadex G 型葡聚糖凝胶的数据见附表 6。

附表 6　常用凝胶的种类型号及性能

种类及主要用途	化学组成	部分型号	颗粒大小（目数）	分离性能（Da）	溶胀时间（h） 20～25℃	90～100℃
葡聚糖凝胶（Sephadex G-）	由葡聚糖和甘油基通过醚桥交联而成	G-10	60～200	<700	3	1
		G-15	60～200	<1500	3	1
		G-25	50～400	100～5000	3	1
		G-50	50～400	500～30000	3	1
		G-75	60～400	1000～8000	24	3
		G-100	120～400	1000～15000	72	3
		G-150	120～400	1000～30000	72	5
		G-200	120～400	1000～60000	72	5
聚丙烯酰胺凝胶（Bio-gel）	由丙烯酰胺和双丙烯酰胺共聚而成	P-2	50～400	200～1800	4	2
		P-4	50～400	800～4000	4	2
		P-6	50～400	1000～6000	4	2
		P-10	50～400	1500～20000	4	2
		P-30	50～200	2500～40000	12	3
		P-60	50～200	3000～60000	12	3
		P-100	50～200	5000～100000	24	5
		P-150	50～200	15000～150000	24	5
		P-200	50～200	50000～20000	48	5
		P-300	50～200	60000～400000	48	5

续表

种类及主要用途	化学组成	部分型号	颗粒大小（目数）	分离性能（Da）	溶胀时间（h）20~25℃	90~100℃
琼脂糖凝胶（Sepharose gio-gel）	由 D-半乳糖和 3、6 脱水的 L-半乳糖连接而成，为中性琼脂糖	A0.5m	50~400	<10000~500000		
		A1.5m	50~400	<10000~1500000		
		A5m	50~400	10000~5000000		
		A15m	50~400	10000~15000000		
		A50m	50~400	100000~50000000		
		A150m	50~200	1000000~150000000		

2. 凝胶的溶胀 G 系交联葡聚糖凝胶亲水性强，只能在水中溶胀（仅有少量的有机溶剂也可以使之溶胀），有机溶剂或含有机溶剂较多的水溶液会改变其孔隙，使之收缩失去或降低凝胶的分离能力。在水中溶胀时如在室温则需要较长时间，才能达到充分溶胀的程度，但可煮沸到100℃，以缩短其溶胀时间。溶胀时要将凝胶浸泡在过量的水或缓冲液中。在整个溶胀过程中应避免剧烈地搅拌，尤其不能使用电磁搅拌，以免破坏了它的颗粒结构以及产生许多碎末，而影响洗脱时的流速。

3. 凝胶的回收与保存 凝胶的再生最好不要在柱上进行（有些凝胶可以在位清洗），可将凝胶在 0.5mol/L 氯化钠及 0.5mol/L 氢氧化钠的混合溶液中浸泡；一般约需 30 分钟以上，然后用蒸馏水洗至中性，最后用缓冲液平衡，即可恢复使用。

经常使用的凝胶，一般加入一些抗菌剂放在普通冰箱中，即可保存较长的时间。如确实在相当长的时间里不准备使用时，则以保存干凝胶为好。处理时可先用较浓的氯化钠浸泡（如0.5mol/L），再用 0.5mol/L 的氢氧化钠处理并用蒸馏水洗至中性，然后用递增百分比浓度的乙醇分多次作脱水处理。一般可从 30% 的乙醇开始，每次均应让凝胶在乙醇中多浸泡一些时间。在无水乙醇处理后，最后再用乙醚处理一次，以加速乙醇的挥发。处理后的凝胶宜在 80℃ 以下的温度烘干。在进行凝胶的回收时，如在每一步操作时，均使用布氏漏斗抽滤，可大大地加快整个回收过程。

八、常用蛋白质分子量标准参照物

附表7 常用蛋白质分子量标准参照物

高分子量标准参照 名称	M_r	中分子量标准参照 名称	M_r	低分子量标准参照 名称	M_r
肌球蛋白	212000	磷酸化酶 B	97000	碳酸酐酶	31000
β-半乳糖苷酶	116000	牛血清清蛋白	66200	大豆胰蛋白酶抑制剂	21000
磷酸化酶 B	97400	谷氨酸脱氢酶	55000	马心肌球蛋白	16000
牛血清清蛋白	66200	卵清蛋白	42700	溶菌酶	14000
过氧化氢酶	57000	醛缩酶	40000	肌球蛋白（F_1）	8100
醛缩酶	40000	碳酸酐酶	31000	肌球蛋白（F_2）	6200

高分子量标准参照		中分子量标准参照		低分子量标准参照	
名　称	M_r	名　称	M_r	名　称	M_r
		大豆胰蛋白酶抑制剂	21000	肌球蛋白（F_3）	2500
		溶菌酶	14000		

九、常用蛋白质与核酸换算关系

附表8　常用蛋白质与核酸换算关系

重量换算	分光光度值与核酸浓度的换算	蛋白质质量与摩尔数的转换
$1\mu g = 10^{-6} g$ $1ng = 10^{-9} g$ $1pg = 10^{-12} g$ $1fg = 10^{-15} g$	$1A_{260}$ 双链 DNA $\approx 50\mu g/ml$ $1A_{260}$ 单链 DNA $\approx 33\mu g/ml$ $1A_{260}$ 单链 RNA $\approx 40\mu g/ml$	100pmol 分子量 100000 蛋白质 $\approx 10\mu g$ 100pmol 分子量 50000 蛋白质 $\approx 5\mu g$ 100pmol 分子量 10000 蛋白质 $\approx 1\mu g$ 氨基酸的平均分子量 = 126.7 Da
DNA 分子质量与摩尔数		**蛋白质与 DNA 换算**
$1\mu g$ 100bp DNA = 1.52pmol = 3.03pmol 末端 $1\mu g$pBR$_{322}$ DNA = 0.36pmol $1pmol$ 1000bp DNA = 0.66μg $1pmol$pBR$_{322}$ = 2.8μg 1kb 双链 DNA（钠盐）$\approx 6.6 \times 10^5$ Da 1kb 单链 DNA（钠盐）$\approx 3.3 \times 10^5$ Da 1kb 单链 RNA（钠盐）$\approx 3.4 \times 10^5$ Da		1kb DNA ≈ 333 个氨基酸编码容量 $\approx 3.7 \times 10^4 Mr$ 蛋白质 10000Mr 蛋白质 ≈ 270bpDNA 30000Mr 蛋白质 ≈ 810bpDNA 50000Mr 蛋白质 ≈ 1.35kb 100000Mr 蛋白质 ≈ 2.7kbDNA

十、常用限制性内切酶位点及缓冲溶液

（一）常用限制性内切酶位点

附表9　常用限制性内切酶位点

常用限制性内切酶	盐浓度	识别顺序	常用限制性内切酶	盐浓度	识别顺序
*Bam*HI	中	G↓GATCC	*Bgl* Ⅱ	低	A↓GATCT
*Eco*RI	高	G↓AATTC	*Eco*R Ⅴ	高	GAT↓ATC
Hind Ⅲ	中	A↓AGCTT	*Nco* Ⅰ	高	C↓CATGG
Kpn Ⅰ	低	GGTAC↓C	*Sin* Ⅰ	低	G↓G ($\begin{smallmatrix}AT\\TA\end{smallmatrix}$) CC
Nde Ⅰ	中	CA↓TATG	*Sma*BI	低	TAC↓GTA
Pst Ⅰ	中	CTGCA↓G	*Sph* Ⅰ	中	GCATG↓C
Sac Ⅰ	低	CCGC↓GG	*Sat* Ⅱ	低	CCGC↓GG
Sal Ⅰ	高	G↓TCGAC	*Xho* Ⅰ	高	C↓TCGAG
Sca Ⅰ	中	AGT↓ACT	*Xma* Ⅰ，*Sma* Ⅰ	低	C↓CCGGG
Xba Ⅰ	高	T↓CTAGA			

（二）常用限制性内切酶缓冲溶液

附表 10　常用限制性内切酶缓冲溶液

10×低盐缓冲液	10×中盐缓冲液	10×高盐缓冲液
	0.5mol/L NaCl	1mol/L NaCl
100mmol/L Tris – HCl（pH 7.5）	100mmol/L Tris – HCl（pH 7.5）	500mmol/L Tris – HCl（pH 7.5）
100mmol/L MgCl$_2$	100mmol/L MgCl$_2$	100mmol/L MgCl$_2$
100mmol/L DTT	10mmol/L DTT	10mmol/L DTT

说明：各种限制性内切酶缓冲液常配制成10倍浓缩液。根据各酶所需的盐浓度请参阅厂家使用说明，不同的酶的酶解条件不同，同一种酶由于不同厂家的产品纯度不同，酶解条件也有差异。

十一、分子生物学实验常用培养基的配制方法

附表 11　分子生物学实验常用培养基的配制方法

名　称	配制方法
1. 100mg/ml 氨苄西林	称量5g 氨苄西林置于50ml 离心管中，加入40ml 灭菌水，充分混合溶解后，定容至50ml，用0.22μm 滤膜过滤除菌，小份分装（1ml/份）后，−20℃保存
2. 24mg/ml IPTG	称量1.2g IPTG 置于50ml 离心管中，加入40ml 灭菌水，充分混合溶解后，定容至50ml，用0.22μm 滤膜过滤除菌，小份分装（1ml/份）后，−20℃保存
3. 20mg/ml X – Gal	称取1g X – Gal 置于50ml 离心管中，加入40ml DMF（二甲基甲酰胺），充分混合溶解后，定容至50ml，小份分装（1ml/份）后，−20℃保存
4. LB 培养基	称量蛋白胨10g，酵母提取物5g，NaCl 10g 置于1L 烧杯中，加入约800ml 的去离子水，充分搅拌溶解，滴加5N NaOH（约0.2ml），调节 pH 值至7.0，加去离子水将培养基定容至1L，高温高压灭菌后，4℃保存
5. LB/Amp 培养基	称量蛋白胨10g，酵母提取物5g，NaCl 10g 置于1L 烧杯中，加入约800ml 的去离子水，充分搅拌溶解，滴加5mol/L NaOH（约0.2ml），调节 pH 值至7.0，加去离子水将培养基定容至1L，高温高压灭菌后，冷却至室温，加入1ml 氨苄西林（100mg/ml）后均匀混合，4℃保存
6. TB 培养基	配制磷酸盐缓冲液（0.17mol/L KH$_2$PO$_4$，0.72mol/L K$_2$HPO$_4$）100ml，灭菌。称取蛋白胨12g，酵母提取物24g，甘油4 ml，置于1L 烧杯中，加入约800ml 的去离子水，充分搅拌溶解；加去离子水将培养基定容至 1L 后，高温高压灭菌；待溶液冷却至60℃以下时，加入100ml 的上述灭菌磷酸盐缓冲液，4℃保存
7. TB/Apm 培养基	配制磷酸盐缓冲液（0.17mol/L KH$_2$PO$_4$，0.72mol/L K$_2$HPO$_4$）100ml。溶解2.31g KH$_2$PO$_4$和2.54g K$_2$HPO$_4$于90ml 的去离子水中，搅拌溶解后，加去离子水定容至100ml，高温高压灭菌；称取蛋白胨12g，酵母提取物24g，甘油4ml 置于1L 烧杯中，加入约800ml 的去离子水，充分搅拌溶解，加去离子水将培养基定容至1L 后，高温高压灭菌；待溶液冷却至60℃以下时，加入100ml 的上述灭菌磷酸盐缓冲液和1ml 氨苄西林（100mg/ml），均匀混合后4℃保存

续表

名　称	配制方法
8. SOB 培养基	配制 250mmol/L KCl 溶液：在 90ml 的去离子水中溶解 1.86g KCl 后，定容至 100ml；配制 2mol/L MgCl₂ 溶液：在 90ml 的去离子水中溶解 19g MgCl₂后，定容至 100ml，高温高压灭菌；称取置于蛋白胨 20g，酵母提取物 5g，NaCl 0.5g 1L 烧杯中，加入约 800ml 的去离子水，充分搅拌溶解，量取 10ml 250mmol/L KCl 溶液，加入到烧杯中，滴加 5mol/L NaOH 溶液（约 0.2ml），调节 pH 至 7.0，加入去离子水将培养基定容至 1L；高温高压灭菌后，4℃保存。使用前加入 5ml 灭菌的 2mol/L MgCl₂ 溶液
9. SOC 培养基	配制 1mol/L 葡萄糖溶液：将 18g 葡萄糖溶于 90ml 去离子水中，充分溶解后定容至 100ml，用 0.22μm 滤膜过滤除菌；向 100ml SOB 培养基中加入除菌的 1mol/L 葡萄糖溶液 2ml，均匀混合；4℃保存
10. 2×YT 培养基	称取蛋白胨 16g，酵母提取物 10g，NaCl 5g 置于 1L 烧杯中，加入约 800ml 的去离子水，充分搅拌溶解，滴加 1mol/L KOH，调节 pH 至 7.0，加去离子水，将培养基定容至 1L，高温高压后，4℃保存
11. Φb×broth 培养基	称取蛋白胨 20g，酵母提取物 5g，MgSO₄·7H₂O 5g 置于 1L 烧杯中，加入约 800ml 的去离子水，充分搅拌溶解，滴加 1mol/L KOH，调节 pH 至 7.5，加水离子水将培养基定容至 1L，高温高压后，4℃保存
12. NZCYM 培养基	称取酵母提取物 5g，酪蛋白氨基酸（Casamino Acid）1g，胺 10g，NaCl 5g，MgSO₄·7H₂O 2g 置于 1L 烧杯中。加入约 800ml 的去离子水，充分搅拌溶解，滴加 5mol/L NaOH 溶液（约 0.2ml），调节 pH 至 7.0，加去离子水将培养基定容至 1L，高温高压后，4℃保存
13. NZYM 培养基	NZYM 培养基除不含酪蛋白氨基酸外，其他成分与 NZCYM 培养基相同
14. NZM 培养基	NZM 培养基除不含酵母提取物酵母提取物外，其他成分与 NZYM 培养基相同
15. 一般固体培养基	按照液体培养配方，准备好液体培养基，在高温高压灭菌前，加入下列试剂中的一种。配制：Agar（琼脂：铺制平板用）15g/L；Agar（琼脂：配制顶层琼脂用）7g/L；Agarose（琼脂糖：铺制平板用）15 g/L；Agarose（琼脂糖：配制顶层琼脂用）7g/L。高温高压灭菌后，戴上手套取出培养基，摇动容器使琼脂或琼脂糖充分混匀（此时培养基温度很高，小心烫伤）；待培养基冷却到 50~60℃时，加入热不稳定物质（如抗生素），摇动容器充分混匀；铺制平板（30~35ml 培养基/90mm 培养皿）
16. LB/Amp/X–Gal/IPTG 平板培养基	称取置于 1L 烧杯中。蛋白胨 10g，酵母提取物 5g，NaCl 10g，加入约 800ml 的去离子水，充分搅拌溶解，滴加 5mol/L NaOH 溶液（约 0.2ml），调节 pH 至 7.0；加去离子水将培养基定容至 1L 后，加入 15g Agar，高温高压灭菌后，冷却至 60℃左右；加入 1ml 氨苄西林（100mg/ml）、1ml IPTG（24mg/ml）、2ml X–Gal（20mg/ml）后均匀混合；铺制平板（30~35ml 培养基/90mm 培养基）；4℃保存平板
17. TB/Amp/X–Gal/IPTG 平板培养基	配制：磷酸盐缓冲液（0.17mol/L KH₂PO₄，0.72mol/L K₂HPO₄）100ml；称取蛋白胨 12g，酵母提取物 24g；Glycerol 4ml 置于 1L 烧杯中，加入约 800ml 的去离子水，充分搅拌溶解，加去离子水将培养基定容至 1L 后，加入 15g Agar；高温高压灭菌后，冷却至 60℃左右；加入 100ml 的上述灭菌磷酸盐缓冲液，1ml 氨苄西林（100mg/ml），1ml IPTG（24mg/ml），2ml X–Gal（20mg/ml）后均匀混合；铺制平板（30~35ml 培养基/90mm 培养基）；4℃保存平板

参 考 文 献

[1] 张龙翔. 生化实验方法和技术. 2版. 北京：高等教育出版社，1997.

[2] 徐秀兰，何执中，吴梧桐. 生物化学实验指导. 北京：中国医药科技出版社，1994.

[3] 汪家政. 蛋白质技术手册. 北京：科学出版社，2001.

[4] 史伟，禹婷. 蛋白质的层析分离. 内蒙古农业科技，2011（1）.

[5] 何秀兰，何执中，吴梧桐. 生物化学实验指导. 北京：中国医药科技出版社，1994.

[6] D. R. 马歇克，J. T. 门永，R. R. 布格斯，等. 蛋白质纯化与鉴定实验指南. 北京：科学出版社，1999.

[7] 郭尧君. 蛋白质电泳实验技术. 北京：科学出版社，2001.

[8] 陈雅蕙等. 生物化学实验原理和方法. 北京：北京大学出版社，2005.

[9] 夏其昌，曾嵘. 蛋白质化学与蛋白质组学. 北京：科学出版社. 2004.

[10] J. 萨姆布鲁克，E. F. 弗里奇，T. 曼尼阿蒂斯. 分子克隆实验指南. 3版. 北京：科学出版社，2002.

[11] 白玲，霍群. 基础生物化学实验. 2版. 上海：复旦大学出版社，2008.

[12] 张剑，赵雷敏，康林霞. 碱性蛋白酶活力分析方法研究. 日用化学工业，2012，42（3）.

[13] 邹承鲁. 细胞色素C的简易制备方法及其若干性质. 生理学报. 1955，19：3 − 4，361.

[14] 陈来同. 生物化学产品制备技术（1）. 北京：科学技术文献出版社. 2003.

[15] 高焕春，吕晓玲，李文英. 鸡蛋清溶菌酶提取工艺及其应用初探. 天津：天津轻工业学院学报. 1996，1：37 − 40.

[16] 郇延军. 蛋清中溶菌酶的提取. 无锡轻工业大学学报，1997，16（2）：59 − 62.

[17] 赵玉萍，张灏，杨严俊. 溶菌酶测定方法的改进. 食品科学，2002，23（3）：116 − 119.

[18] Hung − Min Chang, Ching − Chuan Yang, Yung − Chung Chang. Rapid Separation of Lysozyme from Chicken Egg White by Reductants and Thermal Treatment. J Agric Food Chem. 2000，48，161 − 164.

[19] 余瑞元，袁明秀，陈丽蓉，等. 生物化学实验原理和方法. 2版. 北京：北京大学出版社. 2011.

[20] 陈钧辉，李俊，张太平，等. 生物化学实验. 4版. 北京：科学出版社. 2008.

[21] 许激扬. 生物化学实验与指导. 2版. 北京：中国医药科技出版社. 2009.